Handbook of Pharmaceutical Science

Handbook of Pharmaceutical Science

Editor: Rodrik Ledger

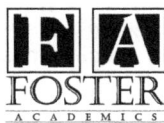

FOSTER
ACADEMICS

www.fosteracademics.com

www.fosteracademics.com

FA
FOSTER
ACADEMICS

Cataloging-in-Publication Data

Handbook of pharmaceutical science / edited by Rodrik Ledger.
    p. cm.
Includes bibliographical references and index.
ISBN 978-1-63242-831-8
1. Pharmacology. 2. Drugs. 3. Pharmacy. 4. Pharmaceutical industry. I. Ledger, Rodrik.
RM301.12 .H36 2019
615--dc23

Foster Academics,
118-35 Queens Blvd., Suite 400,
Forest Hills, NY 11375, USA

ISBN 978-1-63242-831-8 (Hardback)

Contents

Preface

This book has been a concerted effort by a group of academicians, researchers and scientists, who have contributed their research works for the realization of the book. This book has materialized in the wake of emerging advancements and innovations in this field. Therefore, the need of the hour was to compile all the required researches and disseminate the knowledge to a broad spectrum of people comprising of students, researchers and specialists of the field.

Pharmaceutical science refers to a set of interdisciplinary fields of study that are concerned with the design, delivery, action and disposition of pharmaceutical drugs. There is an application of inorganic chemistry, physical chemistry, analytical chemistry, biochemistry, cell biology, molecular biology, anatomy, physics, epidemiology and several other fields of science in pharmaceutical science. Pharmaceutical sciences may be divided into pharmacology, pharmaceutics, pharmaceutical chemistry and pharmacognosy. Together these disciplines encompass the design of drug formulation for optimum stability and delivery, study of the physiological and biochemical effects of drugs on human beings, synthesis of new drug molecules, etc. The book aims to shed light on some of the unexplored aspects of pharmaceutical science and the recent researches in this field. The various studies that are constantly contributing towards advancing technologies and evolution of this field are examined in detail. As this field is emerging at a rapid pace, the contents of this book will help the readers understand the modern concepts and applications of the subject.

At the end of the preface, I would like to thank the authors for their brilliant chapters and the publisher for guiding us all-through the making of the book till its final stage. Also, I would like to thank my family for providing the support and encouragement throughout my academic career and research projects.

Editor

Silencing of High Mobility Group Isoform I-C (HMGI-C) Enhances Paclitaxel Chemosensitivity in Breast Adenocarcinoma Cells (MDA-MB-468)

Behzad Mansoori[1,2]**, Ali Mohammadi**[1]**, Samira Goldar**[1]**, Dariush Shanehbandi**[1]**, Leila Mohammadnejad**[1]**, Elham Baghbani**[1]**, Tohid Kazemi**[1]**, Saeed Kachalaki**[1]**, Behzad Baradaran**[1]*****

[1] *Immunology Research Center, Tabriz University of Medical Sciences, Tabriz, Iran.*
[2] *Student Research Committee, Tabriz University of Medical Sciences, Tabriz, Iran.*

Keywords:
· *HMGI-C* (High mobility group protein isoform I-C)
· Small interference RNA (siRNA)
· Breast adenocarcinoma
· Paclitaxel

Abstract

Purpose: HMGI-C (High Mobility Group protein Isoform I-C) protein is a member of the high-mobility group AT-hook (HMGA) family of small non-histone chromosomal protein that can modulate transcription of an ample number of genes. Genome-wide studies revealed up regulation of the HMGI-C gene in many human cancers. We suggested that HMGI-C might play a critical role in the progression and migration of various tumors. However, the exact role of HMGI-C in breast adenocarcinoma has not been cleared.

Methods: The cells were transfected with siRNAs using transfection reagent. Relative HMGI-C mRNA and protein levels were measured by quantitative real-time PCR and Western blotting, respectively. The cytotoxic effects of HMGI-C siRNA, Paclitaxel alone and combination on breast adenocarcinoma cells were determined using MTT assay. The migration after treatment by HMGI-C siRNA, Paclitaxel alone and combination were detected by wound-healing respectively.

Results: HMGI-C siRNA significantly reduced both mRNA and protein expression levels in a 48 hours after transfection and dose dependent manner. We observed that the knockdown of HMGI-C led to the significant reduced cell viability and inhibited cells migration in MDA-MB-468 cells *in vitro*.

Conclusion: These results propose that HMGI-C silencing and Paclitaxel treatment alone can inhibit the proliferation and migration significantly, furthermore, synergic effect of HMGI-C siRNA and Paclitaxel showed higher inhibition compared to mono treatment. Taken together, HMGI-C could be used as a promising therapeutic agent in the treatment of human breast adenocarcinoma. Therefore HMGI-C siRNA may be an effective adjuvant in human breast adenocarcinoma.

Introduction

Breast cancer is the most common cancer diagnosed among women in the worldwide, accounting for nearly 1 in 3 cancers, also it is the second cause of cancer death among women fallowing lung cancer.[1] Despite the great improvements in the clinical and therapeutic techniques in recent years, many advanced breast cancer patients still die of the postoperative recurrence and metastasis of disease. One of the primary reasons for ineffective therapies for these patients is our lack of understanding about the complete and accurate molecular mechanisms involved in carcinogenesis, progression and invasion of breast cancer. Therefore, the innovation of new treatment modalities to overcome these ineffective therapies are necessary.[2] Effectiveness of siRNA in cancer treatment has been specified by: potential and high efficiency, knock downing in the advanced stages of growth and low cost compared to the other methods of gene therapy,[3-5]

and high specificity contrasted to the other cancer therapy methods such as operation and chemotherapy.[6,7]

HMGI-C protein, also known as HMGA2 protein, belongs to the family of nuclear non-histone phosphoproteins called high mobility group A (HMGA). These proteins have a relatively small molecular weight about 12 kDa and contain three basic short sequences, called the AT-hook. These basic sequences bind to AT-rich regions of the minor groove of B-form DNA. HMGA proteins are involved in many fundamental cellular processes, including mitosis, cell-cycle control, cell division, regulation of transcription (by binding transcription factors such as NF-kB, ATF-2/c-Jun, Elf-1, Oct-2, Oct-6, SRF, NF-Y, PU-1, RAR), differentiation and cellular aging.[8,9]

HMGA protein family is relatively over expressed, where cells proliferate rapidly, as in the early embryo. *HMGA1* genes are expressed in the tissues of

*****Corresponding author:** Behzad Baradaran, Email: Behzad_im@yahoo.com

parenchymal organs and proliferating epithelial cells,[10] whereas the HMGI-C gene highly expressed in all mesenchymal cell condensations and in mesenchymal derivatives.[11] Expression of *HMGA* genes are suppressed in differentiated cells and the HMGI-C gene is under expressed in adult human tissues, other than embryonic tissues.[12,13]

Over expression of HMGI-C gene was observed in many human malignancies such as non-small lung cancers,[14] pancreatic carcinoma,[15] epithelial ovarian cancers,[16] colorectal cancer,[17] retinoblastomas,[18] squamous cell carcinomas,[19] myeloproliferative disorder[20] and it has also been found to participate in EMT.[21,22]

In this study we investigated whether the down-regulation of HMGI-C level by siRNA could sensitize breast adenocarcinoma cells to Paclitaxel. To this end, we examined the effects of either HMGI-C specific siRNA or Paclitaxel treatments alone versus the combination, on invasion and survival invitro, in MDA-MB-468 cell line.

Materials and Methods
Materials
Human HMGI-C siRNA, goat polyclonal anti-HMGI-C antibody, monoclonal b-actin antibody, siRNA transfection reagent and siRNA transfection medium were purchased from Santacruz biotechnology (California, USA). Rabbit anti-goat antibody was purchased from Cytomatin gene company (Isfahan, Iran), rabbit anti-mouse anti-body was purchased from Razi institute. Paclitaxel was purchased from activis (Milan, Italy).QRT-PCR master mix was purchased from Takara bio Inc. (Shiga, Japan).

Cell culture
The human breast adenocarcinoma cell line, MDA-MB-468 was purchased from Pasture institute (Tehran, Iran). The MDA-MB-468 breast cells were maintained in RPMI-1640 culture medium supplemented with 10% heat-inactivated fetal bovine serum (FBS), antibiotics (100 IU/ml penicillin, 100 μg/ml streptomycin) (Gibco, USA) at 37 °C in a 95% humidified atmosphere containing 5% CO_2. Cells were grown on sterilized culture dishes and were passaged every 3 days following 0.25 % trypsin/EDTA (Gibco, USA) digestion.

siRNA transfection
MDA-MB-468 cells were cultured at a density of 2×10^5 cells/ml of six-well plates and transfected at 60-80% confluency. siRNA transfection (at a final concentration of 80 pmol in all experiments) was performed using siRNA transfection reagent (Santacruz biotechnology, USA) according to the manufacturer's recommendations. Briefly, siRNA and siRNA transfection reagent were diluted in siRNA transfection medium (Santacruz biotechnology, USA) separately. The diluted solutions were then mixed and incubated for 15-30 min at room temperature. Subsequently, the mixtures were added to each well containing cells and transfection medium.

After 5-7 hr transfection, RPMI medium containing final FBS concentration of 20% was added into transfected wells. After 48 hr of incubation, down-regulation of HMGI-C was measured using qRT-PCR. Then, Western blot was utilized to test the target protein to ensure the transfection efficiency. The suppression of HMGI-C expression was then assessed by quantitative real-time PCR (qRT-PCR) and Western blotting.

Real-time quantitative PCR
Total- RNA was extracted using AccuZolTM reagent (Bioneer, Daedeok-gu, Daejeon, Korea) as described by the manufacturer's protocol. The mRNA was reverse-transcribed into cDNA from 1 μg of total RNA by use of MMLV reverse transcriptase (Promega, Madison, WI, USA) and oligo-dT primer according to the manufacturer's instructions. The expression level of HMGI-C mRNA was carried out by qRT-PCR using SYBR Premix Ex Taq (Takara Bio, Otsu, Shiga, Japan) and Rotor- GeneTM 6000 system (Corbett Life Science, Mortlake, NSW, Australia). The reaction system of PCR was: 12 μl of SYBR green reagent, 0.2 μM of each primer, 1 μl of cDNA template, and 6 μl of nuclease-free distilled water. All pair primer sequences were blasted using the primer-blast software on the NCBI website (http://www.nchi.nlm.nih.gov) prior to the experiment. The primer sequences were as follows: forward, 5'-TGGGAGGAGCGAAATCTAAA-3', reverse, 5'-TGGTATTCAGGTCTTTCATGG-3', for HMGI-C, and forward, 5'-TCCCTGGAGAAGAGCTACG-3', and reverse, 5'-GTAGTTTCGTGGATGCCACA-3', for β-actin. The initial denaturation step at 95°C for 10 min was followed by 45 cycles at 95°C for 10 sec, 59°C for 30 sec and 72°C for 20 sec. β-actin was used as the reference gene. The relative levels of gene expression were calculated by the $2^{-\Delta\Delta Ct}$ method. All qRT-PCR reactions were performed in triplicate.

Western blot analysis
Briefly, total protein from cells was extracted using RIPA buffer (25 mM Tris HCl pH 7.6, 150 mM NaCl, 1% NP-40, 1% sodium deoxycholate, 0.1% SDS) containing protease inhibitor cocktail (Roche Diagnostics GmbH). Suspensions were centrifuged at 14,000 rpm for 10 min at 4°C and cellular debris was discarded. Protein concentrations were quantified using NanoDrop (Thermo scientific, Wilmington, USA). Fifty micrograms of each protein sample were mixed with protein sample buffer (10% Glycerol, 50 Mm Tris pH 8.6, 2% SDS, 1% Bromophenol blue, and 100 mM DTT) and the samples were incubated for 5 min in a boiling water bath, then separated on 12.5% SDS-polyacrylamide gel electrophoresis. After transferring separated proteins to an activated polyvinylidine diflouride (PVDF) membranes, we blocked the membranes with 0.5% tween 20 in PBS/Tween-20 (0.05%, v/v) for 24 hr at 4°C. Following on, the membranes were probed 1 hr at room temperature with primary goat poly clonal antibodies against HMGI-C (1:2000, Santacruze biotechnology,

California, USA) and β-actin (1:5000, Santacruze biotechnology, California, USA) diluted in 3% BSA in PBS. After four washes with a buffer containing PBS and 0.05% Tween-20, membranes were incubated with appropriate horseradish peroxidase-linked Rabbit anti-goat secondary antibody (1:5,000, cytomatin gene, Isfahan, Iran) and rabbit anti-mouse antibody (Razi institute, Tehran, Iran) diluted in PBS and 0.05% Tween-20 for 1 hr at room temperature. Subsequently, the membranes were washed and protein bands visualized using enhanced BM chemiluminescence blotting substrate POD (Roche Diagnostics GmbH, Mannheim, Germany) and autoradiography films (Estman Kodak, Rochester, NY, USA). Signals were measured using NIH ImageJ 1.63 Software.

Cytotoxicity assay
Cytotoxicity of the treatments was measured using a methylthiazol tetrazolium (MTT) assay kit (Sigma). The experiment was subdivided into eight groups: 80 pmol HMGI-C siRNA, Paclitaxel in 6 different doses around IC50 and combination of 80 pmol HMGI-C siRNA with 6 different paclitaxel doses. Briefly, cells were cultured at a density of 15×10^3 cells/well in 96-well cell culture plates and then transfected with siRNAs. After 48 hr of incubation, the cells were exposed to different concentrations of paclitaxel (0.39, 0.78, 1.56, 3.25, 6.5 and 12.5 μM). After a total 24 hr of treatment, 50μl of MTT (2mg/ml in PBS) was added to each well and then incubated for a further 4 hr. The formazan crystals were formed by adding 200 μl of the solubilization (DMSO + Sorensen buffer) to each well. After 30 minutes incubation in above-mentioned conditions, the optical density (OD) of each well was measured at a wavelength of 570nm using an ELISA reader (Awareness Technology, Palm City, FL, USA) and all experiments were performed in triplicate.

Combination effect analysis
The combination effect between HMGI-C siRNA and paclitaxel were evaluated, based on the principles described by Chou and Talalay.[23] For each combination experiment, a coefficient of drug interaction (CDI) number was calculated using the following formula: CDI=SAB /(SA×SB), were introduced SA as paclitaxel, SB as HMGI-C siRNA and SAB as combination treatment survival rate, relative to the control. Combination effects were assessed after 48 hr of treatment. This method of analysis generally defines CDI<1 as synergistic, CDI=1 as additive and CDI>1 as antagonistic effects, respectively.

Migration assay
MDA-MB-468 cells migration was measured by using a wound-healing assay (Scratch). MDA-MB-468 cells (4×10^5 cells/well) were placed for 24 h in 6-well plates and a wound was made by using yellow pipette tip across the cell monolayer to create an open gap, mimicking a wound when the cultured cells reached >90 %

confluence and cell debris were removed by washing with serum-free medium. Then cells on the plate were photographed under the light microscope (time 0) and then incubated for another 48 hr at 37 °C 5% CO2 and allowed to migrate into the wound area. Images of the wound were collected at 0 and 48 hr using a microscope. The migration rate was quantified by measuring the distance between the wound edges. This assay was independently repeated for three times.

Statistical analysis
All results in this study were presented as mean ± standard deviation (SD). Statistical significance of differences between groups was explored by using student T test and One-way ANOVA followed by Dunnett's multiple comparisons using GraphPad Prism software, La Jolla California USA, http://www.graphpad.com. Value of P less than 0.05 was considered significant.

Results
siRNA suppressed HMGI-C mRNA and protein levels in breast adenocarcinoma cells
First, we explored the effect of siRNA on HMGI-C gene expression in MDA-MB468 cells by qRT-PCR and Western blot analysis. Relative HMGI-C gene expression was calculated in relation to the control group, which was considered as 100%. As shown in Figure 1A,1B, 2A and 2B, HMGI-C siRNA led to a marked reduction of HMGI-C mRNA in both dose – dependent mRNA and protein levels (p<0.05; relative to the control). At 24, 48 and 72hr after the transfection, the relative HMGI-C mRNA expression levels were 77.06%, 54.10% and 78.95%, respectively (Figure 1A), and the dose-dependent at 40, 60, 80 pmol of HMGI-C siRNA transfection relative HMGI-C mRNA expression levels were 88.87%, 71.13% and 47.25% (Figure 1B), and HMGI-C protein expression levels were 67.10%, 11.65% and 8.20%, respectively (Figure 2A, 2B) (p<0.05).

HMGI-C siRNA synergistically enhanced the cytotoxic effect of paclitaxel
To assess whether down-regulation of HMGI-C could enhance the sensitivity of the breast adenocarcinoma cells to paclitaxel, HMGI-C siRNA and Paclitaxel alone and combination treatment of paclitaxel and HMGI-C siRNA were investigated on MDA-MB468 cells (Figure 3A, 3B). As shown in Figure 3B, mono treatment with paclitaxel induced cytotoxicity in a dose-dependent way. The results of MTT assay showed that HMGI-C siRNA significantly decreased the cell survival rate to 43.24%, compared with the control group (p<0.05). Moreover, paclitaxel in combination with HMGI-C siRNA further decreased the cell survival rate relative to paclitaxel or HMGI-C siRNA alone (p<0.05). The CDI values were also less than 1 in all concentrations of Paclitaxel, which indicated the synergistic effect between the two agents (Figure 3B).

1A.

1B.

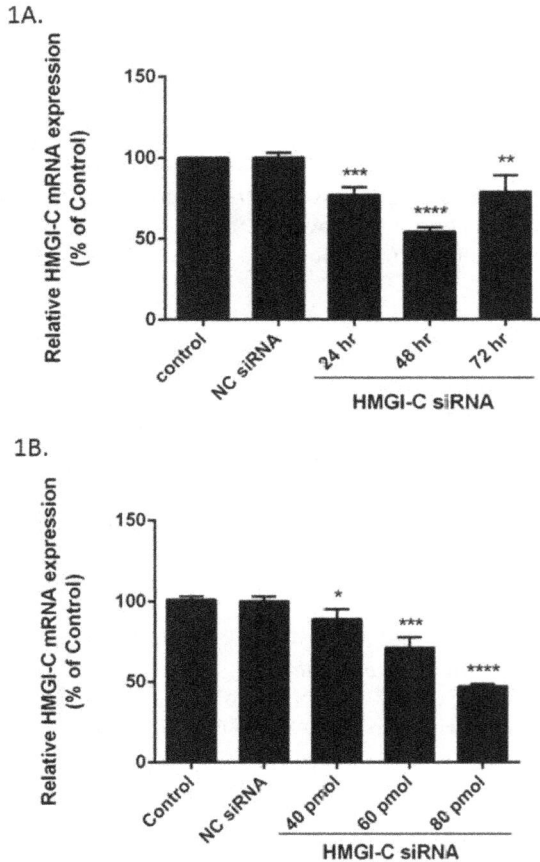

Figure 1. Suppression of HMGI-C mRNA Expression by siRNA in breast adenocarcinoma. (A) MDA-MB-468 cells were transfected with HMGI-C siRNA for 24, 48 and 72 hr. (B) MDA-MB-468 cells were transfected with HMGI-C siRNA with the doses of 40, 60, 80 pmol. Relative HMGI-C mRNA expression was measured by qRT-PCR using $2^{(-\Delta\Delta Ct)}$ method. The results are expressed as mean±SD (n=3); *p<0.05, **p<0.001, *** p= 0.0001 and ****p<0.0001 versus control

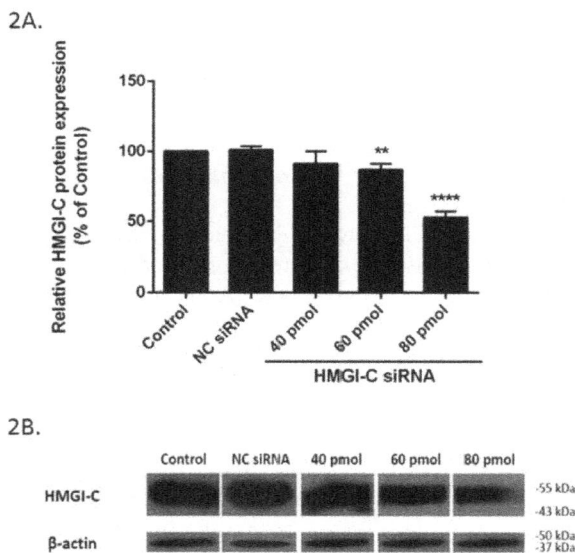

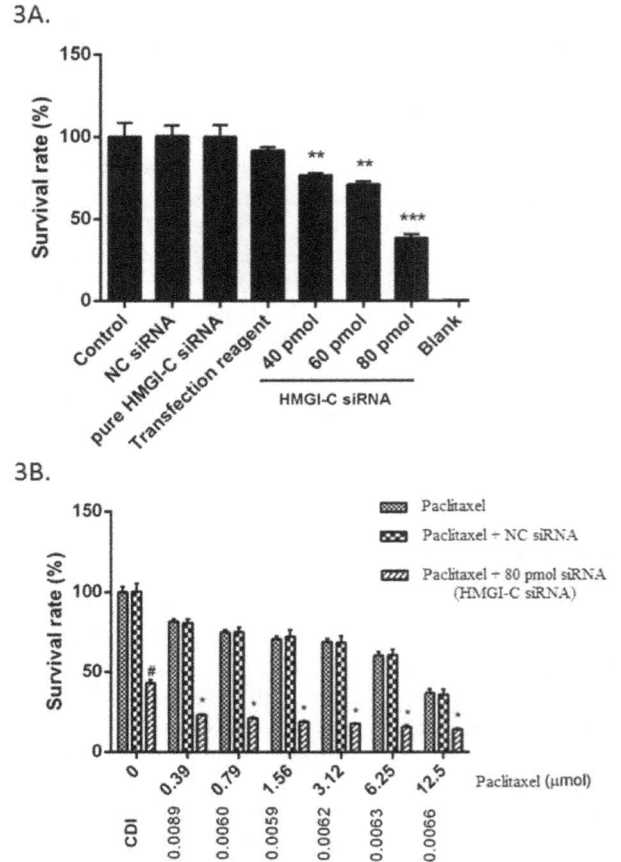

2A.

2B.

Figure 2. HMGI-C Protein Expression in MDA-MB-468 cells Transfected with siRNA. (A) Representative western blot of Beta-actin and HMGI-C proteins from cells transfected with HMGI-C siRNA. (B) The expression level of each band was quantified using densitometry and normalized to the respective Beta-actin. The results are expressed as mean±SD (n=3); **p<0.001 and ****p<0.0001, versus control.

3A.

3B.

Figure 3. Effect of HMGI-C siRNA on the Chemosensitivity of the MDA-MB-468 Cells. (A) 48 hr after transfection with HMGI-C siRNA (40, 60, 80 pmol), cytotoxicity of treatments was determined by MTT assay, **P<0.01 and ***P<0.001, versus control. (B) The cells were treated with Paclitaxel, and combination of paclitaxel and 80 pmol HMGI-C siRNA for 48 hr and then the cytotoxicity of the treatments was determined by MTT assay. The interaction effect between siRNA and Paclitaxel was determined using combination effect analysis and coefficient of drug interaction (CDI) values. The results are expressed as mean±SD (n=3); #p<0.05 versus 80pmol HMGI-C siRNA alone; *p<0.0001 versus control group.

Suppression of HMGI-C inhibited cells migration

Down-regulation of HMGI-C by using siRNA blocks migration of breast adenocarcinoma cells in vitro. Thus, we sought to determine whether siRNA blocks migration and invasion of breast cancer cells in vitro. Wound healing assays were performed to examine whether migration of the MDA-MB-468 cells transfected with HMGI-C siRNA was inhibited. Results showed that the knockdown of HMGI-C with siRNA, or Paclitaxel treatments alone versus the combination blocked the migration of MDA-MB-468 cells (Figure 4B). The number of MDAMB-468 cells with HMGI-C siRNA in 48 hr after treatment was 38.30%, Paclitaxel was 34.57%, and combination of siRNA and Paclitaxel was 24.61% that migrated to the scratched area of that of control (untreated) MDA-MB-468 cells (Figure 4A, 4B) (P < 0.0001). The CDI values were also less than 1 indicated the synergistic effect between the two agents (Figure 4B).

4A.

4B.

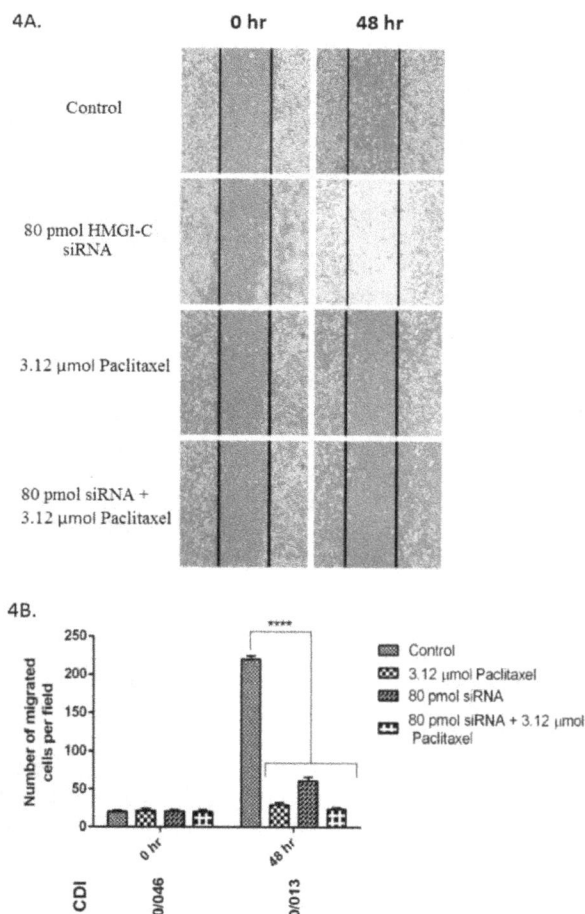

Figure 4. Untreated and treated MDA-MB-468 cells were subjected to scratch wound-healing assays. (A) MDA-MB-468 cells divided in 4 groups including untreated, specific siRNA, Paclitaxel and combination specific siRNA and Paclitaxel. The wound space was photographed at 0 and 48 hr. (B) The number of migrated cells to the wound sides was evaluated and statistically analyzed. Error bars indicate the mean ± SD of three independent experiments (****P < 0.0001).

Discussion

Previous studies showed that HMGI-C increases tumor transformation in different cell types.[24,25] It has been found that HMGI-C overexpression is associated with enhancing tumor growth and invasion, early metastasis, and a poor prognosis, typically seen in pancreatic cancer,[26] papillary thyroid carcinoma,[27] colorectal cancer,[17] ovarian cancer,[28] lung cancer[14] and HG-PSC.[16] Previous studies have demonstrated that, HMGI-C gene suppression leads to increased apoptosis and simultaneously sensitizes the malignant cells to chemotherapeutic agents. In this regards, we utilized RNA interference for specific suppression of HMGI-C in MDA-MB-468 cells to overcome resistance to chemotherapeutic agent, paclitaxel. In the current study we examined the effect of HMGI-C specific siRNA and paclitaxel alone or in combination on MDA-MB-468 breast adenocarcinoma cells cytotoxicity and migration. The results of qRT-PCR and western blot analysis showed that transfection with HMGI-C siRNA could significantly reduce the mRNA levels of HMGI-C and its

translated protein during the 48 hr period in dose dependent manner, suggesting that HMGI-C siRNA could effectively cleave HMGI-C mRNA and blocked its translation to protein.

As our previous study treatment of adenocarcinoma cells with specific HMGI-C siRNA induced apoptosis and cell cycle arrest. The results of MTT assay revealed that pretreatment with HMGI-C siRNA could synergistically reduce the viability of breast malignant cells to paclitaxel, demonstrating that HMGI-C down-regulation could sensitize MDA-MB-468 cells to paclitaxel. we examined the rate of migration through wound-healing (scratch) assay, It was found that migration were significantly inhibited in MDA-MB-468 cell lines after HMGI-C siRNA and paclitaxel alone or in combination treatment compare to control (untreated) group.

In this study, we found that HMGI-C siRNA enhances paclitaxel chemosensitivity and inhibits migration in breast adenocarcinoma cells. Cell cytotoxicity and migration of HMGI-C siRNA transfected, and paclitaxel treated cell lines notably were declined compared to those of untreated cells and the cells that treated with HMGI-C siRNA and paclitaxel individually.

CDI value showed that treatment with HMGI-C siRNA and paclitaxel inhibit cells migration in a synergic manner compared to HMGI-C siRNA group, paclitaxel group and control group (untreated). In similar study, Karami et al. showed specific silencing of survivin expression by siRNA enhanced sensitivity of leukemic cells to etoposide.[29,30] In other studies, they showed MDR1 down-regulation synergistically increased the cytotoxic effects of oxaliplatin and etoposide on oxaliplatin resistant SW480 and etoposide resistant HL-60 cells.[5,31]

In summary, we demonstrated for the first time to our knowledge that, HMGI-C overexpression was sufficient to induce tumor formation and cell migration in MDA-MB-468 cell lines. We postulate that induction of HMGI-C up regulation in early breast adenocarcinoma may be responsible for rapid progression of breast adenocarcinoma. Further characterization of the functional relationship between HMGI-C and HMGI-C-mediated migration target gene regulation will help us understand the tumor genesis of breast adenocarcinoma.

Conclusion

Our data suggest that specific HMGI-C siRNA can inhibit the expression of HMGI-C protein and mRNA in breast adenocarcinoma cells and may potentially be a therapeutic agent for breast cancer metastasis. It can also synergetic effect with paclitaxel and decrease the effective dose of paclitaxel in treatment of breast adenocarcinoma cells.

Acknowledgments

The authors would like to thank IRC team technical assistance. This work was supported by a grant from the Immunology Research Center (IRC), Tabriz University of Medical Sciences (No. 92/74).

Ethical Issues
Not applicable.

Conflict of Interest
Authors declare no conflict of interest in this study.

Abbreviations
siRNA, small interfering RNA; HMGI-C, High mobility group protein isoform I-C; HMGA1, high mobility group A1; HMGA2, high mobility group A1; EMT, *Epithelial-mesenchymal transition*; MDA-MB-468, Breast adenocarcinoma cell line; NF-kB, Nuclear factor kappa-light-chain-enhancer of activated B cells; ATF2, Activating transcription factor 2; ELF1, E74-like factor 1; OCT2, Octamer transcription factor 2; Oct-6, Octamer transcription factor 6; *SRF, Serum response factor;* NF-Y, Nuclear factor Y; RAR, *Retinoic acid receptor*

References
1. DeSantis C, Ma J, Bryan L, Jemal A. Breast cancer statistics, 2013. *CA Cancer J Clin* 2014;64(1):52-62. doi: 10.3322/caac.21203
2. Whelan J. First clinical data on rnai. *Drug Discov Today* 2005;10(15):1014-5. doi: 10.1016/S1359-6446(05)03547-6
3. Fire AZ. Gene silencing by double-stranded rna. *Cell Death Differ* 2007;14(12):1998-2012. doi: 10.1038/sj.cdd.4402253
4. Yazdi Samadi BVM. Genetics a molecular approach. Iran;Tehran University Publishers: Iran: Tehran University Publishers; 1388.
5. Kachalaki S, Baradaran B, Majidi J, Yousefi M, Shanehbandi D, Mohammadinejad S, et al. Reversal of chemoresistance with small interference rna (sirna) in etoposide resistant acute myeloid leukemia cells (hl-60). *Biomed Pharmacother* 2015;75:100-4. doi: 10.1016/j.biopha.2015.08.032
6. Mansoori B, Sandoghchian Shotorbani S, Baradaran B. Rna interference and its role in cancer therapy. *Adv Pharm Bull* 2014;4(4):313-21. doi: 10.5681/apb.2014.046
7. Mansoori B, Mohammadi A, Shir Jang S, Baradaran B. Mechanisms of immune system activation in mammalians by small interfering rna (sirna). *Artif Cells Nanomed Biotechnol* 2015:1-8. doi: 10.3109/21691401.2015.1102738
8. Narita M, Narita M, Krizhanovsky V, Nunez S, Chicas A, Hearn SA, et al. A novel role for high-mobility group a proteins in cellular senescence and heterochromatin formation. *Cell* 2006;126(3):503-14. doi: 10.1016/j.cell.2006.05.052
9. Reeves R. Molecular biology of hmga proteins: Hubs of nuclear function. *Gene* 2001;277(1-2):63-81.
10. Chiappetta G, Avantaggiato V, Visconti R, Fedele M, Battista S, Trapasso F, et al. High level expression of the hmgi (y) gene during embryonic development. *Oncogene* 1996;13(11):2439-46.
11. Hirning-Folz U, Wilda M, Rippe V, Bullerdiek J, Hameister H. The expression pattern of the hmgic

gene during development. *Genes Chromosomes Cancer* 1998;23(4):350-7.
12. Gattas GJ, Quade BJ, Nowak RA, Morton CC. Hmgic expression in human adult and fetal tissues and in uterine leiomyomata. *Genes Chromosomes Cancer* 1999;25(4):316-22.
13. Rogalla P, Drechsler K, Frey G, Hennig Y, Helmke B, Bonk U, et al. Hmgi-c expression patterns in human tissues. Implications for the genesis of frequent mesenchymal tumors. *Am J Pathol* 1996;149(3):775-9.
14. Meyer B, Loeschke S, Schultze A, Weigel T, Sandkamp M, Goldmann T, et al. Hmga2 overexpression in non-small cell lung cancer. *Mol Carcinog* 2007;46(7):503-11. doi: 10.1002/mc.20235
15. Abe N, Watanabe T, Suzuki Y, Matsumoto N, Masaki T, Mori T, et al. An increased high-mobility group a2 expression level is associated with malignant phenotype in pancreatic exocrine tissue. *Br J Cancer* 2003;89(11):2104-9. doi: 10.1038/sj.bjc.6601391
16. Malek A, Bakhidze E, Noske A, Sers C, Aigner A, Schafer R, et al. Hmga2 gene is a promising target for ovarian cancer silencing therapy. *Int J Cancer* 2008;123(2):348-56. doi: 10.1002/ijc.23491
17. Guang-meng XU, Hai-na Z, Xiao-feng T, Mei S, Xue-dong F. Effect of HMGA2 shRNA on the cell proliferation and invasion of human colorectal cancer sw480 cells in vitro. *Chem Res Chinese Univ* 2012;28(2):264-8.
18. Chau KY, Manfioletti G, Cheung-Chau KW, Fusco A, Dhomen N, Sowden JC, et al. Derepression of hmga2 gene expression in retinoblastoma is associated with cell proliferation. *Mol Med* 2003;9(5-8):154-65.
19. Miyazawa J, Mitoro A, Kawashiri S, Chada KK, Imai K. Expression of mesenchyme-specific gene hmga2 in squamous cell carcinomas of the oral cavity. *Cancer Res* 2004;64(6):2024-9.
20. Andrieux J, Demory JL, Dupriez B, Quief S, Plantier I, Roumier C, et al. Dysregulation and overexpression of hmga2 in myelofibrosis with myeloid metaplasia. *Genes Chromosomes Cancer* 2004;39(1):82-7. doi: 10.1002/gcc.10297
21. Lee YS, Dutta A. The tumor suppressor microrna let-7 represses the hmga2 oncogene. *Genes Dev* 2007;21(9):1025-30. doi: 10.1101/gad.1540407
22. Thuault S, Tan EJ, Peinado H, Cano A, Heldin CH, Moustakas A. Hmga2 and smads co-regulate snail1 expression during induction of epithelial-to-mesenchymal transition. *J Biol Chem* 2008;283(48):33437-46. doi: 10.1074/jbc.M802016200
23. Chou TC, Talalay P. Quantitative analysis of dose-effect relationships: The combined effects of multiple drugs or enzyme inhibitors. *Adv Enzyme Regul* 1984;22:27-55.
24. Mayr C, Hemann MT, Bartel DP. Disrupting the pairing between let-7 and hmga2 enhances oncogenic

transformation. *Science* 2007;315(5818):1576-9. doi: 10.1126/science.1137999

25. Di Cello F, Hillion J, Hristov A, Wood LJ, Mukherjee M, Schuldenfrei A, et al. Hmga2 participates in transformation in human lung cancer. *Mol Cancer Res* 2008;6(5):743-50. doi: 10.1158/1541-7786.MCR-07-0095

26. Hristov AC, Cope L, Reyes MD, Singh M, Iacobuzio-Donahue C, Maitra A, et al. Hmga2 protein expression correlates with lymph node metastasis and increased tumor grade in pancreatic ductal adenocarcinoma. *Mod Pathol* 2009;22(1):43-9. doi: 10.1038/modpathol.2008.140

27. Chiappetta G, Ferraro A, Vuttariello E, Monaco M, Galdiero F, De Simone V, et al. Hmga2 mrna expression correlates with the malignant phenotype in human thyroid neoplasias. *Eur J Cancer* 2008;44(7):1015-21. doi: 10.1016/j.ejca.2008.02.039

28. Wu J, Liu Z, Shao C, Gong Y, Hernando E, Lee P, et al. Hmga2 overexpression-induced ovarian surface epithelial transformation is mediated through regulation of emt genes. *Cancer Res* 2011;71(2):349-59. doi: 10.1158/0008-5472.CAN-10-2550

29. Karami H, Baradaran B, Esfahani A, Estiar MA, Naghavi-Behzad M, Sakhinia M, et al. Sirna-mediated silencing of survivin inhibits proliferation and enhances etoposide chemosensitivity in acute myeloid leukemia cells. *Asian Pac J Cancer Prev* 2013;14(12):7719-24.

30. Karami H, Baradaran B, Esfehani A, Sakhinia M, Sakhinia E. Down-regulation of mcl-1 by small interference rna induces apoptosis and sensitizes hl-60 leukemia cells to etoposide. *Asian Pac J Cancer Prev* 2014;15(2):629-35.

31. Montazami N, Kheir Andish M, Majidi J, Yousefi M, Yousefi B, Mohamadnejad L, et al. Sirna-mediated silencing of mdr1 reverses the resistance to oxaliplatin in sw480/oxr colon cancer cells. *Cell Mol Biol (Noisy-le-grand)* 2015;61(2):98-103.

2

Surface Solid Dispersion and Solid Dispersion of Meloxicam: Comparison and Product Development

Mayank Chaturvedi[1], Manish Kumar[2]*, Kamla Pathak[3], Shailendra Bhatt[2], Vipin Saini[2]

[1] Department of Pharmaceutics, Rajiv Academy for Pharmacy, Chattikkara, Mathura, India.
[2] Department of Pharmaceutics, M M College of Pharmacy, Maharishi Markandeshwar University,Mullana, Ambala-133207, Haryana, India.
[3] Department of Pharmaceutics, Pharmacy College Saifai, Uttar Pradesh University of Medical sciences, Saifai, Etawah , 206130, Uttar Pradesh, India.

Keywords:
· Surface solid dispersion
· Solid dispersion
· Dissolution
· Orodispersible tablet

Abstract

Purpose: A comparative study was carried out between surface solid dispersion (SSD) and solid dispersion (SD) of meloxicam (MLX) to assess the solubility and dissolution enhancement approach and thereafter develop as patient friendly orodispersible tablet.

Methods: Crospovidone (CPV), a hydrophilic carrier was selected for SSD preparation on the basis of 89% in- vitro MLX adsorption, 19% hydration capacity and high swelling index. SD on the other hand was made with PEG4000. Both were prepared by co-grinding and solvent evaporation method using drug: carrier ratios of 1:1, 1:4, and 1:8. Formulation SSDS3 (MLX: CPV in 1:8 ratio) made by solvent evaporation method showed $t_{50\%}$ of 28 min and 80.9% DE_{50min} which was higher in comparison to the corresponding solid dispersion, SDS3 ($t_{50\%}$ of 35min and 76.4% DE_{50min}). Both SSDS3 and SDS3 were developed as orodispersible tablets and evaluated.

Results: Tablet formulation F3 made with SSD3 with a disintegration time of 11 secs, by wetting time= 6 sec, high water absorption of 78%by wt and cumulative drug release of 97% proved to be superior than the tablet made with SD3.

Conclusion: Conclusively, the SSD of meloxicam has the potential to be developed as fast acing formulation that can ensure almost complete release of drug.

Introduction

Dissolution of solid dosage forms in gastrointestinal fluids is a precondition for the delivery of the drug to the systemic circulation following oral administration. The parameters that predominantly influence drug dissolution are the solubility of drug and surface area of particle.[1] An increasing problem of poorly water soluble drug requisites obtaining a satisfactory dissolution within the gastrointestinal tract that is necessary for good bioavailability. To improve the aqueous solubility of poorly water soluble drug various techniques have been utilized such as complexation with the polymer, salt formation, addition of surfactant, prodrug and others. Solid dispersion is a frequently used technique to improve the aqueous solubility of drug where one or more active ingredient(s) is uniformly dispersed in an inert water soluble carrier matrix. Amorphization of drug, improved wettability and decrease in particle size are the main mechanisms for enhanced dissolution.[2]

In spite of several advantages of solid dispersions, the water soluble carriers used for their preparation produce soft and tacky mass which is difficult to handle especially in tablet making.[3,4] Additionally, at high concentrations such carriers may decrease dissolution due to high viscosity in the boundary layer close to the dissolving surface.[5] These problems can be mitigated by surface solid dispersion that uses water insoluble hydrophilic carriers and the drug is deposited on the surface of carrier.[6] Such excipients include sodium starch glycolate, crospovidone, potato starch, silicon dioxide, croscarmellose sodium, pre-gelatinized starch and microcrystalline cellulose. Drug release from these carriers depends on the porosity, particle size and surface area of the carrier. When in contact with water, the carrier immediately disperses allowing rapid release of the drug. The dissolution and bioavailability of poorly water soluble drug is expected to improve extensively by surface solid dispersion technique.[7] This technique when coupled with product development into orodispersible tablets is expected to further enhance the solubility of the drug. The advantages of mouth dissolving dosage/ orodispersible tablets are increasingly being recognized in both, industry and academics. The increasing popularity of these dosage

Corresponding author: Manish Kumar, Email: manish_singh17@rediffmail.com forms is in part owing to various factors such as fast disintegration, good mouth feels, easy to handle, easy to swallow and effective taste.[8,9]

Meloxicam a non-steroidal anti-inflammatory and antipyretic agent has low aqueous solubility that delays its absorption from the gastrointestinal tract. The efforts to enhance the solubility and correspondingly the dissolution are widely reported in literature. These include the solid dispersions using hydrophilic carriers,[10] skimmed milk,[11] PEG 4000 by dropping method[12] poloxamer 188 using kneading method,[13,14] PEG 6000[15] polyvinyl pyrrolidone using solvent evaporation method,[16] various polymers[17] and PEG 6000 by fusion melt method.[18] As specified these systems are constrained with the certain limitations, the present work was aimed to develop surface solid dispersions of MLX and compare it with its solid dispersion for assessing the dissolution characteristics. Secondly to develop patient friendly dosage form and evaluate it.

Materials and Methods

Meloxicam was supplied as gift sample from Unimark Pharmaceuticals Ltd., Ahmadabad, India. Crospovidone and sodium starch glycolate were gifted sample from International Specialility Product Technologies Ltd. USA. PEG 6000 was obtained from CDH, New Delhi and N, N-dimethylformamide from Qualikems Fine Chemicals, New Delhi. Microcrystalline cellulose, mannitol and sodium saccharin were procured from Ranbaxy Fine chemicals Pvt.Ltd. Mumbai.

Equilibrium solubility

An excess amount of MLX was added to 25 mL conical flasks containing different amounts of carriers CPV and sodium starch glycolate in double distilled water separately. The flasks were placed in mechanical shaker at 37±0.5°C for 48 h. At the end of 48 h the samples were filtered through Whatman filter paper and analyzed spectrophotometrically at 363 nm (Shimadzu, Pharmaspec1700, Kyoto, Japan).

In vitro adsorption

In vitro adsorption of drug on the carriers CPV and sodium starch glycolate was analyzed by dissolving 10 mg of MLX in 100ml double distilled water. The carriers were dispersed separately into this solution and stirred continuously by magnetic stirrer at room temperature. Samples were taken at regular intervals of 0, 20, 40, 60, 80, 100 and 120 min and assayed for unadsorbed drug at 363nm. Percent drug adsorbed was determined and plotted against time.[7]

Hydration capacity

One gram of the carrier was placed in 10 mL pre-weighed centrifuge tubes. Sufficient distilled water was added to make up the volume to 10 mL and the suspension was shaken vigorously for 5 min. The suspension was allowed to stand for 10 min and then excess water was removed by centrifugation at 4000rpm for 10 min and tube with sediment was then reweighed.[19] The hydration capacity was calculated by Equation 1.

$$Hydration\ capacity = \frac{weight\ of\ tube\ with\ sediment\ -\ weight\ of\ empty\ tube}{weight\ of\ sample\ on\ dry\ basis} \times 100 \qquad \text{Equation 1}$$

Swelling studies

Water uptake and swelling index of the carriers CPV and sodium starch glycolate were determined by method reported[19] using indigenously developed apparatus. Weighed quantity of the carrier was subjected to the graduated arm A and double distilled water was poured in graduated arm B to a level corresponding to the height of powder pile in arm A. The level of swelling medium was maintained constant during the entire experiment. The changes in the volume (cm^3) of the sample were recorded at different time intervals up to 2 h and swelling index was calculated by the following formula (Equation 2):

$$Percent\ swelling\ index = \frac{Final\ volume\ -\ Initial\ volume}{Initial\ volume} \times 100$$

$$\text{Equation 2}$$

Preparation of surface solid dispersion and solid dispersion

Both SSDs and SDs were prepared by co-grinding and solvent evaporation technique, using 1:1, 1:4 and 1: 8 drug: carrier ratios. In the former method, the drug with carrier was co-grounded in a glass mortar-pestle for 30 min. The mixture was sieved through mesh (# 60) and collected for further evaluation. In solvent evaporation method, the drug was dissolved in dimethylformamide followed by dispersion of carrier into it. The mixture was heated at 60°C in a thermostatically controlled water bath till the solvent was completely evaporated and the mass so obtained was kept in a desiccator until used for the further studies.

Evaluation of SSD and SD

Drug content and Equilibrium solubility

SSD equivalent to 10 mg of MLX was weighed accurately and dissolved in 10 mL of methanol. The stock solution was diluted with double distilled water and analyzed spectrophotometrically. Similar procedure was used to determine the drug content of SD. The equilibrium solubility of drug in its SSD and SD forms was determined by the method described earlier.

In vitro dissolution

The *in vitro* dissolution studies for pure meloxicam, SSD and SD were carried out in triplicates, in USP Apparatus II using 900 mL of double distilled water at 37±0.5°C at 100 rpm. Samples equivalent to 10 mg of meloxicam were filled in capsules (size 0) and subjected to the study. Aliquots of 5 mL were withdrawn at specified time intervals of 0, 20, 40 and 60 min and filtered through Whatman filter paper. An equal volume of fresh dissolution medium was replaced to maintain the volume of dissolution medium. The filtered samples were analyzed and used to determine % cumulative drug dissolution with respect to time.

Statistical analysis of in vitro dissolution data
Model independent parameters were calculated to select the optimized system. Percent dissolution efficiency (% DE) was computed to compare the relative performance of the polymers in surface solid dispersion and solid dispersions. The magnitude of % DE was computed as the percent ratio of area under the dissolution curve up to time t (yx.dt), to that of area of the rectangle described by 100% dissolution at the same time (y100xt). It was calculated by Equation 3.

$$\% \, DE = \frac{\int_0^t y \, x \, dt}{y100 \, xt} \times 100 \qquad \text{Equation 3}$$

On the basis of the above interpretation, best among the related group were selected for further studies.

Powder properties
The SSDs and SDs were subjected to a range of powder properties determination. Angle of repose was determined using cylinder method.[20] Apparent bulk density (ρ_b) was determined by pouring weighed amount of powder into a 50 cc graduated cylinder. The bulk volume (V_b) was noted and divided by the powder weight to get the bulk density. The tapped density was determined by subjecting the powder to 50 tapping at height of 1 inch. The tapped volume (V_t) was divided by weight of the powder to get tapped density (ρ_t). The compressibility index which is calculated as follows (Equation 4):

$$CompressibilityIndex = \frac{V_b - V_t}{V_b} \times 100 \qquad \text{Equation 4}$$

The value of compressibility index below 15% indicates a powder with good flow characteristics,[20] whereas above 25% indicates poor flow. Next, Hausner ratio which is an indirect index of ease of powder flow was calculated by dividing tapped density by bulk density.

FTIR
Further to confirm the identity of drug FTIR studies was carried out using Fourier transform infrared spectrophotometer (FTIR-8400S, Shimadzu, Kyoto, Japan). Pure meloxicam and KBr powder was dried in hot air oven for half an hour at 50 °C, ensuring the removal of moisture. Then the drug was mixed with KBr in the ratio of 9:1 and triturated, afterwards it was exposed to infrared rays. The scanning range of 500-4000cm^{-1} was used with 1 cm^{-1} resolution to obtain the IR spectra of this sample.

Differential Scanning Calorimetry
The samples were sealed in aluminium pans and analyzed using a DSC Q-200 V 24.4 Build 116 of TA instruments, USA. Both the sample and reference (alumina) are kept at the same temperature and the heat flow required maintaining the equality in temperature was measured. 5 to 10 mg of sample was sealed in aluminium pan and analyzed using a differential scanning calorimeter focused on the melting temperatures. A scanning rate of 10°C/min from 30°C to 300°C under nitrogen purge was applied.

Orodispersible tablet
The tablets of both optimized SD and SSD formulations were prepared by direct compression method. The ingredients were weighed (Table 1) and except the lubricant, were mixed in a polybag for 15 min.
At the end of mixing period magnesium stearate was incorporated and mixing was continued for another 5 min. Tablets were compressed on single punch Tablet machine and evaluated.

Table 1. Formulation design for orodisperable tablet of meloxicam surface solid dispersions (SSDS) and solid dispersion (SDS)

Formulation code	SSDS3 mixture (equivalent to 10mg drug)	SDS3 mixture (equivalent to 10mg drug)	Mannitol (mg)	Crospovidone (mg)	Sodium saccharine Flavor (mg)	Microcrystalline cellulose
F1	90	–	35	–	2	q.s
F2	90	–	35	5	2	q.s
F3	90	–	35	10	2	q.s
F4	–	90	35	–	2	q.s
F5	–	90	35	5	2	q.s
F6	–	90	35	10	2	q .s

Tablet evaluation
Thickness and Hardness
For thickness determination tablets were selected randomly from each batch and thickness was measured

using Vernier Caliper (Mitotoyo, Japan). The hardness of six tablets was determined using Pfizer tester (Hicon® Grover Enterprises, New Delhi, India) and the results are expressed as average ± SD.

Content uniformity
Ten tablets of each formulation were crushed in a glass pestle mortar. A powder weight equivalent to 10 mg of MLX was dissolved in 100 ml phosphate buffer, pH 7.4 and filtered. One milliliter solution was diluted to 10 ml and assayed for drug content.

Weight variation
Twenty tablets of each batch were selected randomly and weighed. The average weight was calculated, not more than 2 of individual weight deviated from the average weight by more than the percentage as per pharmacopoeial limits (Indian Pharmacopoeia 2007) and not deviated more than twice that percentage.

Disintegration time
The disintegration time of the tablets was determined in phosphate buffer, pH 6.8 at 37±0.5 °C as per IP monograph (2007) via Tablet disintegration test machine (Hicon® Grover Enterprises, New Delhi, India). Six tablets were placed on the wire mesh just above the surface of the buffer media as a disintegrating medium present in the tube of disintegration test apparatus. The time required for each tablet to completely disintegrate and all the granules to go through the wire mesh were recorded. Results are expressed as an average of three determinations.

Friability
Friability of the tablets was determined using Roche Friabilator test apparatus (Hicon® Grover Enterprises, New Delhi, India). Preweighed sample of 10 tablets was placed in the Friabilator and subjected to 100 revolutions with an operating speed of 25rpm. Tablets were dedusted using a soft muslin cloth and reweighed to calculate friability.

Water absorption ratio
A piece of tissue paper folded twice was placed in small petri-dish containing 6 mL of water. A tablet was put on the paper and the time required for complete wetting was recorded. The wetted tablet was then weighed. Water absorption ratio (R), was determined by using Equation 5.

$$R = \frac{(W_a - W_b)}{W_b} \times 100 \qquad \text{Equation 5}$$

Where, W_b = weight of tablet before water absorption and W_a = Weight of tablet after water absorption

In vitro release
The release profiles of meloxicam orodispersible tablets made with SSD3 and SD3 (F1-F6) were determined using the dissolution test apparatus USP II set with a paddle speed of 50 rpm. Dissolution was tested in 900 ml of phosphate buffer, pH 6.8 maintained at 37±0.5°C. An aliquot sample of 5 mL was withdrawn, at 0, 5, 10, 15, 20 and 30 min and filtered through Whatman filter paper.

An equal volume of fresh medium, which was prewarmed at 37°C replaced into the dissolution medium after each sampling to maintain the constant volume throughout the test. The samples were analyzed spectrophotometrically.

Results
The results of *in vitro* adsorption plots of MLX on CPV and sodium starch glycolate revealed similarity in the pattern of adsorption wherein the abundant free adsorption sites led to higher initial adsorption that later on slowed down. However, the extent of adsorption of MLX on CPV was slightly higher (89%) than on sodium starch glycolate (83%). This may be due to higher larger particle size of the former that provided more surface-area for adsorption of MLX.[18] Another determinant property of the carrier was the hydration capacity that was found to be 18% for CPV and 13% for sodium starch glycolate (Table 2).

Table 2. Swelling index profile of Crospovidone and Sodium starch glycolate

Time in (hr)	crospovidone	Sodium starch glycolate
0	0	0
30	150	110
60	275	189
120	350	230

This is because CPV exhibits its action by swelling as well as wicking which is caused due to its capillary action and porosity while sodium starch glycolate does so only by swelling phenomenon.[21] Furthermore, the equilibrium solubility of MLX was higher in presence of CPV rather than sodium starch glycolate. The study elaborated the percent enhancement solubility of the drug with sodium starch glycolate was 300% and 335% with crospovidone due to high interfacial activity of the former.

The drug content of SDs prepared by co-grinding method (SDC1 – SDC3) varied from 89.2 - 96.6 and those prepared by solvent evaporation method (SDS1 – SDS3) varied from 90.2 – 96.3 respectively while the drug content of prepared SSDs by co-grinding method (SSDC1 – SSDC3) varied from 91.9 - 96.0 and that prepared from solvent evaporation (SSDS1 – SSDS3) varied from 89.1 – 97.9 respectively.

The percentage enhancement in solubility of MLX via SSDs ranged from 58.56% – 192.66 % while the percentage enhancement in solubility of MLX via SDs was much lower in the range of 5.09% – 56.83 % (Figure 1).

The pure drug showed poor dissolution characteristics in comparison to *in vitro* dissolution profiles of SSDs (Figure 2a) and SDs (Figure 2b).

Dissolution efficiency and $t_{50\%}$ were determined for SSDs and SDs and are shown in Table 3.

The powder properties of SSDS3 and SDS3 are tabulated in Table 4 and Figure 3.

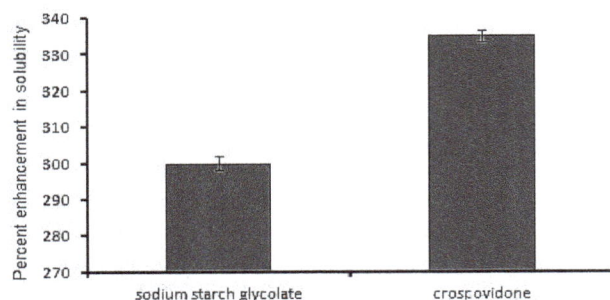

Figure 1. Comparative percent enhancement n solubility of meloxicam with crospovidone and sodium starch glycolate

Table 3. Model independent parameters of Surface solid Dispersion and solid dispersion

Batch code	$t_{50\%}$	%DE_{50min}
SSDC1	48	53.1
SSDC2	35	71.7
SSDC3	32	72.1
SSDS1	38	74.8
SSDS2	45	75.4
SSDS3	28	80.9
SDC1	43	69.3
SDC2	40	71.6
SDC3	38	73.8
SDS1	45	71.5
SDS2	42	72.8
SDS3	35	76.4

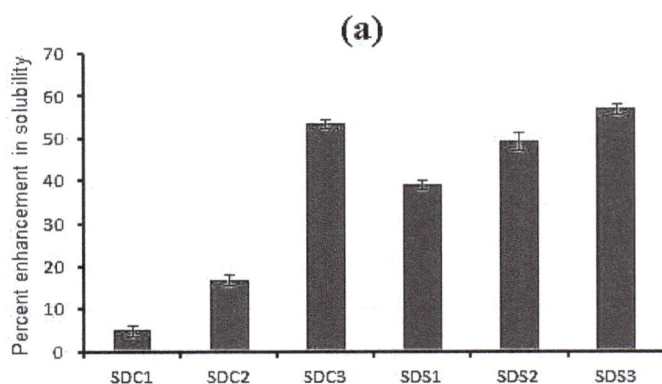

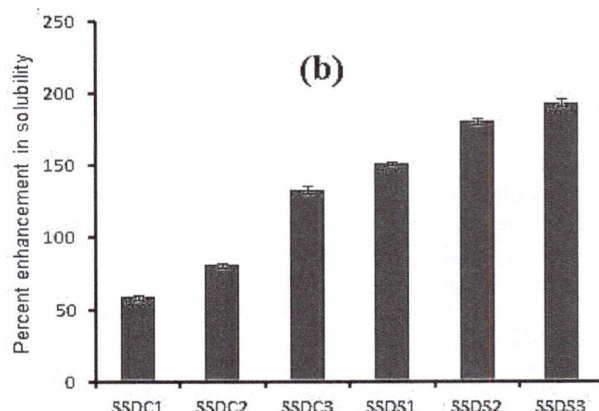

Figure 2. Comparative percent enhancement in solubility of meloxicam with prepared (a) solid dispersion and (b) surface solid dispersion

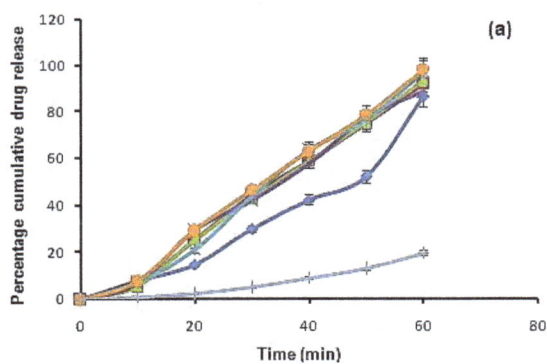

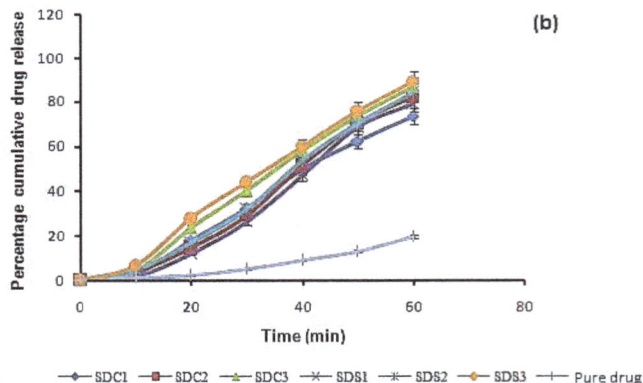

Figure 3. Comparative *in vitro* dissolution profile of (a) SSD's and (b) SD's with respect to pure drug

Table 4. Micromeritics properties

Parameters	SSDS3	SDS3
Angle of Repose (º)	21.79±0.9	41.2±1.99
Loose density	0.325 g/mL	C.472 g/mL
Tapped Density	0.357 g/mL	C.658 g/mL
Carr's Compressibility index	8.82%± 1.2	28.26 %±2.1
Particle Size (μm)	204.68±15.1	321.36±35.34
Hausner's ratio	1.096±0.5	1.394±1.1

The angle of repose (21.79±0.9°) of SSDS3 was much lower than of SDS3 (41.2±1.99 °). This suggests excellent flow property of SSD (<25°) while poor flow characteristics were deduced for SDS3 that will require incorporation of flow activators in SDs in manufacturing lines. Good flow characteristics of SSDS3 can also be interpreted by low Carr's compressibility index of 8.82%±1.2 which lies in the range for excellent particle flow (5-15%)[22] in comparison to 28.26±2.1 for SDS3 (poor flow in 23-35). Furthermore, the Hausner's ratio of SSDS3 was 1.09 ±0.5, which is less than 1.25 and indicated good flow property while SDS3 had a value higher than 1.25 confirming poor flow property of the latter.

The major IR peaks for MLX observed at 3136 (-N-H-stretching), 1639 (-C=O- stretching), 1280-1392 (-CN stretching), 1392-1176 (S=O stretching), 838 (-C-H-aromatic ring stretching) and were retained in SSDS3 spectrum (Figure 4).

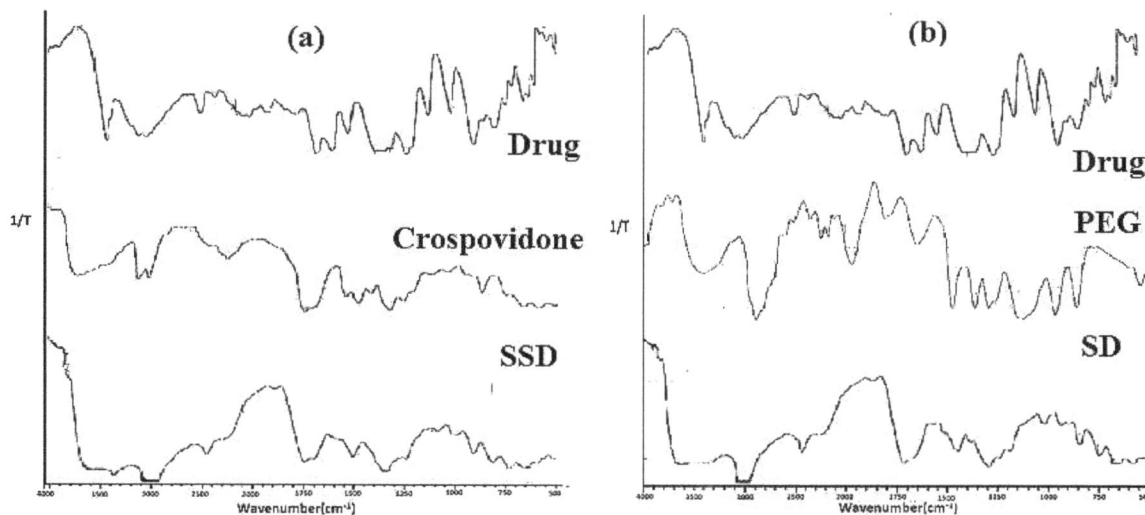

Figure 4. Comparative FTIR spectra of (a) Surface solid dispersion (b) Solid dispersion

The DSC thermogram of MLX (Figure 5a) showed a sharp endothermic peak at 260°C corresponding to its melting point. The thermogram of CPV (Figure 5b) exhibited a broad endothermic peak at 78.60°C with peak onset from 40.48°C. The thermogram of SSDS3 (Figure 5c) showed peaks characteristic of CPV with no additional peaks and most importantly the retention of less intense MLX peaks indicated adsorption of drug over carrier CPV. The DSC in Figure 5d and 5g referred to the physical mixture of SSDS3 and SDS3 respectively in which the peak characteristics of both drug and carriers was observed with no shifting and addition of new peaks. While that of PEG6000 (Figure 5e) showed peak characteristics at 61.5°C. The DSC of SDS3 (Figure 5f) showed peak characteristics of PEG at 60.4 with the loss of peak characteristics of drug indicating the penetration of drug inside carrier PEG6000.

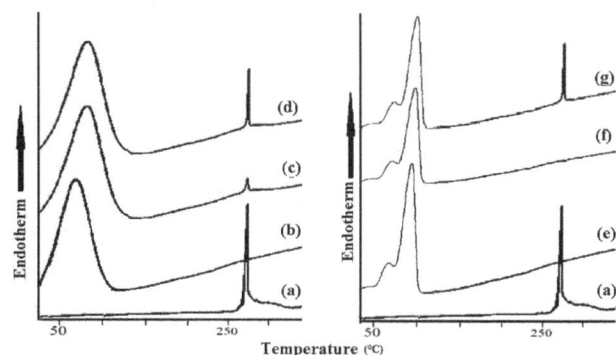

Figure 5. Comparative DSC analysis of (a) pure drug(Meloxicam) (b) Crospovidone (c) Surface solid dispersion (d) Physical mixture of optimized SSD (e) PEG 6000 (f) Solid dispersion (g) Physical mixture of optimized SD

Optimized formulation SSDS3 and SDS3 were developed as orodispersible tablet and evaluated. A total of six formulations were developed and evaluated for weight, diameter, thickness, hardness, friability, wetting time, disintegration time and water absorption ratio and the results are compiled in Table 5. Formulation F1, F2 and F3 weighed 148.2±1.2, 148.8±1.1 and 148.1±1.4 respectively and each having a diameter of 10.3 mm. The thickness of formulation F1, F2, F3 was 5.3 mm, 5.4 mm, 5.6 mm respectively. Hardness of tablets was measured and was found to be 3.15±0.13, 3.27±.09 and 3.32±.05 kg/cm^2. Friability of F1 was 0.7%, F2 was 0.7% and that of F3 was 0.5%.

In vitro release profiles of F1 – F6 were compared with the marketed formulation as shown in Figure 6. Formulation F3 (Figure 6a) shows 97% drug release in 30 min while marketed formulation showed only 42% drug release in 30 min.

Discussion

In vitro adsorption study was aimed to evaluate the water holding capacity of the carrier materials that can affect dissolution of drug and disintegration of dosage form (in this case the tablet). Similarly, the swelling study showed 350 and 230 times swelling for CPV and sodium starch glycolate respectively in 120 h. CPV is reported as carrier with swellable adsorbent group and hence increases the solubility of poorly soluble drugs. A water insoluble but rapidly swellable synthetically cross linked homopolymer of N-vinyl-2-pyrrolidone provides efficient stearic hindrance for nucleation and crystal growth was provided by repeating units in crospovidone due to its anti-plasticizing effect. Thus, CPV with porous and granular high surface area, and high interfacial activity enhanced the solubility of MLX. Thus crospovidone with superior in vitro-drug adsorption property, hydration capacity, swelling index and solubility enhancing effect was selected for the preparation of SSD rather than sodium starch glycolate.[22]

Table 5. Evaluation Parameters of SSDS3 Orodispersible Tablet

Parameter	F1	F2	F3	F4	F5	F6
Weight (mg)	148.2±1.2	148.8±1.1	148.1±1.4	147.2±1.2	148.8±1.1	149.1±1.4
Tablet diameter (mm)	10.3	10.3	10.3	10.2	10.2	10.2
Tablet thickness (mm)	5.3	5.4	5.6	5.4	5.5	5.6
Disintegration Time (sec)	24.66±1.54	18±1.41	11.33±1.52	25.66±1.54	17±1.41	12.25±1.52
Hardness (kg/cm²)	3.15±C.13	3.27±.09	3.32±.05	3.45±0.14	3.47±1.0	3.48±.05
Wetting Time (sec)	14.33±0.57	11.33±058	6±0.9	18.33±0.57	15.33±058	12±0.9
Water absorption ratio (%)	65±1.3	69±2.1	78±1.77	55±1.5	60±2.2	68±1.76
Friability (%)	0.7	0.7	0.5	0.7	0.6	0.5
% Drug content	97.28	97.67	98.34	95.28	96.67	97.34

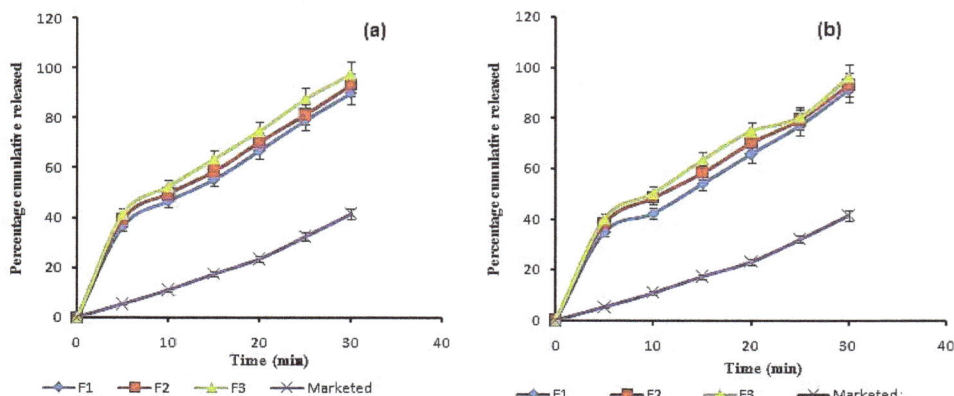

Figure 6. Comparative in vitro release profile of (a) SSDS3(F1- F3) orodispersible and (b) SDS3 (F4-F6) orodispersible formulation with respect to marketed formulation

Grossly, speaking the SSDs contained insignificantly higher drug content rather than SD's and the method of preparation had no prominent effect on drug content.

SSDs showed marked increase in solubility rather than SDs due to distribution of drug on the surface of water insoluble carriers that facilitated diffusion of drug molecules in the dissolution media readily while in SDs that drug gets entrapped inside the carrier and the release of drug molecules is hindered in comparison to SSDs. The solubility enhancement for both systems was analogous to the drug carrier ratio of 1:1<1:4<1:8 due to better wettability with increased drug carrier ratio. Furthermore, solvent evaporation method employed for preparing SSDs and SDs showed higher enhancement in solubility than co-grinding method employed. Solvent evaporation method is advantageous over co-grinding method, since evaporation of solvent leads to finer amorphization of drug particles on the carrier that increases the interfacial area of contact between the drug particles and dissolution medium.[22]

SSD's showed enhanced dissolution characteristics in comparison to SD's as in SSD's water insoluble carriers were used which become hydrated in presence of water and get rapidly swell by water intake. Thus the dissolution got enhanced as the drug particles adsorbed on the carriers get wet and dissolve readily while in SD's penetration of drug inside carrier leads to decrease in dissolution characteristics when compared with SSD's. SSDS3 showed maximum dissolution among SSDs and SDS3 amongst SDs co-relatable to higher amount of carrier in each category. These results are in good agreement with the results obtained with equilibrium solubility studies that demonstrated enhancement in solubility on increase in the concentration of carrier.

Clearly SSDS3 showed minimum $t_{50\%}$ of 28 min and maximum $\%DE_{50min}$ of 80.9% which among all SSDs while best performing SDS3 showed $t_{50\%}$ of 35min and $\%DE_{50min}$ of 76.4% among the SDs.

Though SSDS3 affirmed superiority, SDS3 was also selected for development of tablet formulation to analyze the effect of formulation variables on the performance, if any. Higher dissolution capacity of SSDS3 can be explained by analyzing the mechanisms involved. In surface solid dispersion the drug gets adsorbed on the surface of carrier and when the carrier swells enormously, it releases the drug molecules in the release medium quickly, but in case of solid dispersion; molecular/ particulate matrix is formed between drug and carrier.[21,23] When in dissolution medium, the water soluble carrier is released from the matrix initially followed by drug molecules, thus slow dissolution is observed in comparison to SSD. In the present study, the SSD made with crospovidone had high swelling index that resulted in the breaking of the crust layer formed by the adsorbed drug molecules resulting in fracture formation of crust. This resulted in increased rate of release of drug molecules adsorbed over carrier.

All Micromeritics results demonstrate good powder properties of SSDS3 over SDS3. The obvious reason is the use of water insoluble carrier in SSD that do not produce soft and tacky powder as seen with SDs. This is definitely advantageous aspect in the manufacturing facilities.

MLX crystals appeared to be entrapped into the particles of the carrier. FT-IR results indicate no evidence of chemical interactions between the drug and carrier crospovidone). Similarly, the signals of drug at 1689(-C=O- stretching), 1176 (symmetric S=O stretching), 1278 (-CN stretching of drug), 838 (-C-H-aromatic ring stretching) were recorded in SDS3 evidenced absence of chemical interaction between MLX and PEG6000. DSC indicated the mechanistic difference in the formation of SSD and SD using two different carriers CPV and PEG 6000 respectively. Thus, from DSC of physical mixtures, it can be concluded that drug and carrier in both SD and SSD showed no interaction.

The comparison was also done by taking three formulations made from SDS3 solid dispersions and it was observed that formulation F4–F6 showed 81-89% drug release within 30 min. which is much higher than marketed formulation but smaller than formulation F1-F3. So formulation F3 with 10 mg drug equivalent SSDS3 formulation with highest amount of CPV showed maximum release of drug among all six and marketed formulation, and had suitable properties for formulation of fast dissolving orodispersible tablet of meloxicam.

Conclusion

Comparing SSD and SD of meloxicam, SSD showed higher dissolution enhancement than SD and the effect was extrapolated to the orodispersible tablets also. Hence SSD proved to be an important tool to enhance the dissolution rate of poorly water soluble drugs. SSD can be defined as a variant of solid dispersion but there is mechanistic difference between these two and SSD can be considered advantageous. Hence, surface solid dispersion technology can be successfully utilized for product development of drugs exhibiting dissolution rate limited absorption.

Acknowledgments
The authors are thankful to Torrent Pharmaceutical Ltd. Ahmadabad, India for providing gift of drug sample. We are grateful to financially supported by Rajiv Academy for Pharmacy, Mathura, UP, India.

Ethical Issues
Not applicable.

Conflict of Interest
Authors declare no conflict of interest in this study.

References

1. Sharma DK, Joshi SB. Solubility enhancement strategies for poorly water-soluble drugs in solid dispersions: a review. *Asian J Pharm* 2007;1(1):9-19.
2. Dhirendra K, Lewis S, Udupa N, Atin K. Solid dispersions: A review. *Pak J Pharm Sci* 2009;22(2):234-46.
3. Schulz M, Fussnegger B, Bodmeier R. Adsorption of carbamazepine onto crospovidone to prevent drug recrystallization. *Int J Pharm* 2010;391(1-2):169-76. doi: 10.1016/j.ijpharm.2010.03.015
4. Lalitha Y, Lakshmi PK. Enhancement of dissolution of nifedipine by surface solid dispersion technique. *Int J Pharm Pharm Sci* 2011;3(3):41-6.
5. Williams AC, Timmins P, Lu M, Forbes RT. Disorder and dissolution enhancement: Deposition of ibuprofen on to insoluble polymers. *Eur J Pharm Sci* 2005;26(3-4):288-94. doi: 10.1016/j.ejps.2005.06.006
6. Aly AM. Preparation of rapidly disintegrating Glipizide Tablets by surface solid dispersion through superdisintegrants. *Int J Pharm Sci Nanotech* 2008;1(3):233-42.
7. Rao M, Mandage Y, Thanki K, Sucheta B. Dissolution improvement of simvastatin by surface solid dispersion technology. *Dissolut Technol* 2010;5(13):27-34. doi: 10.14227/DT170210P27
8. Dandagi PM, Mastiholimath VS, Srinivas SA, Godbole AM, Bhagawati ST. Orodispersible Tablets: New-fangled Drug Delivery System-A Review. *Indian J Pharm Educ Res* 2005;39:177-81.
9. Kaur T, Gill B, Kumar S, Gupta GD. Mouth dissolving tablets: A Novel Approach to Drug Delivery. *Int J Curr Pharm Res* 2011;3(1):1-7.
10. Dehghan MHG, Jafar M. Improving dissolution of Meloxicam using solid dispersions. *Iran J Pharm Res* 2006;4(5):231-8.
11. Seedher N, Bhatia S. Solubility enhancement of COX-2 inhibitors using various solvent systems. *AAPS PharmSciTech* 2003;4(3):E33. doi: 10.1208/pt040333
12. Dahiya S, Pathak K, Sharma R. Development of extended release coevaporates and coprecipitates of promethazine HCl with acrylic polymers: Formulation considerations. *Chem Pharm Bull (Tokyo)* 2008;56(4):504-8. doi: 10.1248/cpb.56.504

13. Dadhich T, Kumar M, Pathak K. Capsulated Surface Solid Dispersion of Loperamide for Targeted Delivery. *Pharm Chem J* 2016;3(4):78-90.

14. Dixit RP, Nagarsenkar MS. *In vitro* and *In vivo* advantage of celecoxib surface solid dispersion and dosage form development. *Indian J Pharm Sci* 2010;69(3):370-7. doi: 10.4103/0250-474X.34545

15. Sinko PJ. Martin's physical pharmacy and pharmaceutical sciences. 5th ed. New Delhi: Lippincott William and Wilkins; 2002.

16. Rowe RC, Sheskey PJ, Owen SC. Handbook of Pharmaceutical Excipients. 5th ed. London: Pharmaceutical Press; 2006.

17. Lalitha Y, Lakshmi PK. Enhancement of dissolution of nifedipine by surface solid dispersion technique. *Int J Pharm Pharm Sci* 2011;3(3):41-6.

18. Balsubramaniam J, Bindu K, Rao VU, Ray D, Haldar R, Brzeczko AW. Effect of superdisintegrants on dissolution of cationic drugs. *Dissolut Technol* 2008;15:18-25. doi: 10.14227/DT150208P18

19. Dhirendra K, Lewis S, Udupa N, Atin K. Solid dispersions: A review. *Pak J Pharm Sci* 2009;22(2):234-46.

20. Kiran T, Shastri N, Ramakrishna S, Sadanandam M. Surface solid dispersion of glimepiride for enhancement of dissolution rate. *Int J Pharm Tech Res* 2009;1:822-31.

21. Charumanee S, Okonoki S, Sirithunyalug J. Improvement of the dissolution rate of piroxicam by surface solid dispersion. *CMU J* 2004;3(2):77-84.

22. Shah RB, Tawakkul MA, Khan MA. Comparative evaluation of flow for pharmaceutical powders and granules. *AAPS PharmSciTech* 2008;9(1):250-8. doi: 10.1208/s12249-008-9046-8

23. Dahima R, Pachori A, Netam S. Formulation and evaluation of mouth dissolving tablet containing amlodipine Besylate solid dispersion. *Int J ChemTech Res* 2010;2(1):706-15.

3

The Inhibitory Effect of Ginger Extract on Ovarian Cancer Cell Line; Application of Systems Biology

Roghiyeh Pashaei-Asl[1,2], Fatima Pashaei-Asl[3], Parvin Mostafa Gharabaghi[4]*, Khodadad Khodadadi[5], Mansour Ebrahimi[6], Esmaeil Ebrahimie[7,8,9,10], Maryam Pashaiasl[4,11,12]*

[1] Department of Anatomy, Medical School, Iran University of Medical Science, Tehran, Iran.
[2] Cellular and Molecular Research Center, Iran University of Medical Sciences, Tehran, Iran.
[3] Molecular Biology Laboratory, Biotechnology Research Center, Tabriz University of Medical Sciences, Tabriz, Iran.
[4] Women's Reproductive Health Research Center, Tabriz University of Medical Sciences Tabriz, Iran.
[5] Genetic Research Theme, Murdoch Children's Research Institute, Royal Children's Hospital, The University of Melbourne, Melbourne, Australia.
[6] Department of Biology, University of Qom, Qom, Iran.
[7] Institute of Biotechnology, Shiraz University, Shiraz, Iran.
[8] School of Biological Sciences, Faculty of Science and Engineering, Flinders University, Adelaide, Australia.
[9] School of Information Technology and Mathematical Sciences, Division of Information Technology, Engineering and the Environment, The University of South Australia, Adelaide, Australia.
[10] School of Animal & Veterinary Science, The University of Adelaide, Australia.
[11] Drug Applied Research Center, Tabriz University of Medical Sciences, Tabriz, Iran.
[12] Department of Anatomical Sciences, Faculty of Medicine, Tabriz University of Medical Sciences, Iran.

Keywords:
· Ovarian cancer
· Ginger extract
· Anticancer
· P53
· Bcl-2
· Systems biology analysis
· Meta-analysis

Abstract

Purpose: Ginger is a natural compound with anti-cancer properties. The effects of ginger and its mechanism on ovarian cancer and its cell line model, SKOV-3, are unclear. In this study, we have evaluated the effect of ginger extract on SKOV-3.

Methods: SKOV-3 cells were incubated with ginger extract for 24, 48 and 72 hours. Cell toxicity assay was performed. Different data mining algorithms were applied to highlight the most important features contributing to ginger inhibition on the SKOV-3 cell proliferation. Moreover, Real-Time PCR was performed to assay p53, p21 and bcl-2 genes expression. For co-expression meta-analysis of p53, mutual ranking (MR) index and transformation to Z-values (Z distribution) were applied on available transcriptome data in NCBI GEO data repository.

Results: The ginger extract significantly inhibited cancer growth in ovarian cancer cell line. The most important attribute was 60 µg/ml concentration which received weights higher than 0.50, 0.75 and 0.95 by 90%, 80% and 50% of feature selection models, respectively. The expression level of p53 was increased sharply in response to ginger treatment. Systems biology analysis and meta-analysis of deposited expression value in NCBI based on rank of correlation and Z-transformation approach unraveled the key co-expressed genes and co-expressed network of P53, as the key transcription factor induced by ginger extract. High co-expression between P53 and the other apoptosis-inducing proteins such as CASP2 and DEDD was noticeable, suggesting the molecular mechanism underpinning of ginger action.

Conclusion: We found that the ginger extract has anticancer properties through p53 pathway to induce apoptosis.

Introduction

Ovarian cancer is the main reason of death from gynaecological malignant tumors, worldwide. Although there are advanced improvements in surgical techniques and accurately designed chemotherapy regimens, reversion remains practically unavoidable in patients with progressive disease.[1,2] Ovarian cancer is the fifth cause of death related to the cancer in women and covers a histologically and genetically a wide range of malignancies, containing those of epithelial, sex cord-stromal and germ cell source.[3] In the year 2016, about 22,280 new cases with ovarian cancer were diagnosed and approximately 14,240 women died because of this cancer in the United States.[4]

*Corresponding authors: Parvin Mostafa Gharabaghi and Maryam Pashaiasl, Email: pm_gharabaghi@yahoo.com, pashaim@tbzmed.ac.ir

There are different kinds of ovarian cancer depend on where the cell type originated. Epithelial cell ovarian cancer (EOC), gonadal-stromal, and germ cell make 90%, 6% and 4% incidence of ovarian cancer in patients, respectively. Epithelial ovarian cancer is derived from the celomic epithelium or mesothelium (epithelial ovarian carcinoma) and others arise from primordial germ cells, ovarian stromal or mesenchyme and sex cord.[5-7] Some factors are associated with a high risk of ovarian cancer, such as old age, nuliparity, family history, infertility and endometriosis; on the other hand, factors such as usage of oral contraceptives, salpingo-oopherectomy, tubal ligation, hysterectomy and breast feeding are known to have a more protective effect.[5,7,8]

Due to the lack of specific symptoms, the most ovarian cancers are diagnosed in the advanced stages. Therefore, the cost of treatment is high and prognosis is poor.[5] The majority of women whose diseases are at high risk (poorly differentiated or presence of malignant cells in as cites fluid) benefit from postoperative chemotherapy. Combination chemotherapy is recommended for these patients.[8] Chemotherapy is useful as an adjunct to surgery in some types of ovarian cancers and may be curative. Unfortunately, some factors such as severe disability, old age, malnutrition or direct organ involvement by primary or metastatic cancer influence the incidence of severe side effects of chemotherapy; therefore, using traditional medicine with chemotherapy not only kills cancer cells but also limits the cancer side effects. Ginger is from the rhizome of Zingiber officinale that has been used in traditional medicine for a long time.[9]

Great progresses in biotechnology and molecular biology have been caused the understanding of the genetics and molecular basis of disease which can help to find strategic therapeutic approaches and novel targeted therapies to manage ovarian cancer. Therefore, it might be possible to choose medications based on the molecular characteristics of tumors and also as basis of personalized medicine. Numerous experimental studies have been conducted in the chemo preventive belongings of ginger and their mechanisms. Their main focus is on antioxidant, neuroprotection, proliferation suppression, cancer prevention, pro-apoptotic and anti-inflammatory activities.[10-16] The result of a study on the major extracts of ginger shows that 6-gingerol inhibits angiogenesis in the human endothelial cells, it also down-regulates cyclin D1 and causes cell cycle arrest in the G1 phase.[17] In addition, 6-gingerol plays a rule in oxidative stress, DNA damage, G2/M cell cycle arrest and also it induces autophagy and activates tumor suppressor proteins including P53 and P21.[18] Despite the anticancer activity of ginger, its mechanisms are still poorly understood.

This study focuses on the effects of the ginger extraction on human ovarian cancer cell line (SKOV-3) to find out if the new ginger extraction is effective in treatment of ovarian cancer. In addition, bioinformatics analysis was applied on these datasets to highlight the most important features contribute to ginger inhibition on the SKOV-3 cell proliferation. The expression of p21 (cyclin-dependent kinase inhibitor 1), p53 (tumor suppressor gene), and Bcl-2 (B-cell lymphoma 2) genes following ginger treatment have been investigated. Also, Systems biology analysis and meta-analysis of deposited expression value in NCBI based on rank of correlation and Z-transformation approach were applied for further investigations about effect of ginger extract treatment on ovarian cancer cell line.

Material and Methods

Cell culture

SKOV-3, human epithelial ovarian cancer cell line was purchased from Pasteur Institute Cell Bank of Iran. The cells were grown as monolayer in 25 cm^2 flask (Orange Scientific) with culture medium (DMEM) (Sigma; Chemical Co., St. Louis, MO, USA) supplemented with 10% heat-inactivated fetal bovine serum (FBS) (Gibco-Life technologies), streptomycin (100 µg/mL), penicillin (100 units/mL) (Sigma), and cultured under standard condition at 37°C in a 5% humidified CO_2 incubator. The medium was exchange twice a week.

Cell proliferation assay

The effect of ginger inhibition on the SKOV-3 cell proliferation was determined by MTT (3-(4,5-Dimethylthiazol-2-yl)-2,5-DiphenyltetrazoliumBromide) assay. The cells were seeded in 96-well tissue culture plates at a density of 3500 cells per well and incubated at 37 °C and 5% CO_2 humidified incubator. After 50% confluency, the cells were treated with the ginger extract (Sigma-Aldrich., W252108) in different concentrations and incubated for 24, 48 and 72 hours in assorted plates. Following the appropriate times, the upper medium was removed and 0.5 mg/ml of MTT (Sigma) solution (PBS and medium) was added to each well and incubated for 4h at 37°C. The medium was removed and the blue formazan crystals were dissolved in 100µl of DMSO. The absorbance was read in a microplate reader (Biotek, model Elx808) at 570 nm. Each experiment was repeated in triplicate format, and results were expressed as means ± SEM.

Attribute weighting

As described before the inhibitory effects of ginger extracts on the SKOV-3 cell proliferation were determined by MTT assay. MTT assay was performed as described above. The absorbance was read by a microplate reader at 570 nm. Each experiment was repeated in triplicate format. In order to identify the most important attributes and to find the possible patterns in features which determine the effect of ginger inhibition on the SKOV-3 cell proliferation by MTT, 10 different algorithms of weighting models were applied on the datasets. Dataset imported into software (RapidMiner 5.0.001, Rapid-I GmbH, Stochumer Str. 475, 44,227 Dortmund, Germany). The attribute weighting models were: weight by information gain, weight by information gain ratio, weight by rule, weight by deviation, weight by chi squared statistic, weight by Gini index, weight by uncertainty, weight by relief, weight by principal component analysis (PCA), and weight by Support Vector Machines (SVM). The algorithms definitions have already been described in our previous paper.[19] Weights were normalized into the interval between 0 and 1 to allow the comparison between different methods.

Decision Tree Models
Decision tree algorithms provide visual explanation of the most important features through depicting an inverted tree with the most important feature as root and other variables as leaves. Various decision trees including Random Forest, Decision Stump Decision, Iterative Dichotomiser 3 (ID3), CHi-Squared Automatic Interaction Detection (CHAID) and Random Tree were applied on dataset. Details of each decision tree model have also been presented before.[19]

RNA extraction and c-DNA synthesis
SKO-V cells were seeded 300000 cells per 6 well. After one day, the cells were treated with 30 µg/ml ginger extract. Forty-eight hours after treatment, the upper medium was removed from monolayer cancer cells and scrapped in 1 ml RNAX-PLUS (Cinagene, Iran). RNA was completely extracted from samples using Cinagene Kit based on the manufacturer's instruction (RNX-Plus Solution, SinaClon, Iran). After purification and quantification, RNA was determined by measuring optical density at 260 and 280 nm by nanodrop (NanoDrop- ND-1000). The cDNA synthesis was performed according to cDNA syntheses kit instruction (Qiagene).

Real-time PCR
Real-time PCR was carried out to detect mRNA expression[20] with some modifications. p53, p21 and bcl-2 mRNA expression were investigated using Cycler IQ5 Multicolor Real-time PCR Detection System (Bio-Rad, USA). For various mRNA, first-strand cDNA was amplified using P53, p21 and bcl2 primers as described in the Table 1. β-actin was used as housekeeping gene. Each experiment was repeated in triplicate format, and the results were expressed as means ±SEM.

Statistics
Statistical analysis was performed with SPSS version 16.0 software and ANOVA test was used to compare between groups. Data are represented as Mean ± SEM. The differences were considered significant when *$P < 0.05$.

Co-expression based meta-analysis and co-expression network construction
For co-expression meta-analysis of p53 (Tp53), mutual ranking (MR) index and transformation to Z-values (Z distribution) were applied on available transcriptome data in NCBI GEO, as previously described.[21] MR index is a more reliable index in meta-analysis, compared to Pearson correlation coefficient, as it is based on rank of correlation and geometric average of the Pearson correlation coefficient rank.[22] Geometric average is a as correlation coefficient are raked in logarithmic manner.[22] Lower amount of MR implies higher correlation and a more strong expression association. To perform co-expression meta-analysis, the deposited transcriptome data in NCBI GEO NCBI were subjected to MR and Z-transformation using COXPRESSdb.[23] to identify the top 100 co-expressed genes with p53 transcription factor with low MR. Calculated MR associations, as meta-analysis co-expression measurement, were used for construction of co-expression network.

Table 1. Primers used for Real time- PCR

Gens	Genes Primer sequence (5' to 3')
P53	Forward:GTTCCGAGAGCTGAATGAGG
	Reverse: ACTTCAGGTGGCTGGAGTGA
P21	Forward: GCTTCATGC CAG CTACTTCC
	Reverse: CCCTTCAAAGTG CCATCTGT
Bcl-2	Forward: GTCATGTGTGTGGAGAGCGT
	Reverse: ACAGTTCCACAAAGGCATCC
β-actin	Forward: CCTTCCTTCCTGGGCATG
	Reverse: TCCTGTCGGCAATGCCAG

Results
The effect of ginger on cellular proliferation
In order to determine the effect of ginger on the SKOV-3 cell lines proliferation, MTT assay was illustrated at 24, 48 and 72 hours after ginger treatment. As shown in Figure 1 and 2 cell growth was inhibited considerably by ginger; consequently, it can be seen in figures, cell proliferation was decreased to 50% ($P < 0.05$) after 48 and 72 hours of treatment. The results from analysis of the data for cell viability assay via MTT demonstrated that at 24h, 48h and 72h time points, the IC50 of ginger for SKOV-3 was approximately 97 µg/ml, 60 µg/ml and 40 µg/ml. respectively.

Attribute weighting
Following normalization, 10 different attribute weighting models (as described in material and methods) were applied on GAD and RSD datasets. Each attribute was weighted between 0 and 1. These weights determined the importance of attributes in effect of new ginger extract concentration on SKOV3 cancer cell line. Attributes which gained weight equal to 0.5 or higher by at least five weighting models were selected. Table 2 shows the most important attributes was 70µg/ml concentration which received weights higher than 0.50, 0.75 and 0.95 by 90%, 80% and 50% feature selecting models. Concentration of 60µg/ml and 50µg/ml variables were the second and third important features, while 40 µg/ml concentration granted the lowest weights by attribute weighting algorithms.

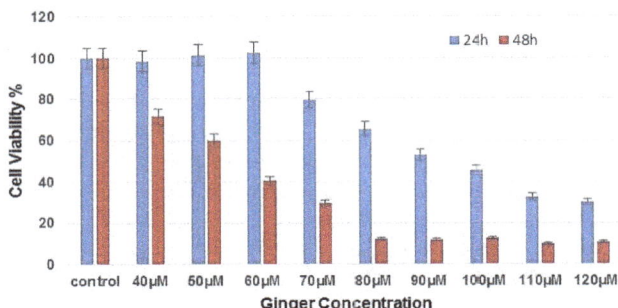

Figure 1. MTT assay was used to assess the effects of ginger in the Proliferation of SKOV-3 Ovarian Cancer Cell Line after 24h and 48h. There are significant differences between treated cells and controls (P<0.05)*.

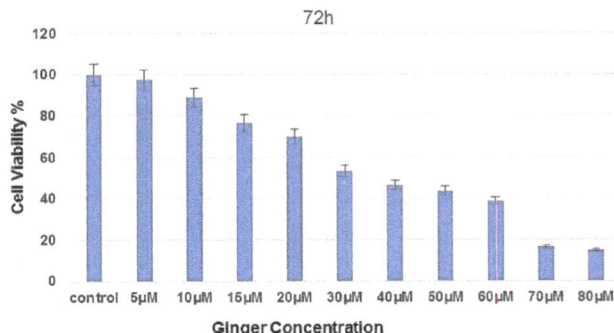

Figure 2. MTT assay was used to assess the effects of ginger on the Proliferation of SKOV-3 Ovarian Cancer Cell Line after 72h. There are significant differences between treated cells and controls (P<0.05)*.

Table 2. 10 different algorithms of weighting models applied on the datasets and new generated datasets

PCA	SVM	Relief	Uncertainty	Gini Index	Chi Squared	Deviation	Rule	Info Gain Ratio	Info Gain	Attribute	Count 0.50	Count 0.75	Count0.95
.79	1.00	.26	.68	1.00	1.00	.80	1.00	1.00	1.00	70µg/ml	9	8	5
.66	.84	.23	1.00	1.00	1.00	.59	1.00	1.00	1.00	50 µg/ml	9	7	5
.86	.65	.40	.68	1.00	1.00	.82	1.00	1.00	1.00	80 µg/ml	9	7	4
1.00	.61	.30	.51	1.00	1.00	1.00	1.00	1.00	1.00	60 µg/ml	9	7	6
.66	.68	.38	1.00	1.00	1.00	.60	1.00	1.00	1.00	90 µg/ml	9	6	5
.53	.72	.39	1.00	1.00	1.00	.44	1.00	1.00	1.00	100µg/ml	8	6	5
.37	.66	.34	.76	1.00	1.00	.26	1.00	1.00	1.00	110µg/ml	7	6	4
.31	.46	.22	.76	1.00	1.00	.23	1.00	1.00	1.00	120µg/ml	6	6	4
.44	.37	.00	.37	1.00	1.00	.36	1.00	1.00	1.00	40µg/ml	5	5	4
.00	.00	1.00	.00	.00	.00	.00	1.00	.00	.00	control	2	2	2

Tree induction algorithms also underlined the significance of features that weighed most in weighting models. Remarkably, decision tree models appointed the same features selected by attribute weighting as the root features to build the trees, as can be seen in Figure 3. The trees were just single branches showing the selected features were so decisive that can be used as cut off criteria.

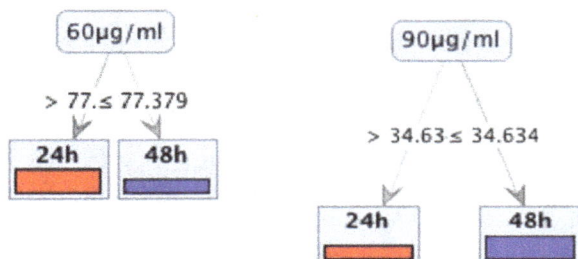

Figure 3. Decision Tree algorithm applied on datasets with Gini Index criterion

P53, P21 and Bcl-2 genes expression in SKOV-3 cells were investigated using RT-PCR analysis (Figurer 4). The genes Ct values were normalized against mRNA level of β-actin as the housekeeping gene and the relative expression for each group was measured. After 48 hours

of ginger treatment, the level of p53 expression was increased.

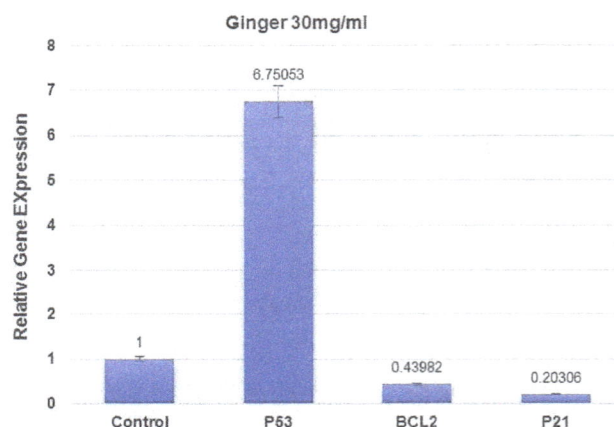

Figure 4. Real Time PCR Analysis: All of data were normalized to β-actin gene expression: Increase in P53 genes expression following ginger (30 µg/ml) treatment following 48h treatment.

Co-expression based meta-analysis of p53 (Tp53) and its co-expression network

Among the studied tumor repressor genes, p53 was the top highly upregulated transcription factor in response to ginger extract, additional systems biology and meta-analysis were performed to unravel possible involved mechanism of ginger action through p53. Here, rank of correlation value was used rather than correlation value due to its reliability in meta-analysis. The top 100 co-expressed genes with p53 (Tp53) sorted based on low MR are presented in Table 3. The co-expression network, derived based on calculated association coefficients, are presented in Figure 5.

Table 3. The top 100 co-expressed genes with p53 (Tp53) sorted based on low mutual ranking (MR) index are presented. Meta-analysis using transcriptomic data in NCBI GEO was used for co-expression meta-analysis. When a gene list is repeatedly observed in indipendent platforms, the coexpressed gene list can be regarded as reliable with high supportability (value=3).

Rank	Gene	Function	Entrez Gene ID	Supportability	MR for TP53 association
0	TP53	tumor protein p53	7157		0
1	YWHAE	tyrosine 3-monooxygenase/tryptophan 5-monooxygenase activation protein, epsilon	7531	1	4
2	RBM14	RNA binding motif protein 14	10432	1	15.9
3	DNAJC14	DnaJ (Hsp40) homolog, subfamily C, member 14	85406	1	20.4
4	APH1A	APH1A gamma secretase subunit	51107	2	41.7
5	NONO	non-POU domain containing, octamer-binding	4841	3	42.5
6	RBBP4	retinoblastoma binding protein 4	5928	2	43.4
7	TAPBP	TAP binding protein (tapasin)	6892	3	44
8	SENP3	SUMO1/sentrin/SMT3 specific peptidase 3	26168	3	45
9	RXRB	retinoid X receptor, beta	6257	2	45.5
10	MAT2A	methionine adenosyltransferase II, alpha	4144	1	46.3
11	DEDD	death effector domain containing	9191	3	49.1
12	MAZ	MYC-associated zinc finger protein (purine-binding transcription factor)	4150	3	49.1
13	FKBP1A	FK506 binding protein 1A, 12kDa	2280	3	51
14	C21orf33	chromosome 21 open reading frame 33	8209	3	59.2
15	WDR1	WD repeat domain 1	9948	3	61.2
16	LRRC41	leucine rich repeat containing 41	10489	2	62.7
17	COLGALT1	collagen beta(1-O)galactosyltransferase 1	79709	3	64.7
18	ARHGAP1	Rho GTPase activating protein 1	392	1	72.5
19	KDELR1	KDEL (Lys-Asp-Glu-Leu) endoplasmic reticulum protein retention receptor 1	10945	3	73.1
20	CALR	calreticulin	811	2	74.2
21	GLE1	GLE1 RNA export mediator	2733	2	75.9
22	ARHGDIA	Rho GDP dissociation inhibitor (GDI) alpha	396	3	77.8
23	PATZ1	POZ (BTB) and AT hook containing zinc finger 1	23598	2	78.6
24	PRR14	proline rich 14	78994	2	80
25	RAB11B	RAB11B, member RAS oncogene family	9230	3	84.5
26	SMARCC1	SWI/SNF related, matrix associated, actin dependent regulator of chromatin, subfamily c, member 1	6599	3	84.7
27	NFYC	nuclear transcription factor Y, gamma	4802	1	85
28	FLOT2	flotillin 2	2319	3	88.6
29	STYX	serine/threonine/tyrosine interacting protein	6815	2	88.7
30	PPP5C	protein phosphatase 5, catalytic subunit	5536	2	95.2
31	TMEM259	transmembrane protein 259	91304	3	96.1
32	EIF5A	eukaryotic translation initiation factor 5A	1984	3	97.6
33	PPP2R5D	protein phosphatase 2, regulatory subunit B', delta	5528	2	98.3
34	MYBBP1A	MYB binding protein (P160) 1a	10514	3	101.4
35	PTBP1	polypyrimidine tract binding protein 1	5725	2	103
36	PHF23	PHD finger protein 23	79142	3	103.6
37	EXOSC6	exosome component 6	118460	1	104.7
38	GTF2I	general transcription factor IIi	2969	1	105.4
39	ZNF672	zinc finger protein 672	79894	2	107.1
40	TRRAP	transformation/transcription domain-associated protein	8295	3	107.3
41	CFL1	cofilin 1 (non-muscle)	1072	3	107.5
42	SAFB	scaffold attachment factor B	6294	3	107.8
43	MPDU1	mannose-P-dolichol utilization defect 1	9526	3	108.3
44	TOMM22	translocase of outer mitochondrial membrane 22 homolog (yeast)	56993	2	108.4
45	MRPL38	mitochondrial ribosomal protein L38	64978	3	109.6
46	MTMR1	myotubularin related protein 1	8776	1	112.2
47	SRSF1	serine/arginine-rich splicing factor 1	6426	3	112.6
48	PFN1	profilin 1	5216	3	114.5
49	EIF2S3	eukaryotic translation initiation factor 2, subunit 3 gamma, 52kDa	1968	3	115
50	FARSA	phenylalanyl-tRNA synthetase, alpha subunit	2193	3	116.6
51	LAMP1	lysosomal-associated membrane protein 1	3916	3	118.4
52	HNRNPH1	heterogeneous nuclear ribonucleoprotein H1 (H)	3187	3	123.3
53	STIP1	stress-induced phosphoprotein 1	10963	2	130.9

Rank	Gene	Function	Entrez Gene ID	Supportability	MR for TP53 association
54	HSF1	heat shock transcription factor 1	3297	3	135.6
55	GANAB	glucosidase, alpha; neutral AB	23193	3	135.7
56	ASB16-AS1	ASB16 antisense RNA 1	339201	2	136
57	LIX1L	Lix1 homolog (chicken) like	128077	3	136.8
58	KLHDC3	kelch domain containing 3	116138	3	137.2
59	DRG2	developmentally regulated GTP binding protein 2	1819	3	139
60	BANF1	barrier to autointegration factor 1	8815	3	139.8
61	AKIRIN2	akirin 2	55122	1	140.8
62	RELA	v-rel avian reticuloendotheliosis viral oncogene homolog A	5970	3	141.5
63	CASP2	caspase 2, apoptosis-related cysteine peptidase	835	2	145.9
64	MAP2K2	mitogen-activated protein kinase kinase 2	5605	3	146.8
65	RANGAP1	Ran GTPase activating protein 1	5905	3	150.6
66	NAP1L4	nucleosome assembly protein 1-like 4	4676	2	151.7
67	MTA1	metastasis associated 1	9112	3	154.1
68	REPIN1	replication initiator 1	29803	2	154.3
69	ZBTB45	zinc finger and BTB domain containing 45	84878	3	155.4
70	PPP2R1A	protein phosphatase 2, regulatory subunit A, alpha	5518	3	156.1
71	CYB5R3	cytochrome b5 reductase 3	1727	2	157.6
72	UBE4B	ubiquitination factor E4B	10277	1	159.4
73	ACLY	ATP citrate lyase	47	3	160.4
74	UBE2G2	ubiquitin-conjugating enzyme E2G 2	7327	0	163.2
75	DNAAF5	dynein, axonemal, assembly factor 5	54919	3	170
76	GDI2	GDP dissociation inhibitor 2	2665	3	170.1
77	BSG	basigin (Ok blood group)	682	3	171.8
78	SLC25A11	solute carrier family 25 (mitochondrial carrier; oxoglutarate carrier), member 11	8402	3	173.4
79	BTBD2	BTB (POZ) domain containing 2	55643	3	173.7
80	C1orf174	chromosome 1 open reading frame 174	339448	2	176.2
81	ABCC1	ATP-binding cassette, sub-family C (CFTR/MRP), member 1	4363	3	178.4
82	DCAF15	DDB1 and CUL4 associated factor 15	90379	2	180.4
83	SLC29A1	solute carrier family 29 (equilibrative nucleoside transporter), member 1	2030	2	181
84	KCTD5	potassium channel tetramerization domain containing 5	54442	1	191.8
85	TBC1D5	TBC1 domain family, member 5	9779	2	192.7
86	SHC1	SHC (Src homology 2 domain containing) transforming protein 1	6464	3	192.9
87	CRTAP	cartilage associated protein	10491	2	194.3
88	NUCKS1	nuclear casein kinase and cyclin-dependent kinase substrate 1	64710	3	197.2
89	STAT2	signal transducer and activator of transcription 2, 113kDa	6773	3	198.6
90	NFRKB	nuclear factor related to kappaB binding protein	4798	2	200.8
91	ANKFY1	ankyrin repeat and FYVE domain containing 1	51479	3	207.5
92	TRAPPC1	trafficking protein particle complex 1	58485	3	208
93	CBFB	core-binding factor, beta subunit	865	2	210
94	NCOA5	nuclear receptor coactivator 5	57727	3	211.2
95	GLYR1	glyoxylate reductase 1 homolog (Arabidopsis)	84656	2	213.7
96	HNRNPU	heterogeneous nuclear ribonucleoprotein U (scaffold attachment factor A)	3192	3	213.9
97	NUCB1	nucleobindin 1	4924	3	214.7
98	NUMA1	nuclear mitotic apparatus protein 1	4926	2	216.3
99	CTNND1	catenin (cadherin-associated protein), delta 1	1500	3	216.6
100	CTNNA1	catenin (cadherin-associated protein), alpha 1, 102kDa	1495	2	217.2

YWHAE (tyrosine 3-monooxygenase) was the top co-expressed genes with P53 according to meta-analysis (Table 3, Figure 5). Interestingly, two apoptosis inducing genes, including DEDD (death effector domain containing) and CASP2 (caspase 2, apoptosis-related cysteine peptidase) are highly co-expressed with P53 which can be induced after ginger application. Based on normalized meta-data derived from expression data of different tissues and cell lines in NCBI GEO (Supplementary 1 and Supplementary 2), we calculated the Pearson correlation, in addition to MR. Highly positive and significant correlation was observed between P53 and CASP2 (Pearson correlation = 94.1%, P-Value = 0.000) and also P53 and DEDD (Pearson correlation = 90%, P-Value = 0.000).

Discussion

In this study, we investigated the effects of the ginger extract on ovarian cancer cell line and used bioinformatics analysis to find out the most accurate and reliable results. Ginger (Zingiber officinale), a natural poly-phenol constituent from rhizomes and ginger root, is extensively used as a spice or a traditional medicine. Researchers have been consistently revealed anti-cancer activities of phenolic substance in vegetables and fruits both in vitro and in vivo.[17,24-27] Recently, different publications reveled the anticancer effect of ginger on various human cancer cell lines such as breast cancer (BC), prostate adeno-carcinoma (PC-3), Hela (Human cervical cancer), lung non-small cancer (A549), and colon cancer.[28-32] Weng and the colleagues reported that 6-Shogaol and 6-gingerol efficiently block invasion and metastasis of hepatocellular carcinoma by different molecular mechanisms.[26]

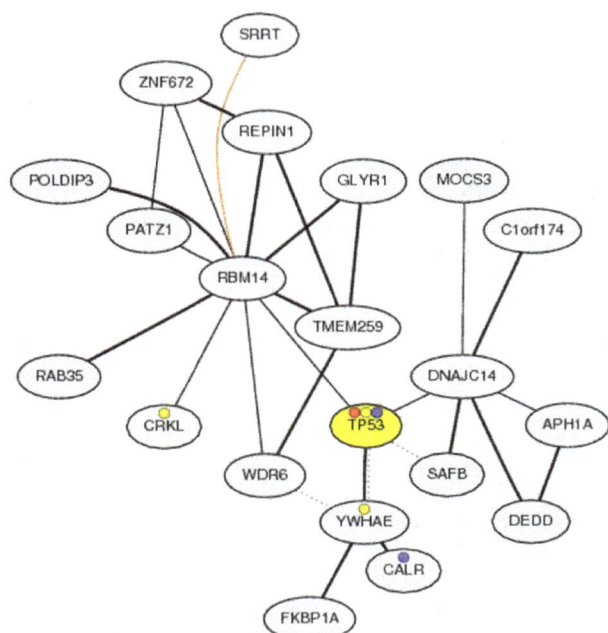

Figure 5. Co-expression network of Tp53, ginger associated transcription factor, derived from co-expression meta-analysis of Tp53 in transcriptomic data of NCBI GEO.

Our studies by MTT assay illustrated that the ginger extract displayed strong cytotoxicity effects on ovarian cancer cell line, SKOV-3. Attribute weighting algorithms weighs the importance of each attribute in distinguishing between different concentrations of ginger; the results showed a few ranges of concentrations, from 50μg/ml to 80μg/ml, gained the highest possible weights and this range can be used to find the best concentration in lab works. Decision tree models also confirmed the above findings and clearly showed that these concentrations are playing crucial roles in suppressing SKOV-3 cancer cell line toxicity.

In order to normal cells are transformed into a fully malignant cancer cells, a set of genetic and epigenetic alterations must be occurred.[33] Genes associated with cell death program is considered crucial for the appropriate function and development of most mammalian organisms. BCL-2 (B-Cell Lymphoma 2), a member of the human Bcl-2 family is one of the main anti-apoptotic genes and seems to be a good target for cancer therapy in the future. They control the status of unreturnable for clonogenic cell survival and thereby affect tumorigenesis and host–pathogen interactions and also regulate animal development.[34-36] Today's clinical trials which target Bcl-2 family proteins or

mRNA are giving hopes for discovering a new group of anticancer drugs.[37] Our studies demonstrated that Bcl-2 has more than 0.4-fold reduction in expression after 48 hours ginger treatment compared to control group. Previously, Wang and colleagues in 2002 demonstrated 6-gingerol effects on apoptosis induction and inhibition of Bcl-2 expression in promyelocytic leukemia HL-60 cell.[38]

Furthermore, we investigated tumor suppressor p53 and cyclin-dependent kinase inhibitor 1 p21 genes in this study to find out their role in SKOV-3 cell death after ginger therapy. In many cell types, inactivation of the p53 gene is the most common alternation explained in ovarian cancer.[39,40] P53 is involved in some cell pathways such as cell cycle arrest, apoptosis, metastasis, invasion, stem cell maintenance, metabolism, cell cycle and DNA repair.[41-43] Moreover, P53-target genes play important roles in cell cycle arrest (e.g., p21) and apoptotic (e.g.; Bax) pathway.[44] p21 is expressed by both p53-dependent and independent mechanisms after stress.[45] In cell cycle arrest pathway, p53 affects p21 expression, thus p21 stimulation inhibits tumor development and causes cell arrest;[45,46] however, it can be activated independently and can have cancer-promoting properties.[47] Therefore, the control of p53's transcriptional activity is critical for novel therapeutic approaches to design drugs for ovarian cancer treatment.[47,48]

Our result showed that the level of p53 expression in the ginger extract treated ovarian cancer cell line was increased about 7-fold compared to the control group (Figure 4). On the other hand, the level of p21 expression was decreased after drug treatment., Therefore, it could be understood that p53 might regulate the cell death in other pathway. Besides, p53 regulates transcription of apoptotic target genes such as Bcl-2 and Bax.[49] Our results revealed bcl-2 gene expression decreased in ginger treated cells, so p53 might stimulate apoptosis through bcl-2 elimination.

Additional, Systems biology analysis and meta-analysis of deposited expression value in NCBI based on rank of correlation and Z-transformation approach unraveled the key co-expressed genes and co-expressed network of P53, as the key transcription factor induced by ginger extract. High co-expression between P53 and the other apoptosis-inducing proteins such as CASP2 and DEDD was noticeable, suggesting the molecular mechanism underpinning of ginger action.

Conclusion

Our study revealed that p53 expression is the main reason for the cytotoxicity effects of ginger in ovarian cancer cells and the cause of cell death in SKOV-3 cells. Bioinformatics analysis help to confirm and get more accurate and reliable results driven from ginger effect on the cell line and p53 expression. The data outlined the key co-expressed genes and co-expressed network of P53, as the key transcription factor induced by ginger extract.

It could be suggested that p53 in new ginger extract treated ovarian cancer cell line stimulates tumor suppression through apoptosis, rather than cell cycle arrest.

Acknowledgments

The authors thank Faculty of Advanced Medical Science of Tabriz University for the support. This work is funded by the Women's Reproductive Health Research Center, Al-Zahra Hospital, Tabriz University of Medical Sciences, Tabriz, Iran.

Ethical Issues
Not applicable.

Conflict of Interest
The authors declare no conflict of interests.

References

1. Yap TA, Carden CP, Kaye SB. Beyond chemotherapy: Targeted therapies in ovarian cancer. *Nat Rev Cancer* 2009;9(3):167-81. doi: 10.1038/nrc2583

2. Dong A, Lu Y, Lu B. Genomic/epigenomic alterations in ovarian carcinoma: Translational insight into clinical practice. *J Cancer* 2016;7(11):1441-51. doi: 10.7150/jca.15556

3. Karnezis AN, Cho KR, Gilks CB, Pearce CL, Huntsman DG. The disparate origins of ovarian cancers: Pathogenesis and prevention strategies. *Nat Rev Cancer* 2017;17(1):65-74. doi: 10.1038/nrc.2016.113

4. Siegel RL, Miller KD, Jemal A. Cancer statistics, 2016. *CA Cancer J Clin* 2016;66(1):7-30. doi: 10.3322/caac.21332

5. Jones HW, Rock JA. Te linde's operative gynecology. 11th ed. US: Lippincott Williams & Wilkins; 2015.

6. Gubbels JA, Claussen N, Kapur AK, Connor JP, Patankar MS. The detection, treatment, and biology of epithelial ovarian cancer. *J Ovarian Res* 2010;3:8. doi: 10.1186/1757-2215-3-8

7. Rice MS, Hankinson SE, Tworoger SS. Tubal ligation, hysterectomy, unilateral oophorectomy, and risk of ovarian cancer in the nurses' health studies. *Fertil Steril* 2014;102(1):192-8 e3. doi: 10.1016/j.fertnstert.2014.03.041

8. Di Saia PJ, Creasman WT. Clinical gynecologic oncology. 8th Edition. Philadelphia, PA: Elsevier/Saunders; 2012.

9. Park EJ, Pezzuto JM. Botanicals in cancer chemoprevention. *Cancer Metastasis Rev* 2002;21(3-4):231-55. doi: 10.1023/a:1021254725842

10. Chrubasik S, Pittler MH, Roufogalis BD. Zingiberis rhizoma: A comprehensive review on the ginger effect and efficacy profiles. *Phytomedicine* 2005;12(9):684-701. doi: 10.1016/j.phymed.2004.07.009

11. Ali BH, Blunden G, Tanira MO, Nemmar A. Some phytochemical, pharmacological and toxicological properties of ginger (zingiber officinale roscoe): A review of recent research. *Food Chem Toxicol* 2008;46(2):409-20. doi: 10.1016/j.fct.2007.09.085

12. Tao QF, Xu Y, Lam RY, Schneider B, Dou H, Leung PS, et al. Diarylheptanoids and a monoterpenoid from the rhizomes of zingiber officinale: Antioxidant and cytoprotective properties. *J Nat Prod* 2008;71(1):12-7. doi: 10.1021/np070114p

13. Shukla Y, Singh M. Cancer preventive properties of ginger: A brief review. *Food Chem Toxicol* 2007;45(5):683-90. doi: 10.1016/j.fct.2006.11.002

14. Rhode J, Fogoros S, Zick S, Wahl H, Griffith KA, Huang J, et al. Ginger inhibits cell growth and modulates angiogenic factors in ovarian cancer cells. *BMC Complement Altern Med* 2007;7:44. doi: 10.1186/1472-6882-7-44

15. Peng F, Tao Q, Wu X, Dou H, Spencer S, Mang C, et al. Cytotoxic, cytoprotective and antioxidant effects of isolated phenolic compounds from fresh ginger. *Fitoterapia* 2012;83(3):568-85. doi: 10.1016/j.fitote.2011.12.028

16. Prasad S, Tyagi AK. Ginger and its constituents: Role in prevention and treatment of gastrointestinal cancer. *Gastroenterol Res Pract* 2015;2015:142979. doi: 10.1155/2015/142979

17. Kim EC, Min JK, Kim TY, Lee SJ, Yang HO, Han S, et al. [6]-gingerol, a pungent ingredient of ginger, inhibits angiogenesis in vitro and in vivo. *Biochem Biophys Res Commun* 2005;335(2):300-8. doi: 10.1016/j.bbrc.2005.07.076

18. Rastogi N, Duggal S, Singh SK, Porwal K, Srivastava VK, Maurya R, et al. Proteasome inhibition mediates p53 reactivation and anti-cancer activity of 6-gingerol in cervical cancer cells. *Oncotarget* 2015;6(41):43310-25. doi: 10.18632/oncotarget.6383

19. Pashaiasl M, Khodadadi K, Kayvanjoo AH, Pashaei-asl R, Ebrahimie E, Ebrahimi M. Unravelling evolution of nanog, the key transcription factor involved in self-renewal of undifferentiated embryonic stem cells, by pattern recognition in nucleotide and tandem repeats characteristics. *Gene* 2016;578(2):194-204. doi: 10.1016/j.gene.2015.12.023

20. Gholizadeh-Ghaleh Aziz S, Pashaei-Asl F, Fardyazar Z, Pashaiasl M. Isolation, characterization, cryopreservation of human amniotic stem cells and differentiation to osteogenic and adipogenic cells. *PloS One* 2016;11(7):e0158281. doi: 10.1371/journal.pone.0158281

21. Ebrahimie M, Esmaeili F, Cheraghi S, Houshmand F, Shabani L, Ebrahimie E. Efficient and simple production of insulin-producing cells from embryonal carcinoma stem cells using mouse neonate pancreas extract, as a natural inducer. *PloS One* 2014;9(3):e90885. doi: 10.1371/journal.pone.0090885

22. Obayashi T, Kinoshita K. Rank of correlation coefficient as a comparable measure for biological significance of gene coexpression. *DNA Res* 2009;16(5):249-60. doi: 10.1093/dnares/dsp016

23. Okamura Y, Aoki Y, Obayashi T, Tadaka S, Ito S, Narise T, et al. Coxpresdb in 2015: Coexpression

database for animal species by DNA-microarray and rnaseq-based expression data with multiple quality assessment systems. *Nucleic Acids Res* 2015;43(Database issue):D82-6. doi: 10.1093/nar/gku1163

24. Mahmoud NN, Carothers AM, Grunberger D, Bilinski RT, Churchill MR, Martucci C, et al. Plant phenolics decrease intestinal tumors in an animal model of familial adenomatous polyposis. *Carcinogenesis* 2000;21(5):921-7.

25. Murakami A, Tanaka T, Lee JY, Surh YJ, Kim HW, Kawabata K, et al. Zerumbone, a sesquiterpene in subtropical ginger, suppresses skin tumor initiation and promotion stages in ICR mice. Int J Cancer 2004;110(4):481-90. doi: 10.1002/ijc.20175

26. Weng CJ, Chou CP, Ho CT, Yen GC. Molecular mechanism inhibiting human hepatocarcinoma cell invasion by 6-shogaol and 6-gingerol. *Mol Nutr Food Res* 2012;56(8):1304-14. doi: 10.1002/mnfr.201200173

27. Kim SO, Chun KS, Kundu JK, Surh YJ. Inhibitory effects of [6]-gingerol on PMA-induced COX-2 expression and activation of NF-κb and p38 MAPK in mouse skin. *Biofactors* 2004;21(1-4):27-31. doi: 10.1002/biof.552210107

28. Karna P, Chagani S, Gundala SR, Rida PC, Asif G, Sharma V, et al. Benefits of whole ginger extract in prostate cancer. *Br J Nutr* 2012;107(4):473-84. doi: 10.1017/S0007114511003308

29. Liu Q, Peng YB, Qi LW, Cheng XL, Xu XJ, Liu LL, et al. The cytotoxicity mechanism of 6-shogaol-treated hela human cervical cancer cells revealed by label-free shotgun proteomics and bioinformatics analysis. *Evid Based Complement Alternat Med* 2012;2012:278652. doi: 10.1155/2012/278652

30. Eren D, Betul YM. Revealing the effect of 6-gingerol, 6-shogaol and curcumin on mPGES-1, GSK-3β and β-catenin pathway in A549 cell line. *Chem Biol Interact* 2016;258:257-65. doi: 10.1016/j.cbi.2016.09.012

31. Sanaati F, Najafi S, Kashaninia Z, Sadeghi M. Effect of ginger and chamomile on nausea and vomiting caused by chemotherapy in iranian women with breast cancer. *Asian Pac J Cancer Prev* 2016;17(8):4125-9.

32. Zhang M, Xiao B, Wang H, Han MK, Zhang Z, Viennois E, et al. Edible ginger-derived nano-lipids loaded with doxorubicin as a novel drug-delivery approach for colon cancer therapy. *Mol Ther* 2016;24(10):1783-96. doi: 10.1038/mt.2016.159

33. Delbridge AR, Grabow S, Strasser A, Vaux DL. Thirty years of BCL-2: Translating cell death discoveries into novel cancer therapies. *Nat Rev Cancer* 2016;16(2):99-109. doi: 10.1038/nrc.2015.17

34. Youle RJ, Strasser A. The BCL-2 protein family: Opposing activities that mediate cell death. *Nat Rev Mol Cell Biol* 2008;9(1):47-59. doi: 10.1038/nrm2308

35. Reed JC. Apoptosis-targeted therapies for cancer. *Cancer Cell* 2003;3(1):17-22. doi: 10.1016/S1535-6108(02)00241-6

36. Cory S, Huang DC, Adams JM. The BCL-2 family: Roles in cell survival and oncogenesis. *Oncogene* 2003;22(53):8590-607. doi: 10.1038/sj.onc.1207102

37. Yip KW, Reed JC. BCL-2 family proteins and cancer. *Oncogene* 2008;27(50):6398-406. doi: 10.1038/onc.2008.307

38. Wang CC, Chen LG, Lee LT, Yang LL. Effects of 6-gingerol, an antioxidant from ginger, on inducing apoptosis in human leukemic HL-60 cells. *In Vivo* 2003;17(6):641-5.

39. Kohler MF, Marks JR, Wiseman RW, Jacobs IJ, Davidoff AM, Clarke-Pearson DL, et al. Spectrum of mutation and frequency of allelic deletion of the p53 gene in ovarian cancer. *J Natl Cancer Inst* 1993;85(18):1513-9. doi: 10.1093/jnci/85.18.1513

40. Elbendary AA, Cirisano FD, Evans AC Jr, Davis PL, Iglehart JD, Marks JR, et al. Relationship between p21 expression and mutation of the p53 tumor suppressor gene in normal and malignant ovarian epithelial cells. *Clin Cancer Res* 1996;2(9):1571-5.

41. Bates S, Vousden KH. Mechanisms of p53-mediated apoptosis. *Cell Mol Life Sci* 1999;55(1):28-37. doi: 10.1007/s000180050267

42. Bieging KT, Mello SS, Attardi LD. Unravelling mechanisms of p53-mediated tumour suppression. *Nat Rev Cancer* 2014;14(5):359-70. doi: 10.1038/nrc3711

43. Kato H, Yoshikawa M, Fukai Y, Tajima K, Masuda N, Tsukada K, et al. An immunohistochemical study of p16, prb, p21 and p53 proteins in human esophageal cancers. *Anticancer Res* 2000;20(1A):345-9.

44. Pant V, Quintás-Cardama A, Lozano G. The p53 pathway in hematopoiesis: Lessons from mouse models, implications for humans. *Blood* 2012;120(26):5118-27. doi: 10.1182/blood-2012-05-356014

45. Gartel AL, Tyner AL. The role of the cyclin-dependent kinase inhibitor p21 in apoptosis. *Mol Cancer Ther* 2002;1(8):639-49.

46. Ahmadian N, Pashaei-Asl R, Samadi N, Rahmati-Yamchi M, Rashidi MR, Ahmadian M, et al. Hesa-a effects on cell cycle signaling in esophageal carcinoma cell line. *Middle East J Dig Dis* 2016;8(4):297-302. doi: 10.15171/mejdd.2016.39

47. Zlotorynski E. Cancer biology: The dark side of p21. *Nat Rev Mol Cell Biol* 2016;17(8):461. doi: 10.1038/nrm.2016.90

48. Vousden KH, Prives C. Blinded by the light: The growing complexity of p53. *Cell* 2009;137(3):413-31. doi: 10.1016/j.cell.2009.04.037

49. Wiman KG. Strategies for therapeutic targeting of the p53 pathway in cancer. *Cell Death Differ* 2006;13(6):921-6. doi: 10.1038/sj.cdd.4401921

4

Melatonin and N- Acetylcysteine as Remedies for Tramadol-Induced Hepatotoxicity in Albino Rats

Elias Adikwu[1]*, Bonsome Bokolo[2]

[1] Department of Pharmacology, Faculty of Basic Medical Sciences, University of Port Harcourt, Choba, Rivers State, Nigeria.
[2] Department of Pharmacology, Faculty of Basic Medical Sciences, Niger Delta University Wilberforce Island, Bayelsa State, Nigeria.

Keywords:
· Tramadol
· Liver
· Toxicity
· Antioxidants
· Pretreatment
· Rat

Abstract

Purpose: The therapeutic benefit derived from the clinical use of tramadol (TD) has been characterized by hepatotoxicity due to misuse and abuse. The implications of drug-induced hepatotoxicity include socio-economic burden which makes the search for remedy highly imperative. The present study investigated the protective effects of melatonin (MT) and n-acetylcysteine (NAC) on TD-induced hepatotoxicity in albino rats.

Methods: Forty five adult rats used for this study were divided into nine groups of five rats each. The rats were pretreated with 10mg/kg/day of NAC, 10mg/kg/day of MT and combined doses of NAC and MT prior to the administration of 15 mg/kg/day of TD intraperitoneally for 7 days respectively. At the termination of drug administration, rats were weighed, sacrificed, and serum was extracted and evaluated for liver function parameters. The liver was harvested, weighed and evaluated for oxidative stress indices and liver enzymes.

Results: Alanine aminotransferase, alkaline phosphatase, aspartate aminotransferase, total bilirubin, conjugated bilirubin, and malondialdehyde levels were significantly ($P<0.05$) increased in rats administered with TD when compared to control. Furthermore, glutathione, superoxide dismutase and catalase levels were decreased significantly ($P<0.05$) in rats administered with TD when compared to control. The Liver of TD-treated rats showed necrosis of hepatocytes. However, the observed biochemical and liver histological alterations in TD-treated rats were attenuated in NAC and MT pretreated rats. Interestingly, pretreatment with combined doses of NAC and MT produced significant ($P<0.05$) effects on all evaluated parameters in comparison to their individual doses.

Conclusion: Based on the findings in this study, melatonin and n- acetylcysteine could be used clinically as remedies for tramadol associated hepatotoxity.

Introduction

Tramadol (TD) is a centrally acting opioid analgesic which is mainly used for the treatment of moderate to severe pain.[1] Its efficiency and potency ranges between weak opioids and morphine.[2] Clinically, hepatotoxity marked by cholelithiasis, cholecystitis, and abnormal liver function tests could occur in more than 1% of patients administered with TD.[3] However, due to its opiate-like and analgesic effects,[4] TD abuse, dependence as well as acute overdose have led to reported cases of hepatotoxicity and even death in humans.[5-8] Studies in animals have reported hepatotoxicity characterized by altered levels of liver function biomarkers[9,10] and histological damage.[11-13] In addition, oxidative stress could be involved in TD-induced hepatotoxicity due to decrease in antioxidant defence and lipid peroxidation observed in treated animals.[14]

N-acetylcysteine (NAC) is a thiol containing molecule that is produced from amino acid cysteine joined to an acetyl group. It is a small molecule which can be easily filtered and has prompt access to intracellular compartments.[15] Studies have shown that it is a source of sulfhydryl groups and is converted in the body to metabolites capable of stimulating glutathione synthesis, promoting detoxification, and acting directly as a free radical scavenger.[16,17] NAC also modulates inflammatory response through signaling pathways that control pro-inflammatory nuclear factor (NF)-κB activation.[18,19] It has a diversity of applications, which include inhibition of xenobiotic-induced toxicities largely because of the chemical properties of the thiol moiety present in its structure. Reports have shown that NAC treatment protects against acetaminophen associated hepatotoxicity in patients,[20] in carbon tetrachloride associated hepatotoxicity in humans,[21] and in experimental animal-induced hepatotoxicity.[22-24]

Melatonin (MT) is the major hormone of the pineal gland, but it has been detected in many other tissues. It is a highly lipophilic and hydrophilic molecule that crosses cell membranes and easily reaches subcellular compartments including mitochondria, where it seems to

*Corresponding author: Elias Adikwu, E mail: adikwuelias@gmail.com

accumulate in high concentrations.[25] Studies have shown that MT could regulate a variety of physiological processes which include endocrine rhythms,[26] reproductive cycle,[27] immunomudulatory and vasomotor effects.[28] MT is able to prevent oxidative stress through its free radical scavenging effect and by directly increasing other antioxidant activities.[29] Furthermore, several MT metabolites which are formed when it neutralizes damaging reactants are themselves free radical scavengers.[30,31] MT is effective against pathological states characterized by an increase in basal rate of reactive oxygen species (ROS) production, and protects liver from oxidative damage in multiple conditions.[32] In view of the above information this study was aimed at investigating the effects of NAC and MT on TD-induced hepatotoxicity in albino rats.

Materials and Methods
Animals
Forty five adult male albino rats, weighing 250±5 g, were used for this study. Rats were housed under continuous observation in appropriate cages at room temperature with a 12-12 h light-dark cycle. The rats were housed five per cage, and fed with commercial standard diet and water *ad libitum*.

Drugs and experimental protocol
Tramadol hydrochloride (TD) used for this study was manufactured by Zahidi Enterprise Mumbai India, while NAC and MT were obtained from Shijiazhuang AO Pharm Import and Export Co Ltd China. All other chemicals used for this study are of analytical grade. TD, (15 mg/kg/day),[33] MT (10mg/kg/day)[34] and NAC (10mg/kg/day)[35] were used for this study. MT was dissolved in 0.1% ethanol and diluted with normal saline.[36,37] Rats were divided into nine (9) groups' 1- IX of five (5) rats each. Rats in group I and II served as placebo and solvent control and were treated intraperitoneally with 0.1% of ethanol and normal saline respectively. Rats in groups III-VI were treated with 15 mg/kg/day of TD, 10mg/kg/day of NAC, 10mg/kg/day MT, and a combination of NAC and MT intraperitoneally for 7 days respectively. Rats in group VII-IX were pretreated with MT, NAC, and combined doses of MT and NAC prior to treatment with TD intraperitoneally for 7 days respectively.

Collection of sample
Rats were sacrificed with diethyl ether; blood was collected via cardiac puncture in anon-heparinized sample container and allowed to clot. It was centrifuged at 1500 rpm for 15 minutes and serum extracted and evaluated for biochemical parameters. The liver was surgically removed weighed and placed in iced beakers. The liver was washed in ice cold KCl solution (1.15% w/v) and then homogenized with 0.1M phosphate buffer (pH 7.2). The homogenate was centrifuged at 15000 rpm for 20 min and evaluated for liver enzymes and oxidative stress indices.

Evaluation of biochemical parameters
Alkaline phosphatase was evaluated as reported by Babson *et al.,* 1966[38] while aspartate aminotransferase and alanine aminotransferase were evaluated as reported by Reitman and Frankel, 1957.[39] Serum conjugated (CB) and total bilirubin (TB) levels were evaluated as reported by Doumas et al., 1979.[40] Superoxide dismutase was evaluated as described by Sun and Zigman, 1978,[41] while catalase was evaluated as reported by Aebi, 1984.[42] Reduced glutathione was assayed according to Sedlak and Lindsay, 1986,[43] while malondialdehyde was evaluated as reported by Buege and Aust,1978.[44]

Results and Discussion
Liver is a key organ actively involved in numerous metabolic and detoxifying functions. Consequently, it continuous exposure to high levels of endogenous and exogenous oxidants which are the by-products of many biochemical pathways could lead to hepatotoxicity.[45,46] Oxidative stress has been reported as one of the possible mechanisms of xenobiotic-induced hepatotoxicity.[47] The present study evaluated the effects of n-acetylcysteine (NAC) and melatonin (MT) on TD -induced hepatotoxicity in albino rats. The present study did not observe significant (p>0.05) changes in body and relative liver weights of rats treated with these agents when compared to control (Table 1). The levels of AST, ALP, ALT, TB, CB and MDA were decreased whereas the levels of SOD, CAT and GSH were increased in MT and NAC treated rats. However, effects on these parameters were not significantly (p>0.05) different when compared to control (Table1 and 2). These observations are consistent with previous reports.[48-50] On the contrary, levels of AST, ALP, ALT, TB, CB and MDA were increased significantly (p<0.05) whereas SOD, CAT and GSH levels were decreased significantly (p<0.05) in TD-treated rats in comparison to control (Table 3-5). Similar observations have been reported in previous studies.[51,52] The microscopic examination of the liver of NAC and MT-treated rats showed normal architecture; however, the liver of TD- treated rats showed necrosis of hepatocytes (Figure 1-4). The observed histological alterations in the liver of TD-treated rats are in conjunction with earlier findings.[53] The increases in AST, ALP, ALT, TB, and CB levels and necrosis of hepatocytes in TD-treated rats are indicators of hepatotoxicity.[53,54] The observed decreases in SOD, CAT and GSH levels in TD-treated rats are pointers to oxidative stress-induced depletions of these antioxidants through the generation of reactive oxygen species. In mammals, a sophisticated antioxidant system, which includes SOD, CAT and GSH are used to maintain redox homeostasis in the liver. When the ROS is excessive, the homeostasis will be disturbed, resulting in oxidative stress, predisposing the liver to oxidative damage.[55] Oxidative stress triggers hepatic damage by inducing irretrievable alteration of lipids, proteins and DNA contents and more importantly, modulating pathways that control normal biological functions.[56,57] The

observed increase in MDA level in TD-treated rats confirms lipid peroxidation because monitoring of MDA levels in different biological systems is an important indicator of lipid peroxidation both *in-vitro* and *in-vivo* for various health disorders.[58] Lipid peroxidation is a chain reaction occurring during oxidative stress leading to the formation of various active compounds including propanedial and 4-hyrdoxynonenal (HNE) resulting in cellular damage.[59] In the present study, supplementations with MT and NAC prior to treatment with TD significantly (p<0.05) decreased AST, ALP, ALT, TB and CB levels when compared to TD-treated rats (Table 3 and 4). Also, supplementation with MT and NAC prior to treatment with TD significantly (p<0.05) increased liver levels of SOD, CAT GSH whereas MDA levels were decreased in comparison to TD-treated rats (Table 5). Furthermore, histological alterations observed in the liver of TD-treated rats were ameliorated in rats supplemented with MT and NAC (Figure 4-7).

Interestingly, supplementation with combined doses of MT and NAC produced significant (p<0.05) effects on AST, ALP, ALT, TB, CB, SOD, CAT, GSH and MDA levels in comparison to their individual doses (Table 3-5). The observed hepatoprotective effects of MT and NAC could be attributed to the inhibition of TD-induced hepatic oxidative stress.[60] The best hepatoprotective effect obtained in rats' supplemented with combined doses of MT and NAC could be attributed to the potentiation of the activity of each other through scavenging and neutralizing oxidative radicals and up-regulating the activities of some endogenous antioxidants. The ameliorative effect of NAC observed in the present study is in agreement with some authors who reported the inhibitory effect of NAC on isoniazid and rifampicin- induced oxidative liver injury in rats.[61] Findings in this study are also consistent with studies that reported the cytoprotective effects of MT in various experimental models of acute liver injury.[62]

Table 1. Effects of n-acetyl cysteine and melatonin on body, relative liver weights   and liver oxidative stress indices of albino Rats

Drugs	Body Weight (g)	Relative Liver Weight (%)	MDA (U/mg protein)	SOD (U/mg protein)	CAT (U/mg protein)	GSH (μmole/mg protein)
Control	255.3 ± 13.9	1.226 ± 0.01	0.25 ± 0.01	14.7 ± 1.36	25.2 ± 2.12	10.8 ± 1.25
NAC	260.7 ± 12.6	1.349 ± 0.06	0.24 ± 0.06	17.7 ± 1.41	27.3 ± 1.06	11.7 ± 0.79
MT	265.1 ± 14.9	1.251 ± 0.09	0.25 ± 0.08	16.2 ± 1.34	25.9 ± 2.21	11.9 ± 0.96
NAC + MT	270.5 ± 15.2	1.239 ± 0.05	0.22 ± 0.06	22.5 ± 2.28	28.3 ± 2.92	12.7 ± 1.03*

NAC= N-acetylcysteine. MT=Melatonin. n=5. Results are expressed as Mean ± SEM

Table 2. Effects of melatonin and n-acetylcysteine on liver function parameters of albino rats

Drugs	SERUM					LIVER		
	AST (U/L)	ALT (U/L)	ALP (U/L)	TB (μmol/L)	CB (μmol/L)	AST (U/L)	ALP (U/L)	ALT (U/L)
Control	34.3 ± 4.05	31.7 ± 2.42	40.0 ± 3.15	8.71 ± 1.09	3.40 ± 0.15	37.2 ± 3.15	42.7 ± 3.10	35.3 ± 2.50
NAC	33.1 ± 3.75	29.9 ± 3.72	38.7± 3.76	7.39 ± 0.11	3.01 ± 0.36	35.2 ± 2.28	40.1 ± 3.18	32.1 ± 3.91
MT	33.1 ± 3.95	31.3 ± 3.96	39.6 ± 4.06	7.33 ± 0.12	3.31 ± 0.12	36.2 ± 3.06	41.6 ± 4.97	34.1 ± 2.02
NAC+ MT	30.0 ± 2.02	29.2 ± 2.06	35.3 ± 3.65	7.23 ± 0.27	2.99 ± 0.18	35.6 ± 2.17	39.3 ± 2.91	31.3 ± 2.06

NAC= N-acetylcysteine. MT=Melatonin. n=5. Results are expressed as Mean ± SEM

Table 3. Effects of melatonin and n-acetylcysteine on tramadol-induced alterations in liver function parameters of albino rats

Drugs	SERUM				
	AST (U/L)	ALT (U/L)	ALP (U/L)	TB (μmol/L)	CB (μmol/L)
Control	34.3 ± 4.05[a]	31.7 ± 2.42[a]	40.0 ± 3.15[a]	8.71 ± 0.19[a]	3.40 ± 0.15[a]
TD	89.5 ± 6.62[b]	98.3 ± 5.42[b]	92.7 ± 8.80[b]	26.6 ± 2.13[b]	12.3 ± 0.16[b]
TD + NAC	52.1 ± 5.16[c]	57.2 ± 4.68[c]	60.3 ± 6.42[c]	14.1 ± 1.22[c]	7.01 ± 0.01[c]
TD + MT	55.3 ± 3.12[c]	60.6 ± 4.01[c]	64.2± 6.02[c]	16.3 ± 1.15[c]	7.51 ± 0.04[c]
TD+ NAC + MT	31.2 ± 2.27[a]	30.0 ± 2.95[a]	31.1± 3.85[d]	9.00 ± 0.12[a]	3.61 ± 0.06[a]

TD= Tramadol. MT= Melatonin. NAC=N-acetylcysteine. n= 5. Results are expressed as mean ± SEM. Values with different superscripts on the same column differ significantly at *p*< 0.05 ANOVA and Tukey's multiple comparison test

Table 4. Effects of melatonin and n-acetylcysteine on body, liver weights and tissue levels of aminotransferases and alkaline phosphatase of tramadol-treated albino rats

Drugs	WEIGHTS		LIVER TISSUE		
	Body Weight (g)	Relative Liver Weight (%)	AST (U/L)	ALT (U/L)	ALP (U/L)
Control	255.3 ± 13.9	1.226 ± 0.01	37.2 ± 3.15[a]	35.3 ± 2.50[a]	42.7 ± 3.10[a]
TD	260.6 ± 10.1	1.237 ± 0.06	80.1 ± 7.15[b]	96.2 ± 4.10[b]	95.4 ± 7.70[b]
TD + NAC	276.1 ± 12.2	1.316 ± 0.21	50.3 ± 3.95[c]	51.7 ± 3.20[c]	63.2 ± 4.97[c]
TD + MT	270.3 ± 10.5	1.212 ± 0.14	53.7 ± 2.10[c]	57.2 ± 2.91[c]	65.7 ± 4.02[c]
TD+NAC+ MT	285.8 ± 14.7	1.343 ± 0.06	30.1± 1.72[d]	37.1 ± 1.96[a]	41.3 ± 3.98[a]

TD= Tramadol. MT= Melatonin. NAC=N-acetylcysteine. n= 5. Results are expressed as mean ± SEM. Values with different superscripts on the same column differ significantly at $p < 0.05$ ANOVA and Tukey's multiple comparison test

Table 5. Effects of n-acetylcysteine and melatonin on liver oxidative stress indices of tramadol-treated albino rats

Drugs	MDA (nmole/mg protein)	SOD (U/mg protein)	CAT (U/mg protein)	GSH (µmole/mg protein)
Control	0.25 + 0.01[a]	14.7± 1.36[a]	25.2 ± 2.12[a]	10.8 ± 1.25[a]
TD	1.15 ± 0.06[b]	3.59 ± 0.27[b]	6.51 ± 0.13[b]	3.21 ± 0.08[b]
TD +NAC	0.58 ± 0.01[c]	7.15 ± 0.16[c]	13.1 ± 0.29[c]	5.98 ± 0.16[c]
TD+ MT	0.62 ± 0.03[c]	6.95 ± 0.01[c]	11.3 ± 0.31[c]	5.10 ± 0.13[c]
TD+NAC+MT	0.37 ± 0.05[d]	12.01 ± 0.26[a]	23.0 ± 1.01[a]	9.98 ± 0.15[a]

TD= Tramadol. MT= Melatonin. NAC=N-acetylcysteine. n= 5. Results are expressed as mean ± SEM. Values with different superscripts on the same column differ significantly at $p < 0.05$ ANOVA and Tukey's multiple comparison test

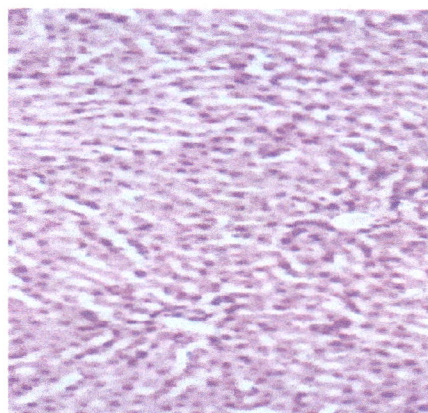

Figure 1. Micrograph of the control liver of rat treated with normal saline for 7 days showing normal liver architecture (Hand E X 200)

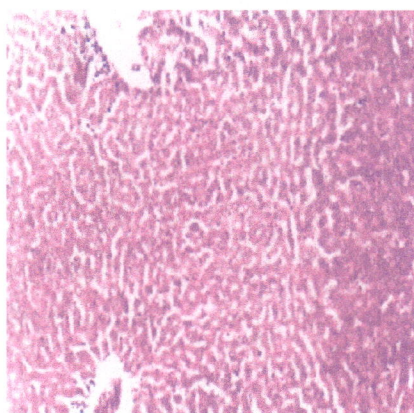

Figure 3. Micrograph of the liver of rat treated intraperitoneally with 10 mg/kg/day of MT for 7 days showing normal architecture (Hand E X 200)

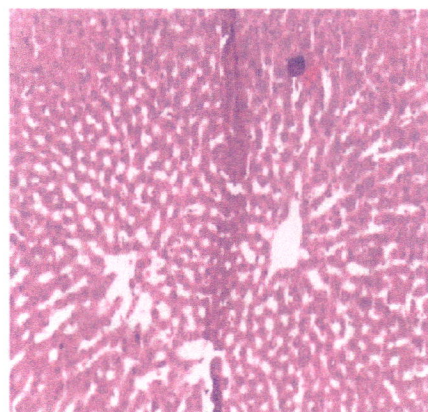

Figure 2. Micrograph of the liver of rat treated intraperitoneally with 10 mg/kg/day of NAC for 7 days showing normal architecture (Hand E X 200)

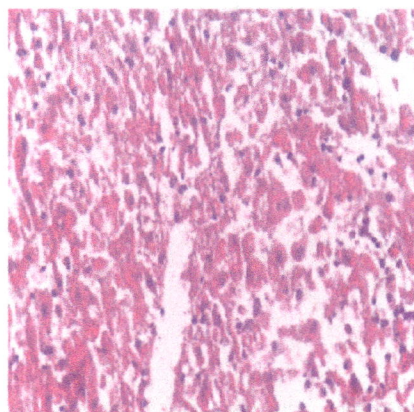

Figure 4. Micrograph of the liver of rat treated with 15 mg/kg/day of TD for 7 days showing hepatocytes necrosis (Hand E X 200)

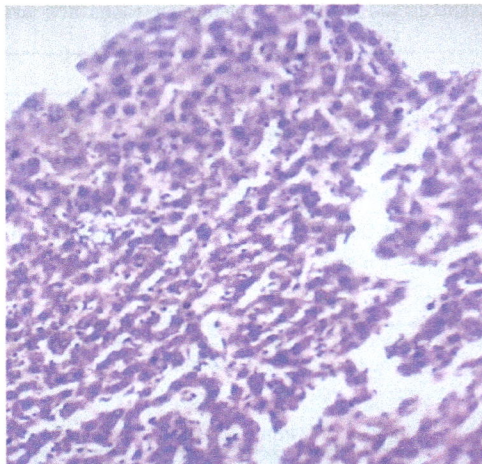

Figure 5. Micrograph of the liver of rat treated with 15 mg/kg/day of TD and10 mg/kg/day of NAC for 7 days showing normal architecture (Hand E X 200)

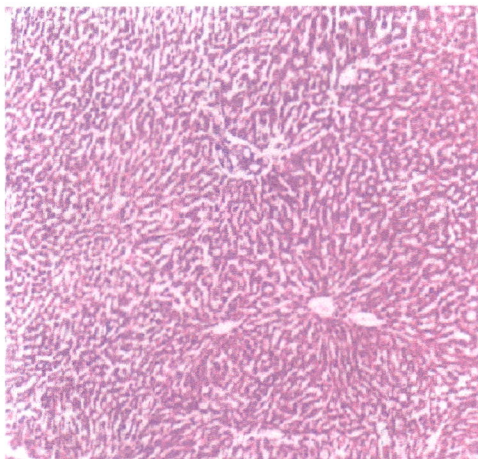

Figure 6. Micrograph of the liver of rat treated with 15 mg/kg/day of TD and10mg/kg/day of MT for 7 days showing normal architecture (Hand E X 200)

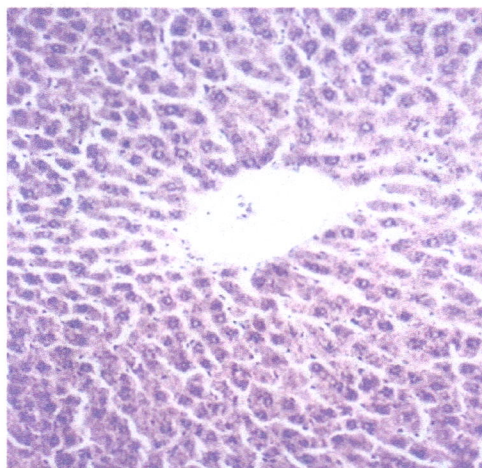

Figure 7. Micrograph of the liver of rat treated with 15 mg/kg/day of TD, 10mg/kg/day of NAC and 10mg/kg/day of MT for 7 days showing normal architecture (Hand E X200)

MT and NAC are free radical scavengers and neutralizers which can inhibit oxidative stress and lipid peroxidation.[63,64] Metabolites of MT, including the major hepatic metabolite 6-hydroxymelatonin, as well as N-acetyl-N-formyl-5-methoxykynuramine and N-acetyl-5-methoxykynuramine have been shown to detoxify radicals.[65,66] In addition, MT may down-regulate pro-oxidant enzymes like nitric oxide synthase (NOS) and lipoxygenases, thus reducing the formation of nitric oxide (NO), superoxide anions, and subsequently peroxynitrite anions.[67,68] MT and NAC can stabilize membranes and increase their resistance toward free radical attack.[69,70] Furthermore, MT and NAC can stimulate the production or regeneration of antioxidants including SOD, CAT and GSH. Studies have shown that NAC and MT experimentally enhanced intracellular glutathione level by stimulating the rate-limiting enzyme required for it synthesis.[71,72] Also, NAC has been reported to prevent xenobiotic-induced hepatotoxicity by inhibiting the hepatic depletion of GSH and up-regulating its activity. Hepatoprotective effect of NAC can also occur through maintaining –SH groups of enzymes and membrane proteins in their reduced state.[73]

Conclusion
The findings in the present study showed the potential of melatonin and n-acetylcysteine as remedies for hepatotoxicity associated with the abuse or clinical use of tramadol.

Acknowledgments
The authors would like to appreciate the technical assistance of Mr Eze Iheukwumere of the Faculty of Pharmacy, Madonna University, Elele, Rivers State.

Ethical Issues
All rats used for this study were handled in accordance with Directive 2010/63/EU of the European Parliament and the Council on the protection of animals used for scientific purposes.

Conflict of Interest
The authors declare no conflict of interests in the authorship and the publication of this research.

References
1. Nossaman VE, Ramadhyani U, Kadowitz PJ, Nossaman BD. Advances in perioperative pain management: Use of medications with dual analgesic mechanisms, tramadol & tapentadol. *Anesthesiol Clin* 2010;28(4):647-66. doi: 10.1016/j.anclin.2010.08.009
2. Miranda HF, Pinardi G. Antinociception, tolerance, and physical dependence comparison between morphine and tramadol. *Pharmacol Biochem Behav* 1998;61(4):357-60. doi: 10.1016/S0091-3057(98)00123-3
3. Product Information: Ultram ER (tramadol). Raritan, NJ: PriCara; 2009.

4. Gutstein HB, Akil H. Opioid Analgesics. In: Brunton LL, Lazo JS, Parker KL, editors. Goodman and Gilman's The Pharmacological Basis of Therapeutics. 11th ed. New York: McGraw-Hill: 2006. PP. 547-90.

5. Senay EC, Adams EH, Geller A, Inciardi JA, Munoz A, Schnoll SH, et al. Physical dependence on Ultram (tramadol hydrochloride): Both opioid-like and atypical withdrawal symptoms occur. *Drug Alcohol Depend* 2003;69(3):233-41. 10.1016/S0376-8716(02)00321-6

6. Lee HJ, Cha KE, Hwang SG, Kim JK, Kim GJ. In vitro screening system for hepatotoxicity: Comparison of bone-marrow-derived mesenchymal stem cells and Placenta-derived stem cells. *J Cell Biochem* 2011;112(1):49-58. doi: 10.1002/jcb.22728

7. Shadnia S, Soltaninejad K, Heydari K, Sasanian G, Abdollahi M. Tramadol intoxication: A review of 114 cases. *Hum Exp Toxicol* 2008;27(3):201-5. doi: 10.1177/0960327108090270

8. Elmanama AA, Abu Tayyem NES, Essawaf HN, Hmaid IM. Tramadol-Induced Liver and Kidney Toxicity among Abusers in Gaza Strip, Palestine. *Jordan J Biol Sci* 2015;8(2):133-7. doi: 10.12816/0027559

9. El-Gaafarawi I, Hassan M, Fouad G El-Komey F. Toxic effects of paroxetine on sexual and reproductive functions of rats. *Egypt J Hosp Med* 2005;21:16-32.

10. Saleem R, Iqbal R, Abbas MN, Zahra A, Iqbal J, Ansari MS. Effects of tramadol on histopathological and biochemical parameters in mice (Mus musculus) model. *Global J Pharmacol* 2014;8(1):14-9.

11. Loughrey MB, Loughrey CM, Johnston S, O'Rourke D. Fatal hepatic failure following accidental tramadol overdose. *Forensic Sci Int* 2003;134(2-3):232-3. doi: 10.1016/S0379-0738(03)00132-4

12. Sevimli ZU, Dursun H, Erdogan F. Histopathologic changes in liver induced by morphine and tramadol. *The Pain Clinic* 2006;18:321-5. doi: 10.1163/156856906778704687

13. El-Wessemy AM. Histopathological and ultrastructural studies on the side effects of the analgesic drug tramadol on the liver of albino mice. *Egypt J Zool* 2008;50:423-42.

14. Elkhateeb A, El Khishin I, Megahed O, Mazen F. Effect of *Nigella sativa Linn* oil on tramadol-induced hepato- and nephrotoxicity in adult male albino rats. *Toxicol Rep* 2015;2:512-9. doi: 10.1016/j.toxrep.2015.03.002

15. Holdiness MR. Clinical pharmacokinetics of N-acetylcysteine. *Clin Pharmacokinet* 1991;20(2):123-34. doi: 10.2165/00003088-199120020-00004

16. De Vries N, De Flora S. N-acetyl-l-cysteine. *J Cell Biochem* 1993;53(S17F):270-7. doi: 10.1002/jcb.240531040

17. Cuzzocrea S, Mazzon E, Costantino G, Serraino I, De Sarro A, Caputi AP. Effects of N-acetylcysteine in a rat model of ischemia and reperfusion injury.

18. Slim R, Toborek M, Robertson LW, Lehmler HJ, Hennig B. Cellular glutathione status modulates polychlorinated biphenyl-induced stress response and apoptosis in vascular endothelial cells. *Toxicol Appl Pharmacol* 2000;166(1):36-42. doi: 10.1006/taap.2000.8944

19. Mansour HH, Hafez HF, Fahmy NM, Hanafi N. Protective effect of N-acetylcysteine against radiation induced DNA damage and hepatic toxicity in rats. *Biochem Pharmacol* 2008;75(3):773-80. doi: 10.1016/j.bcp.2007.09.018

20. Flanagan RJ, Meredith TJ. Use of N-acetylcysteine in clinical toxicology. *Am J Med* 1991;91(3):S131-9. doi: 10.1016/0002-9343(91)90296-A

21. Ochoa Gomez FJ, Lisa Caton V, Saralegui Reta I, Monzon Marin JL. Carbon tetrachloride poisoning. *An Med Interna* 1996;13(8):393-4.

22. Valles EG, de Castro CR, Castro JA. N-acetyl cysteine is an early but also a late preventive agent against carbon tetrachloride-induced liver necrosis. *Toxicol Lett* 1994;71(1):87-95. doi: 10.1016/0378-4274(94)90202-X

23. Remirez D, Commandeur JN, Groot E, Vermeulen NP. Mechanism of protection of lobenzarit against paracetamol-induced toxicity in rat hepatocytes. *Eur J Pharmacol* 1995;293(4):301-8. doi: 10.1016/0926-6917(95)90049-7

24. Al-Mustafa ZH, Al-Ali AK, Qaw FS, Abdul-Cader Z. Cimetidine enhances the hepatoprotective action of N-acetylcysteine in mice treated with toxic doses of paracetamol. *Toxicology* 1997;121(3):223-8. doi: 10.1016/S0300-483X(97)00069-3

25. Reiter RJ, Tan DX. Melatonin: A novel protective agent against oxidative injury of the ischemic/reperfused heart. *Cardiovasc Res* 2003;58(1):10-9. doi: 10.1016/S0008-6363(02)00827-1

26. Forsling ML, Stoughton RP, Zhou Y, Kelestimur H, Demaine C. The role of the pineal in the control of the daily patterns of neurohypophysial hormone secretion. *J Pineal Res* 1993;14(1):45-51. doi: 10.1111/j.1600-079X.1993.tb00484.x

27. Guerrero JM, Reiter RJ. A brief survey of pineal gland-immune system interrelationships. *Endocr Res* 1992;18(2):91-113. doi: 10.1080/07435809209035401

28. Kus I, Akpolat N, Ozen OA, Songur A, Kavakli A, Sarsilmaz M. Effects of melatonin on leydig cells in pinealectomized rat: An immunohistochemical study. *Acta Histochem* 2002;104(1):93-7. doi: 10.1078/0065-1281-00618

29. Adikwu E, Braimbaifa N, Obianime AW. Melatonin and Alpha Lipoic Acid: Possible Mitigants for Lopinavir/Ritonavir- Induced Renal Toxicity in Male Albino Rats. *Physiol Pharmacol* 2015;19(4):232-40.

30. Reiter RJ, Tan DX, Manchester LC, Qi W. Biochemical reactivity of melatonin with reactive

Cardiovasc Res 2000;47(3):537-48. doi: 10.1016/S0008-6363(00)00018-3

oxygen and nitrogen species: A review of the evidence. *Cell Biochem Biophys* 2001;34(2):237-56. doi: 10.1385/CBB:34:2:237

31. Reiter RJ, Tan DX, Terron MP, Flores LJ, Czarnocki Z. Melatonin and its metabolites: new findings regarding their production and their radical scavenging actions. *Acta Biochim Pol* 2007;54(1):1-9.

32. Maldonado MD, Murillo-Cabezas F, Terron MP, Flores LJ, Tan DX, Manchester LC, et al. The potential of melatonin in reducing morbidity-mortality after craniocerebral trauma. *J Pineal Res* 2007;42(1):1-11.   doi: 10.1111/j.1600-079X.2006.00376.x

33. Essam Hafez M, Sahar Issa Y, Safaa Abdel Rahman M. Parenchymatous Toxicity of Tramadol: Histopathological and Biochemical Study. *J Alcohol Drug Depend* 2015;3(5):225. doi: 10.4172/2329-6488.1000225

34. Koksal M, Kurcer Z, Erdogan D, Iraz M, Tas M, Eren MA, et al. Effect of melatonin and n-acetylcysteine on hepatic injury in rat induced by methanol intoxication: A comparative study. *Eur Rev Med Pharmacol Sci* 2012;16(4):437-44.

35. Feldman L, Efrati S, Dishy V, Katchko L, Berman S, Averbukh M, et al. N-acetylcysteine ameliorates amphotericin-induced nephropathy in rats. *Nephron Physiol* 2005;99(1):23-7. doi: 10.1159/000081799

36. Kaplan M, Atakan IH, Aydogdu N, Aktoz T, Puyan FO, Seren G, et al. The effect of melatonin on cadmium-induced renal injury in chronically exposed rats. *Turk J Urol* 2009;35(2):139-47.

37. Adikwu E, Nelson B, Obianime WA. Beneficial effects of melatonin and alpha lipoic acid on lopinavir/ritonavir-induced alterations in serum lipid and glucose levels of male albino rats. *Macedonia Pharm Bull* 2016;62(1):47-55.

38. Babson AL, Greeley SJ, Coleman CM, Phillips GE. Phenolphthalein monophosphate as a substrate for serum alkaline phosphatase. *Clin Chem* 1966;12(8):482-90.

39. Reitman S, Frankel S. A colorimetric method for the determination of serum glutamic oxalacetic and glutamic pyruvic transaminases. *Am J Clin Pathol* 1957;28(1):56-63. doi: 10.1093/ajcp/28.1.56

40. Doumas BT, Perry BW, Sasse EA, Straumfjord JV Jr. Standardization in bilirubin assays: Evaluation of selected methods and stability of bilirubin solutions. *Clin Chem* 1973;19(9):984-93.

41. Sun M, Zigman S. An improved spectrophotometric assay for superoxide dismutase based on epinephrine autoxidation. *Anal Biochem* 1978;90(1):81-9. doi: 10.1016/0003-2697(78)90010-6

42. Aebi H. Catalase *in vitro*. In: Colowick SP, Kaplane NO, editors. *Method in Enzymology*. 12th ed. New York: Academic Press; 1984. P. 121-6.

43. Sedlak J, Lindsay RH. Estimation of total, protein-bound, and nonprotein sulfhydryl groups in tissue with ellman's reagent. *Anal Biochem* 1968;25(1):192-205. doi: 10.1016/0003-2697(68)90092-4

44. Buege JA, Aust SD. Microsomal lipid peroxidation. *Methods Enzymol* 1978;52:302-10. doi: 10.1016/S0076-6879(78)52032-6

45. Ji LL. Antioxidants and oxidative stress in exercise. *Proc Soc Exp Biol Med* 1999;222(3):283-92.

46. Bejma J, Ramires P, Ji LL. Free radical generation and oxidative stress with ageing and exercise: Differential effects in the myocardium and liver. *Acta Physiol Scand* 2000;169(4):343-51. doi: 10.1046/j.1365-201x.2000.00745.x

47. Santos NA, Medina WS, Martins NM, Rodrigues MA, Curti C, Santos AC. Involvement of oxidative stress in the hepatotoxicity induced by aromatic antiepileptic drugs. *Toxicol In Vitro* 2008;22(8):1820-4. doi: 10.1016/j.tiv.2008.08.004

48. Abd El-Motelp BA. Ameliorative effect of n-acetyl cysteine on sodium arsenite induced toxicity and oxidative stress in mice. *World J Pharm Res* 2014;3(2):1746-59.

49. Abdel-Wahab WM. AlCl3-Induced Toxicity and Oxidative Stress in Liver of Male Rats: Protection by Melatonin. *Life Sci J* 2012;9(4):1173-82.

50. Umosen AJ, Ambali SF, Ayo JO, Mohammed B, Uchendu C. Alleviating effects of melatonin on oxidative changes in the testes and pituitary glands evoked by subacute chlorpyrifos administration in Wistar rats. *Asian Pac J Trop Biomed* 2012;2(8):645-50. doi: 10.1016/S2221-1691(12)60113-0

51. Youssef SH, Zidan AHM. Histopathological and Biochemical Effects of Acute and Chronic Tramadol Drug Toxicity on Liver, Kidney and Testicular Function in Adult Male Albino Rats. *J Med Toxicol Clin Forensic Med* 2016;1:2. doi: 10.21767/2471-9641.10007

52. Atici S, Cinel I, Cinel L, Doruk N, Eskandari G, Oral U. Liver and kidney toxicity in chronic use of opioids: an experimental long term treatment model. *J Biosci* 2005;30(2):245-52. doi: 10.1007/bf02703705

53. Awadalla EA, Salah-Eldin AE. Histopathological and Molecular Studies on Tramadol Mediated Hepato-Renal Toxicity in Rats. *J Pharm Biol Sci* 2015;10(6):90-102.

54. Eraslan G, Kanbur M, Silici S. Effect of carbaryl on some biochemical changes in rats: The ameliorative effect of bee pollen. *Food Chem Toxicol* 2009;47(1):86-91. doi: 10.1016/j.fct.2008.10.013

55. Li AN, Li S, Zhang YJ, Xu XR, Chen YM, Li HB. Resources and biological activities of natural polyphenols. *Nutrients* 2014;6(12):6020-47. doi: 10.3390/nu6126020

56. Singal AK, Jampana SC, Weinman SA. Antioxidants as therapeutic agents for liver disease. *Liver Int* 2011;31(10):1432-48.   doi: 10.1111/j.1478-3231.2011.02604.x

57. Feng Y, Wang N, Ye X, Li H, Feng Y, Cheung F, et al. Hepatoprotective effect and its possible

mechanism of coptidis rhizoma aqueous extract on carbon tetrachloride-induced chronic liver hepatotoxicity in rats. *J Ethnopharmacol* 2011;138(3):683-90. doi: 10.1016/j.jep.2011.09.032

58. Zhang Y, Chen SY, Hsu T, Santella RM. Immunohistochemical detection of malondialdehyde-DNA adducts in human oral mucosa cells. *Carcinogenesis* 2002;23(1):207-11. doi: 10.1093/carcin/23.1.207

59. Michiels C, Remacle J. Cytotoxicity of linoleic acid peroxide, malondialdehyde and 4-hydroxynonenal towards human fibroblasts. *Toxicology* 1991;66(2):225-34. doi: 10.1016/0300-483x(91)90221-l

60. Hong RT, Xu JM, Mei Q. Melatonin ameliorates experimental hepatic fibrosis induced by carbon tetrachloride in rats. *World J Gastroenterol* 2009;15(12):1452-8. doi: 10.3748/wjg.15.1452

61. Attri S, Rana SV, Vaiphei K, Sodhi CP, Katyal R, Goel RC, et al. Isoniazid- and rifampicin-induced oxidative hepatic injury--protection by N-acetylcysteine. *Hum Exp Toxicol* 2000;19(9):517-22. doi: 10.1191/096032700674230830

62. Tahan V, Ozaras R, Canbakan B, Uzun H, Aydin S, Yildirim B, et al. Melatonin reduces dimethylnitrosamine-induced liver fibrosis in rats. *J Pineal Res* 2004;37(2):78-84. doi: 10.1111/j.1600-079X.2004.00137.x

63. Zafarullah M, Li WQ, Sylvester J, Ahmad M. Molecular mechanisms of N-acetylcysteine actions. *Cell Mol Life Sci* 2003;60(1):6-20. doi: 10.1007/s000180300001

64. Hardeland R. Antioxidative protection by melatonin: Multiplicity of mechanisms from radical detoxification to radical avoidance. *Endocrine* 2005;27(2):119-30. doi: 10.1385/ENDO:27:2:119

65. Tan DX, Manchester LC, Burkhardt S, Sainz RM, Mayo JC, Kohen R, et al. N1-acetyl-N2-formyl-5-methoxykynuramine, a biogenic amine and melatonin metabolite, functions as a potent antioxidant. *FASEB J* 2001;15(12):2294-6. doi: 10.1096/fj.01-0309fje

66. Tan DX, Manchester LC, Terron MP, Flores LJ, Reiter RJ. One molecule, many derivatives: A never-ending interaction of melatonin with reactive oxygen and nitrogen species? *J Pineal Res* 2007;42(1):28-42. doi: 10.1111/j.1600-079X.2006.00407.x

67. Bettahi I, Pozo D, Osuna C, Reiter RJ, Acuna-Castroviejo D, Guerrero JM. Melatonin reduces nitric oxide synthase activity in rat hypothalamus. *J Pineal Res* 1996;20(4):205-10. doi: 10.1111/j.1600-079X.1996.tb00260.x

68. Zhang H, Akbar M, Kim HY. Melatonin: An endogenous negative modulator of 12-lipoxygenation in the rat pineal gland. *Biochem J* 1999;344(2):487-93. doi: 10.1042/bj3440487

69. Garcia JJ, Reiter RJ, Guerrero JM, Escames G, Yu BP, Oh CS, et al. Melatonin prevents changes in microsomal membrane fluidity during induced lipid peroxidation. *FEBS Lett* 1997;408(3):297-300. doi: 10.1016/S0014-5793(97)00447-X

70. Kamalakkannan N, Rukkumani R, Aruna K, Varma PS, Viswanathan P, Padmanabhan V. Protective Effect of N-Acetyl Cysteine in Carbon Tetrachloride-Induced Hepatotoxicity in Rats. *Iran J Pharmacol Ther* 2005;4(2):118-23.

71. Zhao C, Shichi H. Prevention of acetaminophen-induced cataract by a combination of diallyl disulfide and N-acetylcysteine. *J Ocul Pharmacol Ther* 1998;14(4):345-55. doi: 10.1089/jop.1998.14.345

72. Rodriguez C, Mayo JC, Sainz RM, Antolin I, Herrera F, Martin V, et al. Regulation of antioxidant enzymes: A significant role for melatonin. *J Pineal Res* 2004;36(1):1-9. doi: 10.1046/j.1600-079X.2003.00092.x

73. Wagner PD, Mathieu-Costello O, Bebout DE, Gray AT, Natterson PD, Glennow C. Protection against pulmonary O2 toxicity by N-acetylcysteine. *Eur Respir J* 1989;2(2):116-26.

5

Nanoparticles of Chitosan Loaded Ciprofloxacin: Fabrication and Antimicrobial Activity

Zahra Sobhani[1,2], **Soliman Mohammadi Samani**[3]*, **Hashem Montaseri**[1], **Elham Khezri**[1]

[1] *Department of quality control, Faculty of pharmacy, Shiraz University of Medical Science, Shiraz, Iran.*

[2] *Center for nanotechnology in drug delivery, Faculty of pharmacy, Shiraz University of Medical Science, Shiraz, Iran.*

[3] *Department of pharmaceutics, Faculty of pharmacy, Shiraz University of Medical Science, Shiraz, Iran.*

Keywords:
· Chitosan
· Ciprofloxacin
· MIC
· Nanoparticle
· Tripolyphosphate

Abstract

Purpose: Chitosan is a natural mucoadhesive polymer with antibacterial activity. In the present study, chitosan (CS) nanoparticles were investigated as a vehicle for delivery of antibiotic, ciprofloxacin hydrochloride.

Methods: Ionotropic gelation method was used for preparation chitosan nanoparticles. The effects of various factors including concentration of CS, concentration of tripolyphosphate (TPP), and homogenization rate on the size of nanoparticles were studied. The effects of various mass ratios of CS to ciprofloxacin hydrochloride on the encapsulation efficiency of nanoparticles were assessed.

Results: The particles prepared under optimal condition of 0.45% CS concentration, 0.45% TPP concentration and homogenizer rate at 6000 rpm, had 72 nm diameter. In these particles with 1:0.5 mass ratio of CS to ciprofloxacin hydrochloride, the encapsulation efficiency was 23%. The antibacterial activity of chitosan nanoparticles and ciprofloxacin-loaded nanoparticles against *E.coli* and *S.aureus* was evaluated by calculation of minimum inhibitory concentration (MIC). Results showed that MIC of ciprofloxacin loaded chitosan nanoparticles was 50% lower than that of ciprofloxacin hydrochloride alone in both of microorganism species. Nanoparticles without drug exhibited antibacterial activity at higher concentrations and MIC of them against *E.coli* and *S.aureus* was 177 and 277 µg/ml, respectively.

Conclusion: Therefore chitosan nanoparticles could be applied as carrier for decreasing the dose of antibacterial agents in the infections.

Introduction

Management of infectious disease can be improved by prolonging the contact time of antibiotics with the microorganism surface. The continuous search for potential antimicrobial agent has led to identification of antimicrobial biomaterials that are based on polymers or their composites.[1,2] Chitosan [poly B-(1–4)-2-amino-2-deoxy-d-glucose] as a poly cationic biopolymer has high antimicrobial activity.[3,4] This natural polysaccharide possesses useful properties such as non-toxicity, biodegradability, low price, high biocompatibility and non-antigenicity.[3-10] The proposed mechanism for its antimicrobial action is binding to the negatively charged bacterial cell wall, with consequent destabilization of the cell envelope and altered permeability, followed by attachment to DNA with inhibition of its replication.[1,11,12] Additionally through its positive ionic interactions with the negative charges of the cell surface membranes the drug can be exposed to microorganisms for a longer time.[11,13,14] Furthermore, it has been shown that chitosan and its derivatives can act as antibacterial agents against both Gram-negative and Gram-positive bacteria.[14] Regarding to these points, the potency of antibacterial agents against microorganisms may be increased by loading them into the chitosan nanoparticles. Nanoparticulate drug delivery systems may improve therapeutic efficacy through enhancing the antibiotic concentration in the microorganism without increasing the dose of administrated antibiotic.[15]

In the present work we developed ciprofloxacin-loaded chitosan nanoparticles and evaluated their physicochemical properties. After that, the antibacterial activity of selected formulation with appropriate physicochemical specifications against ciprofloxacin susceptible bacteria including *Escherchia coli* as a Gram-negative strain and *Staphylococcus aureus* as a Gram-positive strain was evaluated.

Materials and Methods

Materials

Low molecular weight chitosan (CS) and tripolyphosphate (TPP) was purchased from Sigma Aldrich Co. (USA). Ciprofloxacin hydrochloride was obtained from Exir pharmaceutical Co. Tryptic soy broth culture was purchased from Merck Co. (Germany). *Escherchia coli* (ATCC 25922) and *Staphylococcus aureus* (ATCC 25923) were kindly donated by Doctor Alborzi Clinical

---

*Corresponding author: Soliman Mohammadi Samani, Email: smsamani@sums.ac.ir

Microbiological Research Center. All other reagents were of analytical grade and used as received.

Preparation of ciprofloxacin-loaded chitosan nanoparticles

Chitosan nanoparticles were prepared using ionic gelation method. Nanoparticles were prepared by addition of TPP aqueous solution to the CS aqueous solution (in 1% v/v acetic acid) dropwise under stirring at room temperature, until faint turbidity.[16] Orthogonal experiment was designed for evaluation of the effect of CS concentration, TPP concentration, and stirring speed on the particle size. Three factors and their three levels were shown in Table 1. The resulting experimental design consisted of 9 runs, was shown in Table 2.

Two selected formulations which had the lowest particle size were used to fabricate ciprofloxacin-loaded CS nanoparticles by the same method, except that ciprofloxacin was added into CS solution at different polymer:drug ratio (W:W) prior to the addition of TPP solution.

Table 1. Factors and levels of orthogonal test

Levels	Factors		
	Chitosan Concentration (%)	TPP Concentration (%)	Stirring speed (rpm)
1	0.2	0.3	6000
2	0.3	0.45	9000
3	0.45	0.675	13500

Table 2. Designed formulations of orthogonal experiments

Formulations	Factors		
	Chitosan Concentration (%)	TPP Concentration (%)	Stirring speed (rpm)
1	0.2	0.3	6000
2	0.2	0.45	9000
3	0.2	0.675	13500
4	0.3	0.3	9000
5	0.3	0.45	13500
6	0.3	0.675	6000
7	0.45	0.3	13500
8	0.45	0.45	6000
9	0.45	0.675	9000

Characterizations of nanoparticles

Particle size

Particle size distribution of CS nanoparticles was determined using laser diffraction particle size analyzer (Shimadzu, Model SALD-2101, Japan) at room temperature. The polydispersity index (PDI) of nanoparticles was calculated by the equation 1:

$$\text{Span} = \frac{(D90 - D10)}{D50} \quad \text{(Equation 1)}$$

Where D90, D50 and D10 designates that the particle size for which 90%, 50% and 10% of the particles are smaller than these volumes, respectively.

Drug encapsulation efficiency

The encapsulation efficiency was analyzed according to the procedure reported by Cevher et al. (2006).[5] After drug loading, nanoparticles were separated from the suspension by ultracentrifugation (Hettich, Model Mikro220R, Germany) at 15500 rpm and 4°C for 30 min. The amount of free ciprofloxacin in the supernatant was measured by UV-Vis spectrophotometer (PG instruments, Model T80+, England) at 270 nm. The encapsulation efficiency (EE) was calculated by the equation 2:

$$\text{EE\%} = \frac{(T-F)}{T} \times 100 \quad \text{(Equation 2)}$$

Where F is the free amount of drug in the supernatant and T is total amount of drug added into CS solution. A blank sample was made from nanoparticles without loaded drug but treated similarly as the drug-loaded nanoparticles.

All analyses were carried out in triplicate.

Statistical analysis

Drug encapsulation efficiencies between different formulations were compared. To determine the optimum formulation for further studies, statistical analysis was performed using the Student's t-test. Differences were considered significant at $P < 0.05$.

Differential scanning calorimetric (DSC) analysis

Thermal analysis using a DSC method was used to characterize the thermal behavior of the chitosan, TPP, ciprofloxacin HCl, blank nanoparticles, and drug-loaded nanoparticles employing differential scanning calorimeter (TA Instruments, Model 302, Germany). Samples were accurately weighed into standard aluminum pans and sealed. All samples were run at a heating rate of 10°C/min over a temperature range of 25–300°C under nitrogen atmosphere. An empty pan, sealed in the same way as the sample, was used as a reference.

In vitro drug release

A comparative in vitro drug release study was carried out in three different pH values of 5.0, 6.8 and 7.4 in phosphate buffer solution (PBS). Drug-loaded chitosan nanoparticles, suspended in 5.0 ml PBS was placed in the dialysis membrane (cutoff: 12kDa, Sigma Aldrich, USA, supplier: Kimia Teb Tajhiz, Shiraz, Iran) tied at both ends and immersed in the cell containing 100 ml of PBS. The cell was put into shaker incubator (Farazma, Iran) under the condition of 37°C and 25 rpm. To determine the concentration of drug in the receiving compartment, samples (5ml) were withdrawn from the cell at scheduled time points and replaced by the same volume of fresh pre-warmed PBS solution to avoid saturation phenomena and maintain the sink condition. Samples were analyzed at 270 nm. The release dosage at each moment was calculated and drawn into cumulative release curve.

Assays for antibacterial activity
Determination of minimum inhibitory concentration (MIC)
All glassware used for the tests were sterilized in an autoclave at 121°C for 15 min prior to use. All particles were sterilized by exposing to UV radiation for 60 min prior to the tests.[17]

The minimum inhibitory concentration (MIC) of ciprofloxacin and ciprofloxacin-loaded CS nanoparticles were determined by a turbidometric method using Tryptic soy broth (TSB), against *E.coli* and *S.aureus* strains. Drug concentrations ranging from 31.25-4000 ng/ml for *S.aureus* and 5-640 ng/ml for *E.coli* was used. All cultures were inoculated with final bacterial concentration of 10^5 CFU/ml. After incubating for 24 hours at 37°C, samples were evaluated. The lowest concentration that inhibited the growth of bacteria was considered as the MIC.

To determine the MIC of chitosan nanoparticles without any drugs against *E.coli* and *S.aureus*, different particle concentrations were prepared and aseptically inoculated and incubated for 24 hours at 37°C.

Results
Particle size
The mean size and polydispersity index (PDI) of CS nanoparticles in aqueous medium measured by dynamic laser light scattering showed in Table 3.

Formulations No.4 and No.8 that had lower particle sizes were selected for further studies.

Table 3. Particle size and polydispersity index of CS nanoparticles

No.	Factors			Experimental result	
	CS Conc. (%)	TPP Conc. (%)	Stirring speed (rpm)	Particle size (nm) (mean±SD)	Polydispersity index (mean±SD)
1	0.2	0.3	6000	5.77±117.33	0.208±1.290
2	0.2	0.45	9000	2.64±112	0.056±1.110
3	0.2	0.675	13500	45.13±160	0.225±1.49
4	0.3	0.3	9000	15.00±94	0.016±0.785
5	0.3	0.45	13500	92.66±623.33	0.027±0.710
6	0.3	0.675	6000	2.89±111.67	0.058±1.103
7	0.45	0.3	13500	29.51±338	0.059±0.717
8	0.45	0.45	6000	13.32±71.67	0.057±0.705
9	0.45	0.675	9000	83.74±159.33	0.169±1.001

Abbreviations: CS Conc., chitosan concentration; TPP Conc. tripolyphosphate concentration. Data are presented as means ± standard deviations (n = 3).

Drug encapsulation efficiency
In this section, different polymer:drug ratio (W:W) ranged from 1:0.125 to 1:8 was considered as a variable factor for two selected formulations. The average percent of drug entrapment efficiency of different nanoparticulate formulations was shown in Figure 1.

The drug encapsulation efficiency in formulation No. 8 was greater than other formulations, significantly (p<0.05). This formulation with 1:0.5 polymer:drug ratio (W:W) was selected for further analysis.

Differential scanning calorimetric (DSC) analysis
Ionic gelation between CS and TPP for formation of nanoparticles (Figure 2) and establishing the presence of ciprofloxacin in the particles was analyzed through DSC (Figure 3). In the CS thermogram (Figure 2), a sharp endothermic peak at 152.2°C and an exothermic peak at 301.1°C were in accordance with the literature.[3] TPP showed endothermic peak at 139.6°C; while nanoparicles without any drugs (unloaded particles) had two endothermic peaks at 147.9°C and 216.5°C.

The physical state of the ciprofloxacin HCl inside the nanoparticles was also assessed by thermal analysis. According to the thermograms (Figure 3), ciprofloxacin HCl presented a broad endotherm centered at 160.4°C. In the DSC curves of drug-loaded nanoparticles, characteristic peaks of CS nanoparticles and ciprofloxacin HCl were joint together and seen.

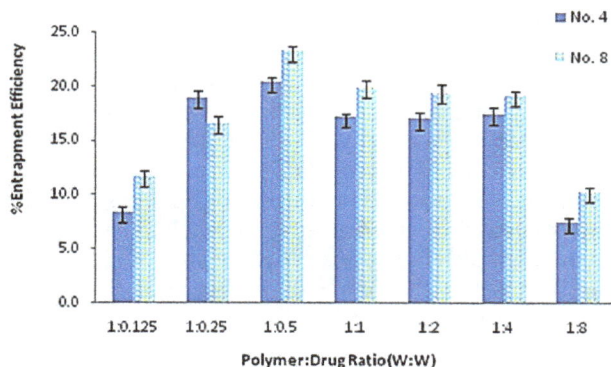

Figure 1. Average percent of drug entrapment efficiency of different nanoparticulate formulations. Data are presented as means ± standard deviations (n = 3).
(Formulation No. 4 has 0.3% chitosan and 0.3% tripolyphosphate, and the stirring speed was 9000rpm. Formulation No 8, has 0.45% chitosan and 0.45% tripolyphosphate, and the stirring speed was 6000rpm.)

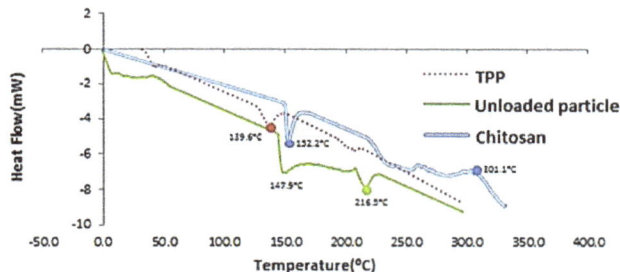

Figure 2. DSC thermogram of Chitosan, TPP (tripolyphosphate) and Unloaded particles.

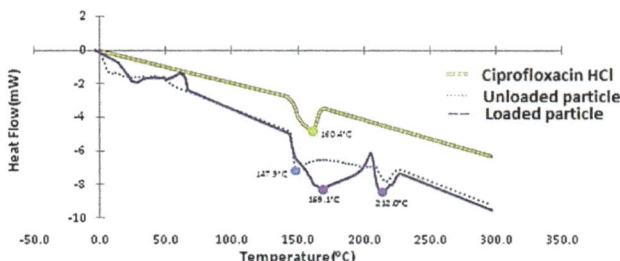

Figure 3. DSC thermogram of ciprofloxacin HCl, unloaded and loaded nanoparticles.

In vitro drug release studies

The release profile of ciprofloxacin HCl from ciprofloxacin-loaded CS nanoparticles at three different pH values were displayed in Figure 4. Released drug from CS nanoparticles was little and through 96 hours less than 12% of drug could be released. By decreasing the pH, the amount of released drug was decreased. The

release of free drug through dialysis membrane was also evaluated and 100% of drug was permeated after 1 hour (data was not shown).

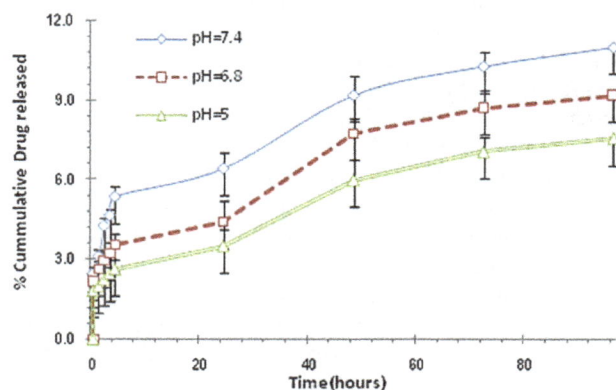

Figure 4. Ciprofloxacin HCl release profile from chitosan nanoparticles at three different pH values. Data are presented as means ± standard deviations (n = 3).

Determination of minimum inhibitory concentration (MIC)

The antibacterial activity of ciprofloxin HCl was compared with that of ciprofloxacin HCl loaded in CS nanoparticles against Gram-positive and Gram-negative bacteria. In both microorganism strains, the MIC value were decreased significantly (Student's t-test, P<0.05) by 50% when charged with ciprofloxacin HCl-loaded CS nanoparticles (80 ng/ml versus 40 ng/ml for $E.coli$ and 500 ng/ml versus 250 ng/ml for $S.aureus$). The MIC values of CS nanoparticles without any drug against $E.coli$ and $S.aureus$ were approximately 177 and 277 µg/ml, respectively.

Discussion

Chitosan is a natural mucoadhesive polymer with antibacterial activity. We prepared nanoparticles of chitosan by ionic gelation method containing ciprofloxacin to evaluate the possible changes in the potency of antibacterial agent. Preparation of ciprofloxacin loaded nanoparticles was performed in some studies, but the antibacterial activity of chitosan loaded ciprofloxacin was not reported elsewhere.[16,18-21] Various concentrations of CS and TPP were examined to get the lowest particle size. The particles prepared under optimal condition of 0.45% CS concentration, 0.45% TPP concentration and homogenizer rate at 6000 rpm had 72 nm diameter. In these particles with 1:0.5 mass ratio of CS to ciprofloxacin hydrochloride, the encapsulation efficiency was 23%. The average drug entrapment efficiency of the nanoparticulate formulations was found to be increased slightly with increasing the amount of drug in polymer:drug ratios (W:W) from 1:0.125 to 1:0.5 (Figure 1). It may be due to the more drugs available which reacted with polymer. In addition, formulation No.8 had more entrapment efficiency in comparison with formulation No.4. Regarding this, No.8 included more polymer concentration (0.45% versus 0.3%) to be reacted. By increasing the amount of drug in the polymer:drug ratio from 1:0.5 to 1:8, the average entrapment efficiency of the nanoparticles was decreased. It may be due to the saturation capacity of nanoparticles. The entrapment efficiency was not high enough in different formulations. The positive charge of both CS and ciprofloxacin HCl, and partial repulsion between them, may cause these observations. In the CS thermogram (Figure 2) a sharp endothermic peak at 152.2°C and an exothermic peak at 301.1°C were related to the melting of polymer and its decomposition, respectively. In analysis between CS, TPP and unloaded particles through DSC, as expected, after the formation of ionic complex between CS and TPP, the different phenomenon from parent materials against heat was received. Endothermic centered peak of ciprofloxacin HCl was also due to the drug melting point.

Molecular weight of chitosan and crosslinking degree in nanoparticles could affect the little released drug from CS nanoparticles (Figure 4). Decrement of released drug through decreasing pH was may be due to the greater ionic interaction of CS with TPP and increasing the crosslinking density of the polymer.

Enhancing the efficacy of antibacterial agents loaded into the polymeric nanoparticles is reported in the numerous studies. These findings are related to many factors, including: facilitated penetration of drug into the bacterial cells, better delivery of the drug to its site of action, and the higher stability of the encapsulated drug into the nanoparticles.[15,18,22] In this study the potency of ciprofloxacin HCl loaded into the CS nanoparticles against *E.coli* as a Gram-negative strain and *S.aureus* as a Gram-positive strain was increased by 50%. Usually Gram-negative bacteria are more resistant to antibiotics than Gram-positive bacteria because of the presence of especially cell wall in their structure. This certain structures limit the penetration of antibiotics to the bacterial cell.[23] Therefore, enhancing the potency of ciprofloxacin HCl especially against *E.coli* as a Gram-negative strain by using CS nanoparticles could be a promising result for clinical studies. Physicochemical properties of ciprofloxacin-loaded chitosan nanoparticles have important effects on the antibacterial activity of the loaded ciprofloxacin. Jeong et al reported that *in vitro* antibacterial activity of ciprofloxacin-encapsulated PLGA nanoparticles against *E.Coli* is relatively lower than free ciprofloxacin.[20] In our work, decreasing the MIC levels in both bacteria may be due to the increasing the penetration of drug by nanoparticles into the bacterial cell that inhibited the bacterial growth. Increasing the antibacterial activity of ciprofloxacin loaded in CS nanoparticles, could not be due to the antimicrobial effect of CS nanoparticles alone, because the CS nanoparticles have inhibitory effect at high concentrations. The MIC value of CS nanoparticles without any drug against Gram-negative strain was lower. The negative charge on the cell wall of the tested Gram-negative bacteria was higher than that on the tested Gram-positive bacteria, leading to more CS adsorbed and higher inhibitory effect against the Gram-negative bacteria.[4] Chung et al reported that chitosan has a stronger effect on the Gram-negative *E. coli* than on the Gram-positive *S. aureus* in terms of the leakage of enzymes.[24]

Conclusion

In summary, ciprofloxacin HCl-loaded chitosan nanoparticles have been prepared and characterized in the present study. The nanoparticles obtained in the present study had small particle size, which may increase the drug penetration into the bacterial cell and improve its antibacterial activity. The results showed that ciprofloxacin HCl-loaded chitosan nanoparticles could inhibit the growth of two strains of Gram-positive and Gram-negative microorganisms markedly. Their MIC values were 50% lower than MIC of free drug itself. It was anticipated that chitosan nanoparticles could be applied broadly as a carrier for antimicrobial agents in medicine for their biocompatibilities and also their antibacterial activity.

Acknowledgments

The authors acknowledge Doctor Alborzi Clinical Microbiological Research Center for providing strains of bacteria.

Ethical Issues

Not applicable.

Conflict of Interest

Authors state that there is no conflict of interest. Financial support of Shiraz university of Medical Sciences is appreciated.

References

1. Das S, Das MP, Das J. Fabrication of porous chitosan/silver nanocomposite film and its bactericidal efficacy against multi-drug resistant (MDR) clinical isolates. *J Pharm Res* 2013;6(1):11-5. doi: 10.1016/j.jopr.2012.11.006

2. Sanpui P, Murugadoss A, Prasad PV, Ghosh SS, Chattopadhyay A. The antibacterial properties of a novel chitosan-ag-nanoparticle composite. *Int J Food Microbiol* 2008;124(2):142-6. doi: 10.1016/j.ijfoodmicro.2008.03.004

3. Gomez-Burgaz M, Torrado G, Torrado S. Characterization and superficial transformations on mini-matrices made of interpolymer complexes of chitosan and carboxymethylcellulose during in vitro clarithromycin release. *Eur J Pharm Biopharm* 2009;73(1):130-9. doi: 10.1016/j.ejpb.2009.04.004

4. Kong M, Chen XG, Xing K, Park HJ. Antimicrobial properties of chitosan and mode of action: A state of the art review. *Int J Food Microbiol* 2010;144(1):51-63. doi: 10.1016/j.ijfoodmicro.2010.09.012

5. Cevher E, Orhan Z, Mulazimoglu L, Sensoy D, Alper M, Yildiz A, et al. Characterization of biodegradable chitosan microspheres containing vancomycin and

treatment of experimental osteomyelitis caused by methicillin-resistant staphylococcus aureus with prepared microspheres. *Int J Pharm* 2006;317(2):127-35. doi: 10.1016/j.ijpharm.2006.03.014

6. Krishna Rao KSV, Ramasubba Reddy P, Lee YI, Kim C. Synthesis and characterization of chitosan–PEG–Ag nanocomposites for antimicrobial application. *Carbohydr Polym* 2012;87(1):920-5. doi: 10.1016/j.carbpol.2011.07.028

7. Li LH, Deng JC, Deng HR, Liu ZL, Li XL. Preparation, characterization and antimicrobial activities of chitosan/Ag/ZnO blend films. *Chem Eng J* 2010;160(1):378-82. doi: 10.1016/j.cej.2010.03.051

8. Liu TY, Chen SY, Li JH, Liu DM. Study on drug release behaviour of CDHA/chitosan nanocomposites-effect of CDHA nanoparticles. *J control release* 2006;112(1):88-95. doi: 10.1016/j.jconrel.2006.01.017

9. Tiyaboonchai W, Limpeanchob N. Formulation and characterization of amphotericin b-chitosan-dextran sulfate nanoparticles. *Int J Pharm* 2007;329(1-2):142-9. doi: 10.1016/j.ijpharm.2006.08.013

10. Wei D, Sun W, Qian W, Ye Y, Ma X. The synthesis of chitosan-based silver nanoparticles and their antibacterial activity. *Carbohydr Res* 2009;344(17):2375-82. doi: 10.1016/j.carres.2009.09.001

11. Anitha A, Deepagan VG, Divya Rani VV, Menon D, Nair SV, Jayakumar R. Preparation, characterization, in vitro drug release and biological studies of curcumin loaded dextran sulphate–chitosan nanoparticles. *Carbohydr Polym* 2011;84(3):1158-64. doi: 10.1016/j.carbpol.2011.01.005

12. Xing K, Chen XG, Kong M, Liu CS, Cha DS, Park HJ. Effect of oleoyl-chitosan nanoparticles as a novel antibacterial dispersion system on viability, membrane permeability and cell morphology of Escherichia coli and Staphylococcus aureus. *Carbohydr Polym* 2009;76(1):17-22. doi: 10.1016/j.carbpol.2008.09.016

13. Chakraborty SP, Sahu SK, Pramanik P, Roy S. In vitro antimicrobial activity of nanoconjugated vancomycin against drug resistant staphylococcus aureus. *Int J Pharm* 2012;436(1-2):659-76. doi: 10.1016/j.ijpharm.2012.07.033

14. Sadeghi AM, Dorkoosh FA, Avadi MR, Saadat P, Rafiee-Tehrani M, Junginger HE. Preparation, characterization and antibacterial activities of chitosan, N-trimethyl chitosan (TMC) and N-diethylmethyl chitosan (DEMC) nanoparticles loaded with insulin using both the ionotropic gelation and polyelectrolyte complexation methods. *Int J Pharm*

2008;355(1-2):299-306. doi: 10.1016/j.ijpharm.2007.11.052

15. Azhdarzadeh M, Lotfipour F, Zakeri-Milani P, Mohammadi G, Valizadeh H. Anti-bacterial performance of azithromycin nanoparticles as colloidal drug delivery system against different gram-negative and gram-positive bacteria. *Adv Pharm Bull* 2012;2(1):17-24. doi: 10.5681/apb.2012.003

16. Jain D, Banerjee R. Comparison of ciprofloxacin hydrochloride-loaded protein, lipid, and chitosan nanoparticles for drug delivery. *J Biomed Mater Res B Appl Biomater* 2008;86(1):105-12. doi: 10.1002/jbm.b.30994

17. Wiarachai O, Thongchul N, Kiatkamjornwong S, Hoven VP. Surface-quaternized chitosan particles as an alternative and effective organic antibacterial material. *Colloids Surf B Biointerfaces* 2012;92:121-9. doi: 10.1016/j.colsurfb.2011.11.034

18. Fawaz F, Bonini F, Maugein J, Lagueny AM. Ciprofloxacin-loaded polyisobutylcyanoacrylate nanoparticles: Pharmacokinetics and in vitro antimicrobial activity. *Int J Pharm* 1998;168(2):255-9. doi: 10.1016/S0378-5173(98)00116-1

19. Fawaz F, Guyot M, Lagueny AM, Devissaguet JP. Ciproflexacin-loaded polyisobutylcyanoacrylate nanoparticles: Preparation and characterization. *Int J Pharm* 1997;154(2):191-203. doi: 10.1016/S0378-5173(97)00138-5

20. Jeong YI, Na HS, Seo DH, Kim DG, Lee HC, Jang MK, et al. Ciprofloxacin-encapsulated poly(dl-lactide-co-glycolide) nanoparticles and its antibacterial activity. *Int J Pharm* 2008;352(1-2):317-23. doi: 10.1016/j.ijpharm.2007.11.001

21. Page-Clisson ME, Pinto-Alphandary H, Ourevitch M, Andremont A, Couvreur P. Development of ciprofloxacin-loaded nanoparticles: Physicochemical study of the drug carrier. *J Control Release* 1998;56(1-3):23-32. doi: 10.1016/S0168-3659(98)00065-0

22. Huh AJ, Kwon YJ. "Nanoantibiotics": A new paradigm for treating infectious diseases using nanomaterials in the antibiotics resistant era. *J Control Release* 2011;156(2):128-45. doi: 10.1016/j.jconrel.2011.07.002

23. Lotfipour F, Nazemiyeh H, Fathi-Azad F, Garaei N, Arami S, Talat S, et al. Evaluation of antibacterial activities of some medicinal plants from north-west iran. *Iran J Basic Med Sci* 2008;11(2):80-5. doi: 10.22038/ijbms.2008.5200

24. Chung YC, Chen CY. Antibacterial characteristics and activity of acid-soluble chitosan. *Bioresour Technol* 2008;99(8):2806-14. doi: 10.1016/j.biortech.2007.06.044

6

Conditioned Medium of Wharton's Jelly Derived Stem Cells Can Enhance the Cartilage Specific Genes Expression by Chondrocytes in Monolayer and Mass Culture Systems

Maryam Hassan Famian[1], Soheila Montazer Saheb[2], Azadeh Montaseri[2]*

[1] *Department of molecular biology, Ahar Branch, Islamic Azad University, Ahar, Iran.*
[2] *Stem Cell Research Center, Tabriz University of Medical Sciences, Tabriz, Iran.*

Keywords:
· Osteoarthritis
· Mesenchymal stem cells
· Wharton's jelly
· Conditioned medium

Abstract

Purpose: Mesenchymal stem cells (MSCs) have been introduced for cell therapy strategies in osteoarthritis (OA). Despite of their capacity for differentiation into chondrocyte, there are some evidences about their life-threatening problem after transplantation. So, some researchers shifted on the application of stem cells conditioned medium. The goal of this study is to evaluate whether Wharton's jelly derived stem cell conditioned medium (WJSCs-CM) can enhance the gene expression profile by chondrocytes in monolayer and mass culture systems.

Methods: Conditioned medium was obtained from WJSCs at fourth passage. Isolated chondrocytes were plated at density of 1×10^6 for both monolayer and high density culture. Then cells in both groups were divided into control (received medium) and experiment group treated with WJ-CM for 3 and 6 days. Samples were prepared to evaluate gene expression profile of collagen II, aggrecan, cartilage oligomeric matrix protein (COMP) and sox-9 using real-time RT-PCR.

Results: After 3 days, Chondrocytes treated with WJSCs-CM expressed significantly higher level of genes compared to the control group in both culture systems. After 6 days, the expression of genes in monolayer cultivated chondrocytes was decreased but that of the mass culture were up-regulated significantly.

Conclusion: WJ-SCs-CM can increase the expression of cartilage-specific genes and can be introduced as a promoting factor for cartilage regeneration.

Introduction

Articular cartilage which covers the joint surfaces is a highly specialized type of connective tissue that predominantly composed of one cell type named chondrocytes scattered in a lattice of extracellular matrix (ECM). In normal cartilage, chondrocytes are responsible for control of constant degradation and re-synthesis of ECM components such as collagen II, aggrecan and cartilage oligomeric matrix protein (COMP).[1] Due to the lack of blood vessels, articular cartilage has limited capacity for self-repair and if its lesions left untreated, consequently progresses toOsteoarthritis (OA).[2] The orthopedic diseases such as Rheumatoid Arthritis (RA) and OA are the major causes of disability and affect about 250 million people worldwide.Osteoarthritis which is the most common form of rheumatoid arthritis, is an active pathological process characterized by ECM degradation that consequently results in joint stiffness, mobility restriction, subchondral bone sclerosis and finally disability.[3,4] The etiology of OA is unknown, but it can occur due to different factors such as aging, obesity, joint trauma and genetic susceptibility.[5] The metabolism of normal articular cartilage is maintained as a result of a delicate balance between synthesis and degradation of ECM components which is regulated by chondrocytes.[1] At the molecular level, onset of OA occurs due to impairment of this precisely controlled mechanism.[6] It has been proved that pro-inflammatory cytokines such as Interleukin-1β (IL-1β) and Tumor necrosis factor-α (TNF-α) which are secreted by synoviocytes and chondrocytes enhance the synthesis of matrix degrading enzymes such as matrix metaloproteinases (MMPs) resulting in collagen and proteoglycan loss.[7] On the other hand, in osteoarthritic cartilage, absence of anabolic growth factors such as TGF-β, BMPs and IGF-1 can make this tissue more susceptible to damage.[1,5] A great number of investigations explored the pivotal roles of these growth factors in acceleration of cartilage formation and integration.[1,8] TGF-β family members have vital function in cell proliferation, migration, control of ECM synthesis, degradation and also have a very important role in cartilage development.[9,10]

*Corresponding author: Azadeh Montaseri, Email: montaseria@tbzmed.ac.ir

Different investigations revealed that enhancement of cartilage repair in *in vivo* conditions, increased proteoglycan synthesis, stimulation of mesenchymal stem cell differentiation into chondrocytes and maintenance of differentiated state of these cells can be occurred in the presence of TGF-β superfamily members.[11,12] Another growth factor with anabolic effects in articular cartilage is insulin like growth factor-1 (IGF-1).[13] It promotes repair of cartilage defects, is able to strongly stimulate matrix synthesis and reverses the catabolic effects of pro-inflammatory cytokines through suppression of IKB-α kinase.[8,14] Recently, medical research focus shifted to the application of stem cells in order to reduce a number of debilitating diseases such as musculoskeletal disorders.[15] During last few years, interest in cell implantation strategies to restore the impaired cartilage has emerged. Autologous chondrocyte implantation (ACI) is the most common cell-based surgical method, but it has some disadvantages such as further injury to the healthy cartilage and *in vitro* dedifferentiation of chondrocytes which is occurred due to increasing the passage numbers required for obtaining sufficient cells for implantation.[16] Compared to the chondrocytes, Mesenchymal stem cells (MSCs) can be isolated and expanded easier with less donor morbidity, are available in large quantities and have the capacity to differentiate into chondrocytes.[17,18] Human umbilical cord (UC) is a rich source for MSCs with characteristics typical to the bone-marrow derived stem cells.[19] This postnatal tissue is easily accessible because normally discarded after birth, so it's a noncontroversial source for MSCs. The mucoid Wharton's jelly also known as intervascular UC tissue, composed of fibroblast-like cells recognized as multipotent MSCs capable to differentiate into chondrocytes in *in vitro* and *in vivo* conditions.[20,21] It has been reported that Wharton's jelly mesenchymal stem cells (WJ-MSCs) can up-regulated the synthesis of cartilage ECM molecules such as hyalorunic acid and glycosaminoglycans and also enhance the SOX-9, COMP, and type II collagen gene expression.[22] Despite the regenerative capacity of Mesenchymal stem cells, normally engrafted cells have poor differentiation and survival rates and it has been reported that administration of this cells for clinical application can induce the risk of cancer. So, it's necessary to find a solution for this hazardous and life-threatening problem.[23] Stem cells secrete a wide spectrum of elements such as trophic, anti-apoptotic and immunomodulatory factors into culture medium (CM) through paracrine activity,[4,23,24] so it seems that stem cell-CM may overcome the obstacles of using them alone.

Taken together, regarding to the presence of trophic factors in the CM of WJ-SCs and the role of them in promotion of cartilage metabolism, the goal of the present study is to investigate whether WJ-SCs-CM can promote the expression of cartilage specific genes such as collagen type II, SOX-9, COMP andaggrecan by chondrocytes.

Materials and Methods
Chondrocyte isolation and culture
Cartilage samples were taken from patients undergoing joint replacement surgery for femoral neck fractures. All patients gave written informed consent andthe institutional review board and medical ethics committee of Tabriz University of Medical Sciences approved the study protocol. For chondrocyte isolation, after 3 times washing with PBS, cartilage samples were cut into 1×1 mm thick pieces using sterile scalpel and then incubated in 1% pronase enzyme for 1 hour. In the next step, samples were incubated by collagenase type II (0.02% solved in medium) in a shaking water bath at $37^{\circ C}$ for 4-6 hours. The digested samples were centrifuged at 1500 rpm/5 min and obtained chondrocytes were seeded at 5×10^5 cells per T75 flasks and incubated at $37^{\circ C}/co_2$ 5%. The first medium change was performed after 24 hours and following medium changes were performed three times per week. After reaching about 70% confluency, cells were passaged.

Harvesting the mesenchymal stem cells from Wharton's jelly
Umbilical cord samples were obtained from women who underwent caesarean section (S/C). Written consent was obtained from all patients and institutional ethical review board of Tabriz University of Medical Sciences, Tabriz, Iran approved the study protocol. Samples were stored aseptically in cold PBS containing antibiotics and transported to the cell culture lab. After 3 times washing, umbilical cord samples inserted into 70% ethanol for 30 seconds and then cut into 2.5-3 cm long pieces and placed in a sterile dish. Then, using a scissor, cord pieces were incised longitudinally and vessels were dissociated. In the next step, delicate Wharton's jelly (WJ) tissue was separated from amniotic layer and later cut into small fragments (1×2 mm) using scalpel. Obtained WJ samples were placed in the T-25 culture flasks with Dulbeco's Modified Eagle Medium (DMEM)containing 20% fetal bovine serum (FBS) and penicillin/streptomycin (P/S) 1%. After about 14 days, stem cells started to crawl from explanted WJ tissues. It should be noted that such cells have been characterized as mesenchymal stem cells by identification of specific cell surface markers on these cells in studies performed by our coworkers.[25] When migrated cells filled about 70% of culture flask, subculture was performed using Trypsin/EDTA (0.05%).

Preparation of supernatant from Wharton's jelly derived stem cell
Fourth passage Wharton's jelly derived mesenchymal stem cells (WJSCs) were used for conditioned medium (supernatant) collection. After reaching about 70% confluency, the supernatant was discarded and the attached cells were washed with PBS. Then, serum-free DMEM was added and cells were incubated for 48 hours. Obtained conditioned medium was centrifuged at 1500 rpm for 5 min for removing any debries. The second centrifugation was done at 3000 rpm for 3 min

and samples were stored at -80°C till further use. Furthermore to compare the secretion of growth factors by WJ-SCs in different passages, cells at passage 1, 2 and 3 were also obtained as described.

Experimental design

Chondrocytes at third passage were used for this evaluation. To understand the effect of WJSC-CM on chondrocytes, cells were seeded at density of 1×10^6 and further divided into control group which received only DMEM culture medium (containing 0.05% FBS) or treated with WJSC-CM for 3 and 6 days. We also evaluated the probable effects of WJ-SCs-CM on chondrocytes cultured in mass culture condition. For this purpose, 1×10^6 millions of cells were centrifuged in 15 ml conical tubes to form cell pellet. Mass-cultivated chondrocytes were also divided into control and treated groups as described for monolayer cells. After this period, samples were prepared for evaluation of the expression of specific cartilage genes, including collagen type II, aggrecan, COMP and sox9 using Real-time PCR.

Enzyme – linked immunosorbent assay (ELISA) for measurement of TGF-β1 and IGF-1 in WJ-SCs-CM:

The concentration of TGF-β1 and IGF-1 in the supernatant of WJSCswas measured by ELISAusing Human TGF-β1 ELISA kit (BOSRER, cat. No: EK0513,CA) and Human IGF-BP-1 ELISA kit (BOSRER, cat. No: EK0382,CA).

According to the manufactur's instruction, samples and standards were incubated at 37°C for 90 min. after addition of biotinylated antibodies (60 min), samples were washed using 0.01 M PBS. In the next step, samples were incubated with Avidin-Biotin-Peroxidase complex, following by addition of TMB color developing agent in dark place for 25-30 min. Finally, absorbance was measured at 450 nm using a microplate reader (ELISA Reader, Tecan, CH-8708, Australia).

Real time RT-PCR

The genetic information for type IIcollagen, Sox-9, aggrecan and cartilage oligomeric matrix protein (COMP) in samples of both control and CM-treated groups was detected by Real-time reverse transcriptase polymerase chain reaction (Real time RT-PCR). Total cellular RNA was extracted using YTA mini kit (Cat.NO: YT9065, Taiwan) according to the manufacture's protocol. Briefly, after centrifugation and supernatant removal, RB Buffer was added to the cell pellet to lyse the cells. Then sample mixture was transferred to the collection tube containing filter column and centrifuged at 14000 rpm/2 min. In the next step, samples were mixed with 70% ethanol. RB mini column was washed at first with wash buffer 1 and subsequently with wash buffer 2. Finally, RNase–free ddH$_2$O was added to the samples and centrifugation at 14000 rpm/2 min was performed to elute RNA. Approximately 1000ng/1 ml of total RNA was used as template for cDNA synthesis using reverse transcription kit (Takara,

RR037I, Japan). The Real time RT-PCR reactions were performed using a (Corbett, 010755, Australia) system with a SYBR Green master mix (Takara, RR820L, Japan) under the condition of 15s at 95°C and different time and annealing temperature for each gene as can be found in Table 1. The primer sequences used for this investigation are also listed in Table 1. The gene expression levels were calculated using Pfaffl formula and β-actin used as internal control. All experiments were done in triplicate.

Table 1. Primer sequences used in Real Time RT-PCR and related annealing temperature.

gene	primer	Annealing temperature
Sox9-F	AGAGAGGACCAACCAGAATTC	57°c for 30 sec
Sox9-R	TGGGTAATGCGCTTGGATAG	57°c for 30 sec
Coll2-F	GGCAATAGCAGGTTCACGTACA	59°c for 30 sec
Coll2-R	CGATAACAGTCTTGCCCCACTT	59°c for 30 sec
Comp-F	TGCAATGACACCATCCCAG	56°c for 30 sec
Comp-R	ACACACACTTTATTTTGTCCTCTC	56°c for 30 sec
ACAN-F	CAACTACCCGGCCATCC	56°c for 30 sec
ACAN- R	GATGGCTCTGTAATGGAACAC	56°c for 30 sec
B actin-F	TCCTCCCTG GAG AAG AGC TA	58°c for 45 sec
B actin-R	TCA GGAGGA GCA ATG ATC TTG	58°c for 45 sec

Statistical analysis

All data are reported as means ± SD. Statistical difference between two groups was determined by Two-way ANOVA and followed by t-test post test. P<0.05 was set as significant.

Results

Enhancement of TGF-β and IGF-1 secretion by increased number of WJ-SCs passages

WJSCs at 4 different cell passages cultured in DMEM medium lacking supplemental serum for 48 hours, then after the amount of TGF-β and IGF-1 were measured. As it can be found from Figure 1 (A and B), by increasing the cell passage number, the level of these growth factors secreted by WJSCs enhanced. There is a significant increase in TGF-β and also IGF-1 concentration between WJSCs at third and fourth passage when compared to the first passage of cells, with P-value of less than 0.001 and 0.0001, respectively.

Effect of WJSCs on chondrocyte gene expression

The mRNA expression level of cartilage-specific genes including collagen type II, Sox-9, Aggrecan and COMP was assessed in monolayer and mass-cultured chondrocytes treated with WJ-SCs-CM for 3 and 6 days. As it has been revealed in Figure 2 (A-D) the expression of all of the above mentioned genes was up-regulated significantly in monolayer chondrocytes after 3 days compared to the control (P<0.00001).There is no significant difference between treated and control chondrocytes in monolayer after 6 days of culture period in the expression of collagen II, aggrecan (ACAN) and COMP genes but that of SOX-9 up-regulated on 6 days

of culture period, too (P<0.001) as can be observed in Figure 2 (A).

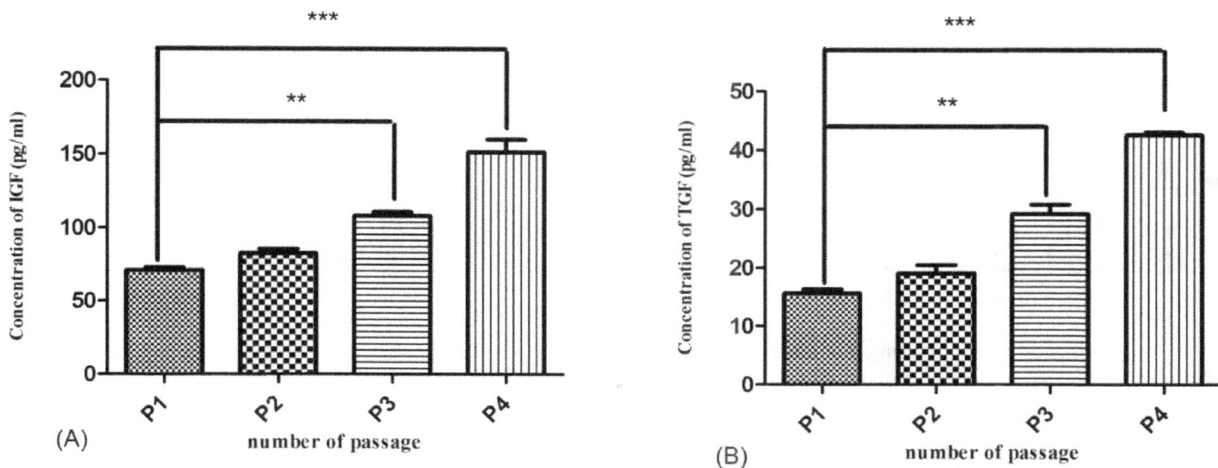

Figure 1. Measurement of IGF-1 (A) and TGF-β (B) secretion by WJ-SCs in different cell passages. **P<0.001, ***P<0.0001

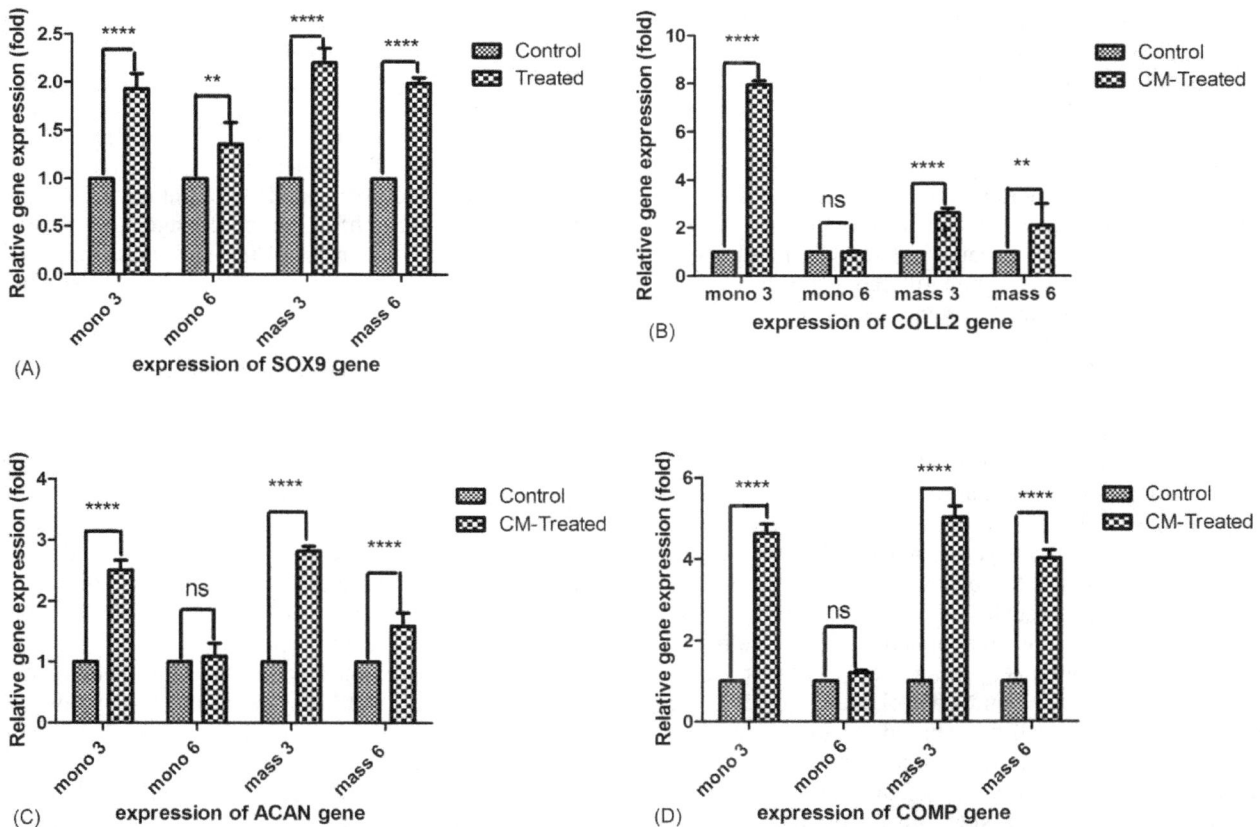

Figure 2. Comparison of cartilage specific gene expression in monolayer and mass cultured chondrocytes on 3 and 6 days. A) Sox-9, B) Collagen type II, C) Aggrecan and D) COMP. Ns: non-significant, **P<0.001, ****P<0.00001

In mass cultivated chondrocytes, the expression of Sox-9, Collagen II, aggrecan and COMP genes was enhanced significantly in chondrocytes treated with WJ-SCs-CM compared to the control cells on both time points as can be found from Figure 2 (A-D).

On the third day of the experiment, as it can be understood from Figure 3 (A) there is no significant difference in expression of Sox-9, aggrecan and COMP in monolayer and mass cultured chondrocytes treated with WJ-SCs-CM, but that of the Collagen type II was significantly increased in monolayer cells in comparison to the mass culture (P<0.00001). After 6 days of culture periodas described in Figure 3 (B)the expression level of

these genes increased significantly in mass cultured chondrocytes treated with WJ-SCs-CM compared to the treated chondrocytes in monolayer culture.

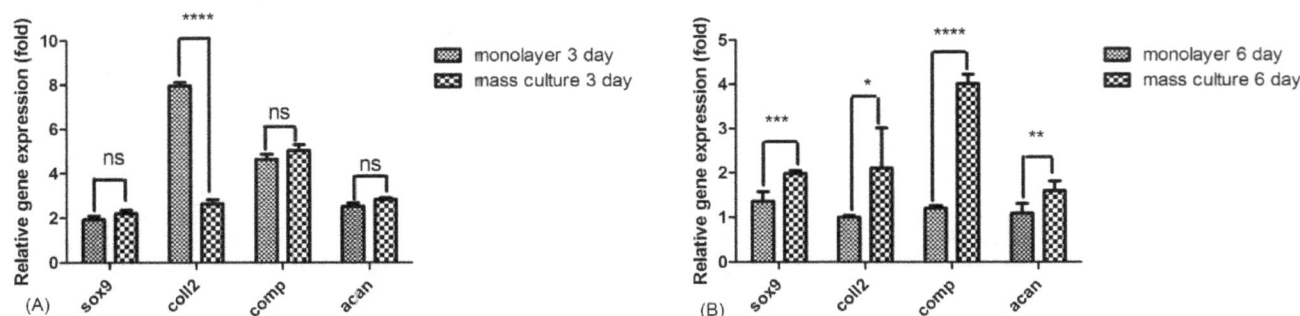

Figure 3. The analysis of the expression of cartilage-specific genes in the chondrocytes cultured in monolayer and mass culture on A) 3 days and B) 6 days of culture period. Ns: non-significant, *p<0.01, **p<0.001, ***p<0.0001 and ****p<0.00001

Discussion

In this study we found that exposure of chondrocytes to the WJ-SCs conditioned medium resulted in up-regulation of cartilage specific genes such as aggrecan, COMP, SOX-9 and Collagen type II in both monolayer and mass culture systems on the third day of culture period, but after 6 days, the expression of these genes up-regulated only in mass culture chondrocytes.

Osteoarthritis is the major cause of disability in the elderly that occurs mostly due to an imbalancebetween synthesis and degradation of cartilage ECM.[26] Strategies for application of mesenchymal stem cells (MSCs) as a feasible cell-based therapy are being investigated for regenerative medicine.[27] MSCs can be obtained from various sources and because of their chondrogenic potential, considered as a hopeful candidate in cartilage regenerative medicine.[28] Stem cells derived from umbilical cord Wharton's jelly show high proliferative capacity, can differentiate into the three germ lineages, are available in large numbers and have prolonged stemness characteristic.[29,30] These advantages combined with their non-controversial nature and non-tumorogenicity make them attractive cell source for cell-based therapy.[15] The exact mechanism by which WJ-SCs exert their function isn't yet completely known but they can affect the other cell's behavior through secretion of specific molecules such as cytokines and growth factors.[27,30] For the clinical application of stem cells, it is necessary to produce these cells under good manufacturing practice and control their biosafety and purity.[27] Recently cell-free based therapy has been introduced to overcome these limitations.

In this study we investigated whether WJ-SCs-CM can enhance the gene expression profile by chondrocytes. The results of this study demonstrate that WJ-SCs-CM can promote the expression of aggrecan, COMP, Collagen type II and SOX-9 in both time points after 3 days.

The master transcription SRY-BOX 9 (SOX-9) which is expressed in chondroprogenitors and mature chondrocytes, is an essential factor for chondrocyte

differentiation.[31,32] SOX-9 regulates the synthesis of cartilage ECM components such as collagen type II and aggrecan and also suppresses the chondrocyte hypertrophy.[32,33] In this study we showed that in the presence of WJ-SCs-CM the expression of sox-9 gene can be up-regulated. The increased expression of sox-9 can explain the up-regulation of other ECM components genes by chondrocytes treated with WJ-SCs-CM.

In this study we also found that treatment of chondrocytes with conditioned medium of WJ-SCs increased the expression of collagen type II gene as an essential element of articular cartilage, on the third day of culture in monolayer chondrocyte but not at the 6 days of culture period. This type of collagen gives tensile strength and provides most of the mechanical properties of cartilage tissue.[21,34] Decreased level of collagen type II by chondrocytes in monolayer condition after 6 days can be contributed to the loss of phenotype of this cells by increasing the time. Cartilage Oligomeric Matrix Protein (COMP) is a non-collagenous protein found in territorial matrix surrounding the chondrocytes and regulates the collagen network in cartilage tissue.[35] Another component of articular cartilage ECM is aggrecan that donates resilience and flexibility to this tissue. During OA process the ECM molecules are degraded enzymatically, so the restoration and repair of articular cartilage requires the re-construction of ECM by synthesis of these macromolecules.[36]

As it has been previously described, the metabolism of normal articular cartilage is regulated by different anabolic growth factors[8] and decrease in these stimuli will disrupt the cartilage integrity.[1] An example for these anabolic stimuli is TGF- β which is expressed in high levels in normal cartilage tissue and have an important role in maintaining the chondrocyte phenotype, ECM synthesis and enhancing the biochemical composition of articular cartilage.[5,37] IGF-1 is another major factor involved in modulating the collagen network, increasing the proteoglycan and collagen synthesis and inhibiting the matrix degradation rate of cartilage tissue.[38,39] In this study we found that the anabolic growth factors including TGF-β and IGF-1 were secreted into the supernatant of WJ-SCs after 48hr of serum starvation and the increased expression of cartilage-specific genes by chondrocytes can be contributed to these factors. Serum deprivation stimulates MSCs for secretion of different factors that are necessary for cell survival and antagonization of toxic condition so it can promote the effectiveness of MSC-CM through higher amount of trophic factors secreted by these cells.[24] As a consequent, application of conditioned medium can bring the paracrine secretion of stem cells without considerations of immune system responses or tumor formation of stem cell transplantation.[23,40]

It has been widely accepted that chondrocyte phenotype is lost during long *in vitro* monolayer culture so culturing of chondrocytes in 3D condition is suggested to support the re-differentiation of these cells.[41] In this study we also used the mass culture of chondrocytes in which the cell-cell and cell-matrix interactions can be established better and then we treated them with WJ-SCs-CM as in monolayer group. It has been revealed for us that the cultivated chondrocytes in mass culture can express SOX-9, Collagen II, aggrecan and COMP in significantly higher amount compared to the monolayer condition. So, the high-density (mass) culture system employed in this study seems to be a prosperous method for retention of chondrocyte phenotype compared to the monolayer culture.

During the process of chondrogenesis, condensation of chondrogenic cells provides a strong cell-cell contact that can be mimicked using mass culture technique.[42] Furthermore the expression of SOX-9 by highly packed chondroprogenitor cells enhance during this phase of chondrogenesis that eventually results in the regulation of cartilage specific matrix components such as collagen II and aggrecan.[43] In line with these data, our study also reported that the expression of chondrocyte genes was significantly higher in mass cultivated cells compared to the monolayer condition when treated with WJ-SCs-CM.

Conclusion

The results presented in this investigation suggest that WS-SCs conditioned medium is a potent, safe and relatively cost-benefit medium for enhancing the expression of cartilage specific genes in both monolayer and mass culture system. Findings of this study also revealed that the expression of genes by WJ-SCs-CM treated chondrocytes in mass culture condition is stronger when compared to the treated monolayer cells.

Acknowledgments

This article is resulted from the research proposal leading to thesis of Maryam Hassan Famian, M.Sc student of genetics and approved by Stem Cell Research center, Tabriz University of Medical sciences, Tabriz, Iran. The authors gratefully acknowledge the research deputy of Tabriz Universityof Medical Sciences for financial support.

Ethical Issues

Not applicable.

Conflict of Interest

The authors declare no conflict of interests.

References

1. Blaney Davidson EN, van der Kraan PM, van den Berg WB. Tgf-beta and osteoarthritis. *Osteoarthritis Cartilage* 2007;15(6):597-604. doi: 10.1016/j.joca.2007.02.005

2. Mobasheri A, Batt M. An update on the pathophysiology of osteoarthritis. *Ann Phys Rehabil Med* 2016;59(5-6):333-9. doi: 10.1016/j.rehab.2016.07.004

3. Hunter DJ, Nevitt M, Losina E, Kraus V. Biomarkers for osteoarthritis: Current position and steps towards further validation. *Best Pract Res Clin Rheumatol* 2014;28(1):61-71. doi: 10.1016/j.berh.2014.01.007

4. Mamidi MK, Das AK, Zakaria Z, Bhonde R. Mesenchymal stromal cells for cartilage repair in osteoarthritis. *Osteoarthritis Cartilage* 2016;24(8):1307-16. doi: 10.1016/j.joca.2016.03.003

5. Mazor M, Lespessailles E, Coursier R, Daniellou R, Best TM, Toumi H. Mesenchymal stem-cell potential in cartilage repair: An update. *J Cell Mol Med* 2014;18(12):2340-50. doi: 10.1111/jcmm.12378

6. Lorenz H, Richter W. Osteoarthritis: Cellular and molecular changes in degenerating cartilage. *Prog Histochem Cytochem* 2006;40(3):135-63. doi: 10.1016/j.proghi.2006.02.003

7. Sandell LJ, Aigner T. Articular cartilage and changes in arthritis. An introduction: Cell biology of osteoarthritis. *Arthritis Res* 2001;3(2):107-13. doi: 10.1186/ar148

8. Montaseri A, Busch F, Mobasheri A, Buhrmann C, Aldinger C, Rad JS, et al. Igf-1 and pdgf-bb suppress il-1β-induced cartilage degradation through down-regulation of nf-κb signaling: Involvement of src/pi-3k/akt pathway. *PloS One* 2011;6(12):e28663. doi: 10.1371/journal.pone.0028663

9. Cals FL, Hellingman CA, Koevoet W, Baatenburg de Jong RJ, van Osch GJ. Effects of transforming growth factor-beta subtypes on in vitro cartilage production and mineralization of human bone marrow stromal-derived mesenchymal stem cells. *J Tissue Eng Regen Med* 2012;6(1):68-76. doi: 10.1002/term.399

10. Horbelt D, Denkis A, Knaus P. A portrait of transforming growth factor beta superfamily signalling: Background matters. *Int J Biochem Cell Biol* 2012;44(3):469-74. doi: 10.1016/j.biocel.2011.12.013

11. Fortier LA, Barker JU, Strauss EJ, McCarrel TM, Cole BJ. The role of growth factors in cartilage repair. *Clin Orthop Relat Res* 2011;469(10):2706-15. doi: 10.1007/s11999-011-1857-3

12. Freyria AM, Mallein-Gerin F. Chondrocytes or adult stem cells for cartilage repair: The indisputable role

of growth factors. *Injury* 2012;43(3):259-65. doi: 10.1016/j.injury.2011.05.035

13. Zhang Z, Li L, Yang W, Cao Y, Shi Y, Li X, et al. The effects of different doses of IGF-1 on cartilage and subchondral bone during the repair of full-thickness articular cartilage defects in rabbits. *Osteoarthritis Cartilage* 2017;25(2):309-20. doi: 10.1016/j.joca.2016.09.010

14. Morales TI. The quantitative and functional relation between insulin-like growth factor-I (IGF) and IGF-binding proteins during human osteoarthritis. *J Orthop Res* 2008;26(4):465-74. doi: 10.1002/jor.20549

15. Watson N, Divers R, Kedar R, Mehindru A, Mehindru A, Borlongan MC, et al. Discarded wharton jelly of the human umbilical cord: A viable source for mesenchymal stromal cells. *Cytotherapy* 2015;17(1):18-24. doi: 10.1016/j.jcyt.2014.08.009

16. Moreira-Teixeira L, Georgi N, Leijten J, Wu L, Karperien M. Cartilage tissue engineering. Cartilage and bone development and its disorders. Karger Publishers; 2011. P. 102-15.

17. Loeser RF, Goldring SR, Scanzello CR, Goldring MB. Osteoarthritis: A disease of the joint as an organ. *Arthritis Rheum* 2012;64(6):1697-707. doi: 10.1002/art.34453

18. Haleem AM, Chu CR. Advances in tissue engineering techniques for articular cartilage repair. *Oper Tech Orthop* 2010;20(2):76-89. doi: 10.1053/j.oto.2009.10.004

19. Arufe MC, De la Fuente A, Mateos J, Fuentes I, De Toro FJ, Blanco FJ. Analysis of the chondrogenic potential and secretome of mesenchymal stem cells derived from human umbilical cord stroma. *Stem Cells Dev* 2011;20(7):1199-212. doi: 10.1089/scd.2010.0315

20. La Rocca G, Lo Iacono M, Corsello T, Corrao S, Farina F, Anzalone R. Human wharton's jelly mesenchymal stem cells maintain the expression of key immunomodulatory molecules when subjected to osteogenic, adipogenic and chondrogenic differentiation in vitro: New perspectives for cellular therapy. *Curr Stem Cell Res Ther* 2013;8(1):100-13. doi: 10.2174/1574888X11308010012

21. Lo Iacono M, Anzalone R, Corrao S, Giuffrè M, Di Stefano A, Giannuzzi P, et al. Perinatal and wharton's jelly-derived mesenchymal stem cells in cartilage regenerative medicine and tissue engineering strategies. *Open Tissue Eng Regen Med J* 2011;4(1):72-81. doi: 10.2174/1875043501104010072

22. Fong CY, Gauthaman K, Cheyyatraivendran S, Lin HD, Biswas A, Bongso A. Human umbilical cord wharton's jelly stem cells and its conditioned medium support hematopoietic stem cell expansion ex vivo. *J Cell Biochem* 2012;113(2):658-68. doi: 10.1002/jcb.23395

23. Kwon SH, Bhang SH, Jang HK, Rhim T, Kim BS. Conditioned medium of adipose-derived stromal cell

culture in three-dimensional bioreactors for enhanced wound healing. *J Surg Res* 2015;194(1):8-17. doi: 10.1016/j.jss.2014.10.053

24. Ando Y, Matsubara K, Ishikawa J, Fujio M, Shohara R, Hibi H, et al. Stem cell-conditioned medium accelerates distraction osteogenesis through multiple regenerative mechanisms. *Bone* 2014;61:82-90. doi: 10.1016/j.bone.2013.12.029

25. Maleki M, Ghanbarvand F, Behvarz MR, Ejtemaei M, Ghadirkhomi E. Comparison of mesenchymal stem cell markers in multiple human adult stem cells. *Int J Stem Cells* 2014;7(2):118-26. doi: 10.15283/ijsc.2014.7.2.118

26. Platas J, Guillén MI, del Caz MD, Gomar F, Mirabet V, Alcaraz MJ. Conditioned media from adipose-tissue-derived mesenchymal stem cells downregulate degradative mediators induced by interleukin-1beta in osteoarthritic chondrocytes. *Mediators Inflamm* 2013;2013:357014. doi: 10.1155/2013/357014

27. Manferdini C, Maumus M, Gabusi E, Paolella F, Grassi F, Jorgensen C, et al. Lack of anti-inflammatory and anti-catabolic effects on basal inflamed osteoarthritic chondrocytes or synoviocytes by adipose stem cell-conditioned medium. *Osteoarthritis Cartilage* 2015;23(11):2045-57. doi: 10.1016/j.joca.2015.03.025

28. Van Buul GM, Villafuertes E, Bos PK, Waarsing JH, Kops N, Narcisi R, et al. Mesenchymal stem cells secrete factors that inhibit inflammatory processes in short-term osteoarthritic synovium and cartilage explant culture. *Osteoarthritis Cartilage* 2012;20(10):1186-96. doi: 10.1016/j.joca.2012.06.003

29. Fong CY, Tam K, Cheyyatraivendran S, Gan SU, Gauthaman K, Armugam A, et al. Human wharton's jelly stem cells and its conditioned medium enhance healing of excisional and diabetic wounds. *J Cell Biochem* 2014;115(2):290-302. doi: 10.1002/jcb.24661

30. Lin HD, Fong CY, Biswas A, Choolani M, Bongso A. Human umbilical cord wharton's jelly stem cell conditioned medium induces tumoricidal effects on lymphoma cells through hydrogen peroxide mediation. *J Cell Biochem* 2016;117(9):2045-55. doi: 10.1002/jcb.25501

31. Akiyama H, Chaboissier MC, Martin JF, Schedl A, de Crombrugghe B. The transcription factor sox9 has essential roles in successive steps of the chondrocyte differentiation pathway and is required for expression of sox5 and sox6. *Genes Dev* 2002;16(21):2813-28. doi: 10.1101/gad.1017802

32. Kondo M, Yamaoka K, Tanaka Y. Acquiring chondrocyte phenotype from human mesenchymal stem cells under inflammatory conditions. *Int J Mol Sci* 2014;15(11):21270-85. doi: 10.3390/ijms151121270

33. Im GI. Regeneration of articular cartilage using adipose stem cells. *J Biomed Mater Res A* 2016;104(7):1830-44. doi: 10.1002/jbm.a.35705

34. Shafaei H, Baghernezhad H. Ultrasound effect on gene expression of sex determining region y-box 9 (sox9) and transforming growth factor β isoforms in adipose stem cells. *Zahedan J Res Med Sci* 2016;18(4):e6465. doi: 10.17795/zjrms-6465

35. Zivanović S, Rackov LP, Zivanović A, Jevtić M, Nikolić S, Kocić S. Cartilage oligomeric matrix protein - inflammation biomarker in knee osteoarthritis. *Bosn J Basic Med Sci* 2011;11(1):27-32.

36. Hemshekhar M, Thushara RM, Kumar SKN, Basappa B, Kemparaju K, Girish KS. Role of cartilage degrading enzymes and their end products in the pathogenesis of inflammatory arthritis. *Inflamm Cell Signal* 2014;1(3):e341. doi: 10.14800/ics.341

37. Makris EA, Gomoll AH, Malizos KN, Hu JC, Athanasiou KA. Repair and tissue engineering techniques for articular cartilage. *Nat Rev Rheumatol* 2015;11(1):21-34. doi: 10.1038/nrrheum.2014.157

38. Mobasheri A, Kalamegam G, Musumeci G, Batt ME. Chondrocyte and mesenchymal stem cell-based therapies for cartilage repair in osteoarthritis and related orthopaedic conditions. *Maturitas* 2014;78(3):188-98. doi: 10.1016/j.maturitas.2014.04.017

39. Davies LC, Blain EJ, Gilbert SJ, Caterson B, Duance VC. The potential of IGF-1 and TGFβ1 for promoting "adult" articular cartilage repair: An in vitro study. *Tissue Eng Part A* 2008;14(7):1251-61. doi: 10.1089/ten.tea.2007.0211

40. Fukuoka H, Suga H, Narita K, Watanabe R, Shintani S. The latest advance in hair regeneration therapy using proteins secreted by adipose-derived stem cells. *Am J Cosmet Surg* 2012;29(4):273-82.

41. Shi Y, Ma J, Zhang X, Li H, Jiang L, Qin J. Hypoxia combined with spheroid culture improves cartilage specific function in chondrocytes. *Integr Biol (Camb)* 2015;7(3):289-97. doi: 10.1039/c4ib00273c

42. Shakibaei M, Seifarth C, John T, Rahmanzadeh M, Mobasheri A. IGF-I extends the chondrogenic potential of human articular chondrocytes in vitro: Molecular association between Sox9 and Erk1/2. *Biochem Pharmacol* 2006;72(11):1382-95. doi: 10.1016/j.bcp.2006.08.022

43. Aigner T, Gebhard PM, Schmid E, Bau B, Harley V, Pöschl E. SOX9 expression does not correlate with type II collagen expression in adult articular chondrocytes. *Matrix Biol* 2003;22(4):363-72. doi: 10.1016/S0945-053X(03)00049-0

7

Development of Nanoemulsion Based Gel Loaded with Phytoconstituents for the Treatment of Urinary Tract Infection and *in Vivo* Biodistribution Studies

Atinderpal Kaur[1], Sonal Gupta[1], Amit Tyagi[2], Rakesh Kumar Sharma[3], Javed Ali[4], Reema Gabrani[1], Shweta Dang[1]*

[1]*Department of Biotechnology, Jaypee Institute of Information Tehnology, A-10, Sector 62, Noida, UP 201307, India.*
[2]*Department of Nuclear Medicine, Institute of Nuclear Medicine and Allied Sciences, Brig SK Mazumdar Marg, Delhi, 110054, India.*
[3]*Division of CBRN Defence, Institute of Nuclear Medicine and Allied Sciences, Brig SK Mazumdar Marg, Delhi, 110054, India.*
[4]*Faculty of Pharmacy, Jamia Hamdard, Hamdard Nagar, New Delhi, 110062, India.*

Keywords:
· Cranberry
· Gamma scintigraphy
· Intravaginal drug delivery
· Polyphenon 60
· Radiolabelling
· Urinary tract infection

Abstract

Purpose: A nanoemulsion based gel containing Polyphenon 60 (P60) and cranberry (CRB) has been developed to deliver via intravaginal route for the treatment of urinary tract infection.

Methods: Polyphenon 60 and cranberry were loaded in a single nanoemulsion gel (NBG) by ultra-sonication method and characterized for particle size, rheological properties, in vitro release and growth curve analysis. P60+CRB NBG were radiolabelled using technetium pertechnetate (^{99m}Tc) to perform *in vivo* pharmacokinetic studies in animals.

Results: The finalized NE had a droplet size of 58±1 nm. *In vitro* release of 90.92 ± 0.6% in 8 hr for P60 and 99.39 ± 0.5% in 6 hr for CRB was observed in simulated vaginal fluid. Growth curve of *E. coli* indicated the inhibitory action of nanoemulsion based gel at the fifth hour of inoculation. Gamma scintigraphy studies on female Sprague-Dawley rats showed transport of nanoemulsion based gel from the vaginal cavity into the systemic circulation. Further, biodistribution studies with radiolabelled P60+CRB NBG showed significant higher uptake of radiolabelled actives by kidney (3.20±0.16) and urinary bladder (3.64±0.29), when administered intravaginally.

Conclusion: The findings suggested ^{99m}Tc-P60+CRB NBG can potentially be transported through vaginal cavity and reach the target organs and showed effective distribution in organs affected in urinary tract infection

Introduction

Urinary tract infection (UTI) is the most common type of infection occurring amongst women caused by *E. coli*. Antibiotic therapy is used as a standard treatment for UTI, however rising rates of reoccurrence and resistance to antibiotics has led to consideration of natural plant products as alternative treatment.[1] Cranberry (CRB), *Vaccinium macrocarpon*, is well known for its use in urinary tract infection (UTI) for many years.[2] CRB is particularly known to exert anti-adhesive effect against P-fimbriated bacteria by releasing certain adhesion factors that do not allow bacteria to adhere on the surface.[3] Green tea catechins (GTCs) are also known to exhibit a range of pharmacological and biological effects like anti-microbial,[4] anti-inflammatory and many more.[5,6] Most of the polyphenols present in green tea are flavanols that can be categorised as catechins[7] and are accountable for anti-microbial activity.[4] GTCs are reported to exert antibacterial action by binding to the outer cell membrane and cause cell leakage leading to ultimate cell lysis/death.[8] However, gram negative bacteria are less susceptible to GTCs due to the presence of an additional lipopolysaccharide layer over their cell membrane.[9]

The combination therapy has been investigated to prevent emergence of resistant strains and to lower down the concentration of individual agents thus minimizing the likelihood of dose-related toxicity.[10] The therapeutic efficacy of natural compounds can be improved by their incorporation in suitable delivery systems. With advances in the field of nano medicine, nanotechnology based formulations are being explored for intravaginal delivery. Nanoemulsions (NEs) have shown to enhance the solubility, evade the enzymatic attack and thus increase the bioavailability and prolong the shelf life by protection against oxidation and hydrolysis.[11] NEs serve as a versatile carrier for drug delivery owing to their lipophillic, hydrophilic and amphiphillic phases.[12] Vaginal formulations for local delivery have been reported.[13] However, the aspect of systemic delivery via vaginal route has not been reported widely; fate and stability of active agents crossing the vaginal mucosa being a major concern. Prolonged residence time of vaginal formulation inside the cavity is desired because of leakage and redistribution of vaginal fluids within the cavity.[13] For systemic delivery, it is of prime

*Corresponding author: Shweta Dang, Email: shweta.dang@jiit.ac.in

importance that formulations either adhere for considerable time or cross the vaginal lining as soon as possible as it is instilled in the vaginal cavity. To overcome these limitations, a chitosan based muco-adhesive polymeric gel of NE was prepared hypothesizing increased drug contact time with infected tissue and improved therapy.[14] Chitosan is a bio-polymer that exhibits good biodegradability, low toxicity and bio-adhesiveness which makes it an appropriate agent to be used in drug delivery systems.[15]

The aim of the present work was to prepare nanoemulsion based gel formulation for GTCs and cranberry powder for intravaginal delivery. A comparative oral vs intravaginal study was planned to study the path and biodistribution of P60+CRB NBG by radiolabelling it with ^{99m}Tc on female Sprague-Dawley rats.

Materials and Methods

Polyphenon 60 or green tea catechins (GTCs) and reagent grade Tween 20 was obtained from Sigma Aldrich (Bangalore, India). Cranberry powder was generously gifted by Naturex, DBS, New Jersey (U.S.A). Oleic acid and glycerol was a product of CDH (P) Ltd, India. Water used was Milli-Q (Millipore, USA).

Animal Preparation

Female Sprague Dawley rats (aged 3-4 months) weighing 180-200 g was obtained from the Central Animal House Facility of INMAS, Delhi, India. Rats were kept at normal room temperature of $25 \pm 5°C$.

Formulation of Polyphenon 60 and Cranberry nanoemulsion

The solubility of polyphenon 60 and cranberry were checked in different oils, surfactants and co-surfactants. The nanoemulsion was prepared by dissolving cranberry in oleic acid as oil phase, tween 20 as surfactant and glycerol as a co-surfactant. P60 was dissolved in milli-Q water to prepare aqueous phase and added drop wise to the oil phase with continuous stirring to form pre emulsion. This pre-emulsion was subjected to high shear homogenization using Tissue Master 125 homogenizer (Omni International, Georgia) at 10,000 rpm for 20 min under ice bath and further subjected to high energy ultra-sonication via Bench Top Ultrasonicator (Model UP400S, 24 KHz 400 W, Hielcher, Ultrasound Technology, Germany) at amplitude of 70% for 286 sec at 0.3s ON and 0.7s OFF cycles. The prepared nanoemulsion was characterized for particle size and zeta potential determination using Malvern Zetasizer (Malvern, Worcestershire, UK). Before determining particle size and zeta potential, the nanoemulsion was diluted with HPLC water at ratio of 1:50 v/v.

Development and characterization of Nanoemulsion based gel

Preparation of Nanoemulsion based Gel

Different concentrations of Chitosan (1%) were mixed in lactic acid (1%) because it provides simulated vaginal medium pH for chitosan to dissolve easily at vaginal pH,[15] and kept overnight to ensure complete hydration and was

then added to NE formulation with continuous mixing using a magnetic stirrer until a homogeneous dispersion was achieved.

Rheological characterization of gels

Chitosan gels were first evaluated in terms of pH and phase separation/turbidity to identify the most suitable gel for vaginal application. pH values were measured by pH meter (Thermo Orion 420A+ Basic pH meter) after dilution of the gel formulation in ultrapure water (1:10, w/v). Formulations were then subjected to rheological characterization by using Modular Compact Rheometer MCR302 (Anton Paar, Austria). The rheological measurements were performed at 37°C, after a 5 min rest time. Viscosity curves were obtained between 0.01 and 100 s^{-1} shear rates to study the flow behaviour of different gels. Storage modulus G' (that describes elastic properties) and loss modulus G'' (that describes viscous properties) were recorded at frequencies ranging between 0.1 and 10 Hz. The loss tangent (tan δ) was calculated as the G'' to G' ratio (measure of the ratio of energy lost to energy stored during gel deformation). All these parameters relate with the stability, spreading and retention properties of prepared gels.

Growth Curve Analysis

The effect of P60+CRB and their formulations on the growth of bacteria over a time period of 20 hr were studied by plotting the bacterial growth curve. To examine the growth curve of bacteria, bacterial cells adjusted to final concentration of 5×10^5 cfu/ml, were exposed to different formulations including aqueous form of P60+CRB, their NE formulation, corresponding placebo (P_{NE}), NE based gel of P60+CRB and corresponding placebo (P_{NBG}), at their respective MIC values that were observed in our previous work[16] as (3.3 mg/ml) for P60 and (10 mg/ml) for CRB, respectively. Each culture was incubated in a shaking incubator at 37°C and absorbance was measured at 595 nm at different time intervals (0, 5, 10, 15 and 20 hr) to obtain growth curve for the bacteria.[17]

In vitro drug release (Ex vivo release profile from porcine vaginal mucosa)

Porcine vaginal mucosa was obtained from a slaughter house and approximately 2.5 cm^2 area was sliced out with sharp blade, excess fat was trimmed and slices of about 450 mm thickness were prepared. These slices were hydrated in simulated vaginal fluid (SVF) (acetate buffer with pH 4.2: was prepared by dissolving sodium acetate 13.6 g and 6 ml until pH 4.2 of acetic acid in 1000 ml of distilled water)[14] until used. 5 mg of gel was applied on vaginal mucosa (2 cm^2 area) that is tied to the lower end of donor compartment. The volume of the receptor compartment was kept 10 ml. The cell was assembled in such a way that the mucosal surface was just flushed with the SVF (pH 4.2) maintained at 37°C and stirred continuously on a magnetic stirrer at 50 rpm. Aliquots of 1 ml were withdrawn at pre-determined time intervals and analyzed for P60 and CRB content after suitable dilutions by UV spectrophotometric method. The volume of fluid was replaced with the same volume of simulated vaginal fluid after each sampling to maintain the sink conditions. The percentage of drug permeated across the vaginal mucosa was calculated as in equation 1.

%Release= {(conc. of drug × Vol. of dissolution media × dilution factor) / Dose} × 100   **(Equation 1)**

In vivo Pharmacokinetic studies

Radiolabeling of aqueous form of P60 and CRB and its nanoemulsion based gel

P60+CRB NBG were radiolabeled by the incorporation of short half-life gamma emitting radionuclide like Technetium-99m (^{99m}Tc). Aqueous form of P60+CRB and its NE based gel were radiolabeled with ^{99m}Tc using direct labelling method.[18] 500 µl of aqueous form of P60 (3 mg) in acetone was taken and mixed with 200 µl of stannous chloride dihydrate solution (2 mg/ml in ethanol). To the resultant mixture (filtered through 0.22 micron nylon filter) 500 µl of ^{99m}Tc (5 mCi) was added with continuous mixing and incubated at 37°C for 30 min. The resultant formulations obtained had 100 µCi/20 µl activities. The radiolabelled P60 was then mixed with CRB NE based gel. The radiolabeling efficiency (%) was determined by using instant thin layer chromatography-silica gel strips (ITLC-SG, Gelman Sciences, Inc., Ann Arbor, MI USA) using acetone as mobile phase. *In vitro* stability of radiolabeled formulation was evaluated and optimized in normal saline as well as in blood plasma.[19] The effect of concentration of stannous chloride and incubation time on radiolabeling efficiency was studied to achieve optimum reaction conditions by using the equation 2.

% Radiolabelling= (Radioactive counts retained in lower half of strip / Total radioactive counts retained in the strip) ×100
(Equation 2)

Gamma scintigraphy imaging

The Sprague-Dawley rats (female, aged 2-3 months) were selected for the study. The rats were anesthetized using 0.4 ml ketamine hydrochloride intraperitonial injection (50 mg/ml). The rats were divided into three groups (3 rats in each group). (n=9)

Group I: Rats were administered with ^{99m}Tc-P60+CRB NBG (orally);

Group II: Rats were administered with ^{99m}Tc-P60+CRB NBG (intra vaginally) and

Group III: Rats were administered with ^{99m}Tc-P60+CRB Aqueous form (intra vaginally).

Each rat was given 0.6 µl radiolabelled NBG containing concentration of (100 µCi/20 µl) equivalent to (3 mg of P60 and 1 mg of CRB in 0.6 µl, respectively) with the help of catheter made up of low density polyethylene tubing (LDEP) of internal diameter 0.1 mm. Anesthetized rats were then placed on the imaging platform and imaging was performed using Single photon emission computerized tomography (SPECT, LC 75-005, Diacam, Siemens AG; Erlanger, Germany) gamma camera.

Biodistribution Studies

The rats were divided into three groups as following: 3 rats per time point per group (n=36)

Group I: Rats administered with ^{99m}Tc-P60+CRB NBG orally

Group II: Rats administered with ^{99m}Tc-P60+CRB NBG intravaginally

Group III: Rats administered with ^{99m}Tc-P60+CRB aqueous intravaginally

Each group contains 12 rats. 3 rats were sacrificed at each time interval of the study. Prior to the administration of formulations, the rats were anesthetized using 0.4 ml ketamine hydrochloride intraperitonial injection (50 mg/ml). Blood samples were collected by retro-orbital vein puncture from each rat at predetermined time points (0.5, 3, 6 and 24 h) post-administration of formulations. The rats were sacrificed by cervical dislocation at different time intervals. Subsequently, urinary tract organs (kidney, spleen and urinary bladder along with ureters) were dissected, washed twice using normal saline, made free from adhering tissue/fluid, and weighed. Radioactivity present in each tissue/organ was measured using shielded well-type gamma scintillation counter. Radio pharmaceutical uptake per gram in each tissue/organ was calculated as a fraction of administered dose using equation 3.

Radioactivity %/g of tissue = (counts in sample × 100) / (wt. of sample × Total counts injected)   (Equation 3)

Pharmacokinetic parameters for P60+CRB NBG formulation were calculated.[20] Kidney and Urinary bladder were selected as target organs and their organ targeting efficiency was calculated using two equations (5 and 6) mentioned below.[21] Drug targeting efficiency (DTE %) represents time average partitioning ratio was calculated as follows:

DTE %={(AUC target organ/ AUC blood) Ivag / (AUC target organ/ AUC blood) oral} × 100   (Equation 4)

Direct transport percentage (DTP %) of target organ was calculated using equation,

DTP %={(Bivag- Bx) / Bivag} × 100   (Equation 5)

Where B_x= (B_{oral}/P_{oral}) × P_{ivag}. B_x is the target organ AUC fraction contributed by systemic circulation following oral administration,

B_{oral} is the AUC_{0-24h} (target organ) following oral administration,

P_{oral} is the AUC_{0-24h} (blood) following oral administration,

B_{ivag} is the AUC_{0-24h} (target organ) following intravaginal administration,

P_{ivag} is the AUC_{0-24h} (blood) following intravaginal administration,

AUC is the area under the curve.

Data Analysis

Results of *in vitro* drug release and biodistribution data were reported as mean± SD (n=3), and the difference between the groups were tested using two-way ANOVA using Graph Pad Prism 5.0 and data analysis tool in Microsoft Excel.

Results

Preparation of P60+CRB Nanoemulsion

Optimized NE was formulated with combined level of drug content 41 mg/ml (P60=11 mg/ml; CRB=30 mg/ml), oil content 5% w/w, emulsifier content 16.4% w/w (Table 1). The time of sonication and amplitude was optimised to be 300 s and 30% respectively. Particle size analysis showed particles with 58 nm size, PDI of 0.2 and zeta potential of -16 mV.

Table 1. Conditions and quantities of drugs and excipients selected for formulation of Nanoemulsion and characterization

Nanoemulsion		
Drug candidate	P60+CRB	Composition
Oil	Oleic Acid	10%
Surfactant	Tween 20	20%
Co-surfactant	Glycerol	3.52%
Aqueous Phase	Mili Q water	66.48%
Label claim	41 mg/ml	P60 = 11 mg/ml
		CRB = 30 mg/ml
Formulation Parameters		
Homogenization Speed		10,000 rpm
Homogenization Time		30 min
Time of Ultrasonication		300 sec
% Amplitude		30%
Charaterization Parameters		
Droplet size		58±1 nm
PDI		0.2±0.015
Zeta potential		-16±0.2 mV

Where, P60: Polyphenon 60; CRB: Cranberry; PDI: Particle distribution index

Development and characterization of Nanoemulsion based gel

Chitosan at three different concentrations was used to prepare the nanoemulsion based Gels (NBG). Chitosan gel (1%), hydrated in lactic acid (1%) was selected primarily based on their clarity and pH value that is close to the physiological (vaginal pH=3.5-4.5) conditions. (Table 2) represented the final composition and pH values of all the prepared chitosan gels.

Table 2. Composition of different gels with their pH values and homogeneity

Ingredients (for 10g of gel)	Formulation codes		
	CH 1%	CH 1.5%	CH 2%
Chitosan (g)	0.10	0.15	0.20
Lactic acid (ml)	1.15	0.15	0.20
Nanoemulsion (ml)	8.85	8.85	8.85
pH	3.2±0.2	3.7±0.2	4.9±0.1
Homogeneity	✓	✓	✓

Where, CH is the different concentration of Chitosan containing formulations

Rheological studies of selected nanoemulsion based gel

The apparent viscosity profiles of all the selected gels are presented in (Figure 1). All three gels presented a non-Newtonian, pseudo-plastic behaviour, which is a characteristic of polymeric systems. Results showed viscosity values from around 141 Pa.s up to 1060 Pa.s at 0.01 s^{-1}, decreasing down to approximately 0.5-2 Pa.s at 100 s^{-1}. (Figure 2) presents its variability for all the three gels along the considered frequency range (0.1 to 10 Hz). Higher elastic component (lower values of tan δ) observed for CH 1.5% gel, could favour its ability to stay in place after being administered.

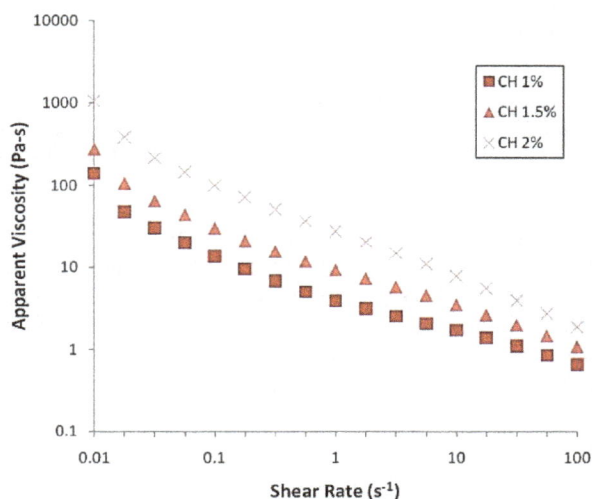

Figure 1. Viscosity profiles as a function of shear rate for tested gels prepared with different concentrations of chitosan CH 1%, CH 1.5%, CH 2%.

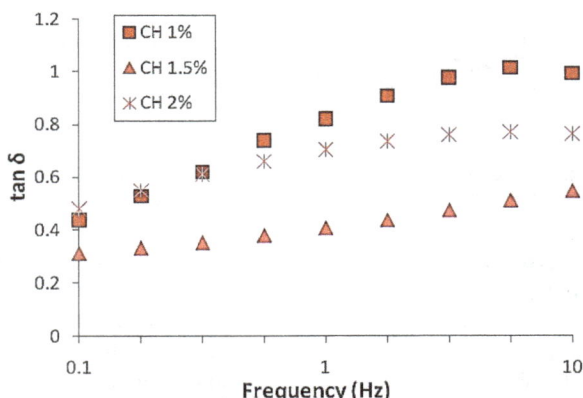

Figure 2. tan δ as a function of frequency for tested gels prepared with different concentrations of chitosan CH 1%, CH 1.5%, CH 2%.

In vitro analysis of nanoemulsion based gel

Drug Release Studies: The *ex- vivo* release profile of prepared nanoemulsion gel was performed in simulated vaginal media using porcine vaginal mucosa. (Figure 3) showed maximum release of 90.92 ± 0.6% in 8 hr for P60, while CRB showed 99.39 ± 0.5% release within 6 hr. This sustained release pattern for both the P60 and CRB from NBG indicated that active was released from the polymeric matrix and gel in the simulated vaginal fluid.

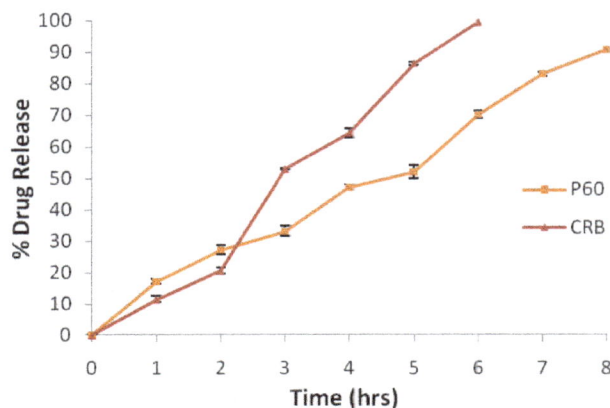

Figure 3. Percentage release of Polyphenon 60 and Cranberry from Nanoemulsion based gel across Porcine Vaginal Mucosa via Franz Diffusion Cell

Antibacterial potential of nanoemulsion based gel with respect to time: The graph (Figure 4) indicates that the aqueous P60+CRB could inhibit the growth of *E. coli* at 15 hr while the NE formulation of P60+CRB and its NBG showed the sudden drop in the turbidity of bacterial culture at the 5th hr of inoculation.

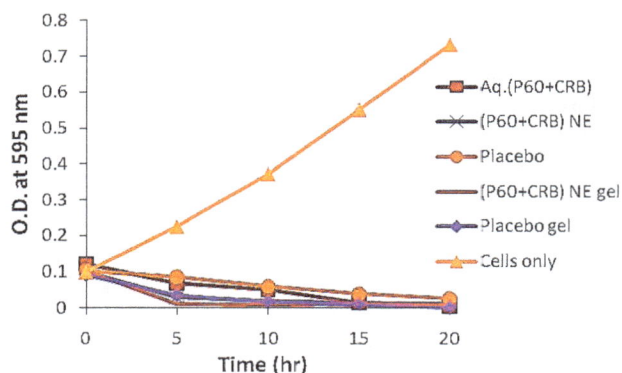

Figure 4. Growth Curve of *E. coli* when exposed to different formulations at 37°C over a time period of 0 hr-20 hr

In vivo pharmacokinetic analysis of nanoemulsion based gel

P60 was radiolabeled using ^{99m}Tc and optimum $SnCl_2.2H_2O$ concentration was found to be 2 mg/ml with an incubation time of 30 min. Radiolabelled P60 was mixed with cranberry NBG to prepare radiolabelled P60+CRB NBG. Maximum labelling efficiency of aq. P60+CRB and P60+CRB-NBG was found to be 95.32 ± 0.15 % and 92.62 ± 0.09 %, respectively. Further the *in vitro* stability of radiolabelled formulation was checked in normal saline and blood serum which was found to be 90.25 ± 0.10 % and 94.64 ± 0.21 % respectively.

Gamma scintigraphy imaging

Among the three groups scintigraphy images as shown in (Figure 5b) post intra-vaginal administered ^{99m}Tc-P60+CRB-NBG rats indicated the rapid distribution and maximum systemic bioavailability of radiolabelled formulation within urinary tract as complete coverage of vaginal mucosa and urinary bladder was seen. While

scintigraphy images of post intra-vaginal administered ^{99m}Tc-P60+CRB rats as shown in (Figure 5c) indicated local distribution and minimal systemic distribution of the formulation. However the scintigraphy images (Figure 5a) of orally administered ^{99m}Tc-P60+CRB-NBG rat showed maximum distribution in GIT as compared to the urinary tract.

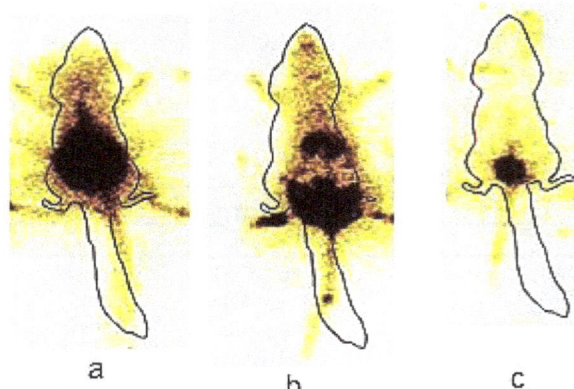

Figure 5. Gamma scintigraphy images of (a) oral ^{99m}Tc-P60+CRB NBG, (b) intra-vaginal ^{99m}Tc-P60+CRB NBG, (c) intra-vaginal ^{99m}Tc-Aq. P60+CRB showing presence of radioactivity in different organs

Biodistribution Analysis

In this analysis distribution of radiolabelled drug in target organs after administration of ^{99m}Tc-P60+CRB NBG and ^{99m}Tc-P60+CRB aqueous form following vaginal and oral administration in Sprague-Dawley rats were compared. The radioactivity in percentage per gram of the total administered dose was estimated at pre-determined time intervals up to 24 hr (Table 3). The concentration of radiolabelled drug in blood at different sampling time points for different formulations was calculated. The analysis indicated that ^{99m}Tc-P60+CRB NBG given intravaginally and orally reached the systemic circulation in 3 hr as compared to the aqueous formulation given vaginally. The percent per gram concentration of ^{99m}Tc-P60+CRB NBG in kidney and urinary bladder were found to be (3.20±0.16) and (3.64±0.29), respectively following the vaginal administration, which was significantly higher as compared to both ^{99m}Tc-P60+CRB NBG administered orally (1.82±0.32) for kidney and (0.91±0.21) for urinary bladder and ^{99m}Tc-P60+CRB aqueous form administered vaginally (1.21±0.28) for kidney and (1.88±0.14) for urinary bladder. Whereas no comparative difference at different time points in concentration of drug in the spleen was observed after administration of radiolabelled drug. The ^{99m}Tc-P60+CRB NBG maintained its concentration systemically up to 24 hr when given vaginally. Pharmacokinetic parameters for the ^{99m}Tc-P60+CRB NBG and ^{99m}Tc-P60+CRB aqueous form were also calculated (Table 4). The target organs showed the $Cmax_{kidney}$ (3.20 %/g) and $Cmax_{urinary\ bladder}$ (3.64 %/g) at 3 hr following vaginal administration as compared to oral administration showed $Cmax_{kidney}$ (2.01 %/g) and $Cmax_{urinary\ bladder}$ (1.08 %/g) at 6 hr was achieved, which may also be attributed to maximum target drug delivery in minimum time following vaginal administration of ^{99m}Tc-P60+CRB NBG. This confirmed that nano sized gel adhered to the mucosa and crossed epithelium to reach the target organs when given vaginally as compared to oral route. The Area Under Curve (AUC) of kidney and urinary bladder after administration of ^{99m}Tc-P60+CRB NBG (intravaginal), was found to be (68.27 hr %/g) and (59.30 hr %/g), respectively, which was significantly higher as compared to AUC_{kidney} (33.22 hr %/g) and $AUC_{urinary\ bladder}$ (56.95 hr %/g) calculated following administration of ^{99m}Tc-P60+CRB NBG (orally) and

AUC_{kidney} (20.95 hr %/g) and $AUC_{urinary\ bladder}$ (23.5 hr %/g) after ^{99m}Tc-P60+CRB aqueous form administered vaginally. DTP% and DTE% were also calculated which represent the percentage of drug directly transported to the target organs via the vaginal pathway using tissue/organ distribution data (Table 5). The results showed the $DTE\%_{kidney}$ (162.98), $DTE\%_{urinary\ bladder}$ (249.15) and $DTP\%_{kidney}$ (38.64), $DTP\%_{urinary\ bladder}$ (59.67) for target organs via vaginal administration of ^{99m}Tc-P60+CRB NBG. The findings suggested that ^{99m}Tc-P60+CRB NBG administered vaginally had better target organ efficiency.

Table 3. Distribution of 99mTc-P60+CRB NBG (orally and Ivag), 99mTc-P60+CRB aqueous form (Ivag) at Different Time Intervals in Sprague-Dawley female Rats.

Formulation and route of drug administration	Distribution of radiolabelled P60+CRB in different organs at different sampling time points				
	ORGAN	0.5 hr	3 hr	6 hr	24 hr
Oral 99mTc-P60+CRB NBG	BLOOD	0.46±0.12	1.49±0.22	2.06±0.17	0.38±0.19
	KIDNEY	0.73±0.21	1.82±0.3	2.01±0.15	0.67±0.19
	URINARY BLADDER	0.23±0.15	0.91±0.21	1.08±0.30	0.42±0.12
	SPLEEN	0.49±0.13	0.99±0.15	1.20±0.22	0.73±0.11
Ivag99mTc-P60+CRB NBG	BLOOD	0.65±0.20	1.69±0.14	2.12±0.25	0.90±0.23
	KIDNEY	1.44±0.25*	3.20±0.16*	3.09±0.35*	1.83±0.18*
	URINARY BLADDER	2.87±0.35*	3.64±0.29*	3.12±0.27*	1.36±0.19*
	SPLEEN	0.32±0.08	1.36±0.13	1.58±0.17	0.82±0.09
Ivag99mTc P60+CRB Aqueous form	BLOOD	0.31±0.10	0.97±0.20	0.84±0.13	0.33±0.10
	KIDNEY	0.46±0.11	1.21±0.28	1.10±0.20	0.60±0.10
	URINARY BLADDER	2.30±0.24	1.88±0.14	0.94±0.09	0.56±0.10
	SPLEEN	0.30±0.10	0.68±0.11	0.52±0.08	0.43±0.1

Each value is the mean ± SD of three estimations. Radioactivity was measured at 0.5 hr, 3 hr, 6 hr and 24 hr. Only statistically significant outcomes at p<0.05 have been reported with *. *The percentage per gram count of radioactivity in kidney and urinary bladder observed after intravaginal administration showed significant difference as compared to radioactivity observed after oral administration of gel and intravaginal administration of aqueous formulation.

Table 4. Pharmacokinetics of 99mTc-P60+CRB NBG (orally and Ivag) and 99mTc-CRB aqueous form (Ivag) at Different Time Intervals in Sprague Dawley Rats.

Formulation and route of administration	ORGAN	Cmax (%/gm)	Tmax (hr)	$AUC_{0-24\ hr}$
Oral 99mTc-P60+CRB NBG	BLOOD	2.26	6	31.925
	KIDNEY	2.01	6	33.22
	URINARY BLADDER	1.08	6	18.6
	SPLEEN	1.20	6	22.62
Ivag99mTc-P60+CRB NBG	BLOOD	2.52	6	40.26
	KIDNEY	3.20*	3	68.27*
	URINARY BLADDER	3.64*	3	59.30*
	SPLEEN	1.58	6	28.19
Ivag99mTc P60+CRB Aqueous form	BLOOD	0.97	3	14.92
	KIDNEY	1.21	3	20.955
	URINARY BLADDER	2.30	0.5	23.52
	SPLEEN	0.68	3	11.64

Only statistically significant outcomes at p<0.05 have been reported with *. AUC: area under the curve, CRB: Cranberry, P60: Polyphenon 60, Ivag: intravaginal, NBG: Nanoemulsion based gel.*The Cmax and AUC of radiolabelled NBG administered via intravaginal route in kidney and urinary bladder showed significant difference as compared to other groups of study.

Table 5. Drug targeting efficiency and direct target organ transport following intravaginal administration of 99Tc-P60+Cranberry Nanoemulsion based gel.

Formulation and route of administration	Target organ	Drug target efficiency (DTE %)	Direct target organ transportation (DTP %)
P60+CRB NBG Ivag	Kidney	162.98	38.64
P60+CRB NBG Ivag	Urinary bladder	249.15	59.67

Where ivag: intravaginal, NBG: Nanoemulsion Based Gel, P60: Polyphenon 60, CRB: Cranberry.

Discussion

Ease of administration, bypass of hepatic metabolism and achieving systemic concentration in therapeutic ranges at lower doses make intravaginal delivery a lucrative route of administration. Cicinelli[22] reported that the vagina has specific blood flow characteristics, either by venous and lymphatic channels or by portal type circulation that allows bypassing the GIT -absorption and liver detoxification and facilitate the transport of drug molecules from vagina to the uterus and systemic circulation.

Lai et al.[23] reported that polymeric nanoparticles of particle size less than 500 nm can distributed in cervical-vaginal regions and rate of transport across the vaginal mucosa depend highly upon the surface properties of nano-carriers. Particles in micro meter range were reported to be too large to cross the mucosa.

Hypothesizing the effect of particle size, nanoemulsions of Green tea and cranberry were prepared in the present study and for enhanced residence time, a bio adhesive gel using chitosan was prepared. As reported by das Neves et al.[24] most of the vaginal formulations were administered to animal models by making a dispersion of the same in PBS; however, aqueous based gel is a feasible and acceptable option for human administration. The gel not only provides a medium to carry the actives, it also provides a three dimensional matrix which can form interlocks with the mucin layers of the cervical–vaginal region. Lin et al.[25] and Abbas et al.[26], reported administration of thermo sensitive gels for PLGA nanoparticles and for delivery of plasmid DNA respectively. In our previous work, we have established synergy between green tea catechins and CRB.[16] Catechins and Proanthocyanidins are two classes of secondary metabolites that are characterized by a common O-heterocyclic structure and are reported to be used as anti-bacterial agents.[27] To prepare CRB and P60 loaded NE system, a set of variables was generated that could result in minimum particle size, PDI and zeta potential. Besides, it would be desirable to encapsulate highest possible content of P60 and CRB with minimum amount of emulsifier. Upon formulating it was observed that both the criteria did not lead to expected particle size range. Therefore, higher content of emulsifier was used so as to solubilise high content of P60 and CRB and got adequately adsorbed on the interface. Similarly, while deciding between % amplitude and time of sonication, preference was given to % amplitude to be kept as minimum to avoid degradation of actives. The optimized NE (closest to the predicted values) was achieved by combining the 41mg/ml (P60=11 mg/ml; CRB=30 mg/ml) drug content, 5% w/w oil content, 16.4% w/w emulsifier content, 31% of amplitude and 286 s time of sonication. . The values of MDS, PDI and zeta potential were found to be in good agreement with the previous findings from literature. Hielscher[28] reported the use of minimum % amplitude while studying the effect of ultrasonication process parameters.

With the aim to enhance the residence time chitosan gels were prepared. Rheological characterization of all three gels presented a non-Newtonian, pseudo-plastic behaviour.[23] Newtonian flow was not observed at varying shear stress values. 1.5% chitosan gel showed higher elastic component (lower values of tan δ).

The sharp drop in turbidity of bacterial culture as exhibited by NBG of P60+CRB could be attributed to nano-sized droplets besides, NH^{3+} groups on protonated chitosan interact electrostatically with negatively charged phospholipids present in cellular membranes of bacteria resulting in leakage of intracellular material. Costa et al.[29] also studied the effect of chitosan at low pH on *E. coli* and showed an increase in inner and outer permeability of *E. coli* cellular membrane. *Ex vivo* release model comprising porcine vaginal mucosa showed maximum release of $90.92 \pm 0.6\%$ in 8 hr for P60 and $99.39 \pm 0.5\%$ release for CRB within 6 hr implying complete release of actives in simulated vaginal media.

To investigate the transport of the optimized ^{99m}Tc-P60+CRB-NBG via vaginal route, gamma scintigraphy and biodistribution studies were conducted. Gamma scintigraphy images showed significant distribution of radiolabelled NBG formulation administered intravaginally as compared to formulation administered orally and aqueous drug administered intravaginally. In a similar study by Mehta et al.[30] pellets (filled into hard gelatin capsule) and cetomacrogol cream, both labeled with Indium-111 DTPA (for gamma scintigraphy) were evaluated for intravaginal distribution and retention over a 24 hr period. From the results it was found that there was complete distribution of creams after 1 hr of administration in the vaginal system and complete coverage of vaginal mucosa was observed. The radiolabelled drug also retained in the vaginal mucosa slightly at 24 hr. Our obtained scintigrams also showed that radiolabelled gel retained for 24 hr after intravaginal administration. A higher uptake of percentage per gram of ^{99m}Tc-P60+CRB-NBG into systemic circulation and target organs, kidney and urinary bladder was observed as compared to ^{99m}Tc- P60+CRB aqueous form after vaginal administration. The DTP% and DTE% was also observed higher, which could be due to mucoadhesive nano emulsion based gel formulation. It is evident from biodistribution results that the ^{99m}Tc-P60+CRB-NBG could cross the vaginal mucosa substantially to reach the organs infected by *E. coli* in Urinary Tract infections. In a similar *in vivo* study performed by Ilem-Ozdemir et al.[31] alendronate was labelled with ^{99m}Tc by direct method and a comparative study was done for intravaginal and intravenous routes. Results suggested that the labeled alendronate could cross the vaginal mucosa and there was an uptake of drug by bone tissues upon intra-vaginal administration. Hanson et al.[32] also investigated the efficacy of metronidazole for bacterial vaginosis when given as a vaginal gel (0.75% twice daily for 5 days) and as oral therapy (500 mg twice daily for 7 days). The efficacy of these two formulations was reported to be similar; however, oral therapy was associated with more gastrointestinal complaints. In another study, Levine & Watson[33] described the pharmacokinetics studies of progesterone gel given via vaginally and oral progesterone. From findings it was suggested that progesterone gel caused greater bioavailability with less relative variability than oral progesterone. Our findings were also in agreement to the findings from previous literature. As hypothesized, vaginal administration of ^{99m}Tc-P60+CRB-NBG exhibited higher systemic absorption as compared to oral administration. This could be due to bypass of GI Tract and first pass metabolism, as P60 and CRB are reported to undergo high first pass metabolism.[34]

The pharmacokinetic parameters calculated were also in agreement with the gamma scintigrams. It can be concluded that NBG for P60+CRB showed enhanced antibacterial activity and owing to the nano-droplet size, the formulation could be transported trans-vaginally from vaginal cavity to the systemic circulation.

Conclusion

Aim of the present work was to prepare NBG encapsulated with P60 and CRB for enhanced antibacterial activity. Optimized oil-in-water NE of P60+CRB was developed that showed a MDS of 58 nm, PDI of 0.2 and zeta potential of -16 mV. To enhance the residence time of the formulation at the site of action, chitosan based gel (1.5%) formulation was developed and characterized for P60+CRB NBG. NBG showed enhanced antibacterial activity (as compared to its aq. and NE counterparts) against *E. coli* as determined via growth curve. *Ex vivo* release studies of P60+CRB NBG performed on porcine vaginal mucosa showed 99% release of P60 after 8 hr while 90% CRB was released after 6 h in simulated vaginal fluid. Preliminary *in vivo* gamma scintigraphy and biodistribution studies were performed by radiolabeling of P60+CRB. Scintigrams indicated the higher uptake of gel from vaginal cavity into the systemic circulation as compared to the aqueous form of P60+CRB which was retained primarily in the vaginal cavity. The pharmacokinetic parameters calculated were also in agreement with the gamma scintigrams. It can be concluded that NBG for P60+CRB showed enhanced antibacterial activity and owing to the nano-droplet size, the formulation could be transported trans-vaginally from vaginal cavity to the systemic circulation.

Acknowledgments

The authors would like to thank the Department of Biotechnology, Government of India for providing financial support to conduct the research work *(DBT project No.BT/PR7215/NNT/28/654/2013)*. The authors are grateful to the Jaypee Institute of Information Technology, Noida, UP (India), for the infrastructural support.

Ethical Issues

Approval to carry out animal studies was obtained from the INMAS Institutional Animal Ethics Committee (IAEC), New Delhi, India, IAEC vide number INM/IAEC/2012/05 and their guidelines were followed throughout the study.

Conflict of Interest

All the authors declared that they have no conflict of interest.

References

1. Gold HS, Moellering RC, Jr. Antimicrobial-drug resistance. *N Engl J Med* 1996;335(19):1445-53. doi: 10.1056/nejm199611073351907
2. Howell AB. Bioactive compounds in cranberries and their role in prevention of urinary tract infections. *Mol Nutr Food Res* 2007;51(6):732-7. doi: 10.1002/mnfr.200700038
3. Lacombe A, Wu VC, Tyler S, Edwards K. Antimicrobial action of the american cranberry constituents; phenolics, anthocyanins, and organic acids, against escherichia coli o157:H7. *Int J Food Microbiol* 2010;139(1-2):102-7. doi: 10.1016/j.ijfoodmicro.2010.01.035
4. Sakanaka S, Aizawa M, Kim M, Yamamoto T. Inhibitory effects of green tea polyphenols on growth and cellular adherence of an oral bacterium, porphyromonas gingivalis. *Biosci Biotechnol Biochem* 1996;60(5):745-9.
5. Reto M, Almeida C, Rocha J, Sepodes B, Figueira M-E. Green tea (camellia sinensis): Hypocholesterolemic effects in humans and anti-inflammatory effects in animals. *Food Nutr Sci* 2014;5(22):2185. doi: 10.4236/fns.2014.522231
6. Gupta S, Sahni JK, Ali J, Gabrani R, Dang S. Development and characterization of green tea loaded microemulsion for vaginal infections. *Adv Materials Lett* 2012;3(6):493-7. doi: 10.5185/amlett.2012.icnano.205
7. Graham HN. Green tea composition, consumption, and polyphenol chemistry. *Prev Med* 1992;21(3):334-50. doi: 10.1016/0091-7435(92)90041-F
8. Taylor PW, Hamilton-Miller JM, Stapleton PD. Antimicrobial properties of green tea catechins. *Food Sci Technol Bull* 2005;2:71-81.
9. Reygaert WC. The antimicrobial possibilities of green tea. *Front Microbiol* 2014;5:434. doi: 10.3389/fmicb.2014.00434
10. Giamarellou H, Bassaris HP, Petrikkos G, Busch W, Voulgarelis M, Antoniadou A, et al. Monotherapy with intravenous followed by oral high-dose ciprofloxacin versus combination therapy with ceftazidime plus amikacin as initial empiric therapy for granulocytopenic patients with fever. *Antimicrob Agents Chemother* 2000;44(12):3264-71. doi: 10.1128/AAC.44.12.3264-3271.2000
11. Talegaonkar S, Azeem A, Ahmad FJ, Khar RK, Pathan SA, Khan ZI. Microemulsions: A novel approach to enhanced drug delivery. *Recent Pat*

Drug Deliv Formul 2008;2(3):238-57. doi: 10.2174/187221108786241679

12. Gao Y, Yuan A, Chuchuen O, Ham A, Yang KH, Katz DF. Vaginal deployment and tenofovir delivery by microbicide gels. *Drug Deliv Transl Res* 2015;5(3):279-94. doi: 10.1007/s13346-015-0227-1

13. Edsman K, Hagerstrom H. Pharmaceutical applications of mucoadhesion for the non-oral routes. *J Pharm Pharmacol* 2005;57(1):3-22. doi: 10.1211/0022357055227

14. El-Kamel A, Sokar M, Naggar V, Al Gamal S. Chitosan and sodium alginate-based bioadhesive vaginal tablets. *AAPS PharmSci* 2002;4(4):E44. doi: 10.1208/ps040444

15. Higgins DM, Skauen DM. Influence of power on quality of emulsions prepared by ultrasound. *J Pharm Sci* 1972;61(10):1567-70. doi: 10.1002/jps.2600611004

16. Gupta S, Bansal R, Maheshwari D, Ali J, Gabrani R, Dang S. Development of a nanoemulsion system for polyphenon 60 and cranberry. *Adv Sci Lett* 2014;20(7-8):1683-6. doi: 10.1166/asl.2014.5579

17. Kim S-H, Lee H-S, Ryu D-S, Choi S-J, Lee D-S. Antibacterial activity of silver-nanoparticles against staphylococcus aureus and escherichia coli. *Korean J Microbiol Biotechnol* 2011;39(1):77-85.

18. Sugiura G, Kuhn H, Sauter M, Haberkorn U, Mier W. Radiolabeling strategies for tumor-targeting proteinaceous drugs. *Molecules* 2014;19(2):2135-65. doi: 10.3390/molecules19022135

19. Zou H, Jiang X, Kong L, Gao S. Design and gamma-scintigraphic evaluation of a floating and pulsatile drug delivery system based on an impermeable cylinder. *Chem Pharm Bull (Tokyo)* 2007;55(4):580-5. doi: 10.1248/cpb.55.580

20. Sharma D, Sharma RK, Sharma N, Gabrani R, Sharma SK, Ali J, et al. Nose-to-brain delivery of plga-diazepam nanoparticles. *AAPS PharmSciTech* 2015;16(5):1108-21. doi: 10.1208/s12249-015-0294-0

21. Kumar M, Misra A, Babbar AK, Mishra AK, Mishra P, Pathak K. Intranasal nanoemulsion based brain targeting drug delivery system of risperidone. *Int J Pharm* 2008;358(1-2):285-91. doi: 10.1016/j.ijpharm.2008.03.029

22. Cicinelli E, Cignarelli M, Sabatelli S, Romano F, Schonauer LM, Padovano R, et al. Plasma concentrations of progesterone are higher in the uterine artery than in the radial artery after vaginal administration of micronized progesterone in an oil-based solution to postmenopausal women. *Fertil Steril* 1998;69(3):471-3. doi: 10.1016/S0015-0282(97)00545-1

23. Li Y, Chen XG, Liu N, Liu CS, Liu CG, Meng XH, et al. Physicochemical characterization and antibacterial property of chitosan acetates. *Carbohydr Polym* 2007;67(2):227-32. doi: 10.1016/j.carbpol.2006.05.022

24. das Neves J, Nunes R, Machado A, Sarmento B. Polymer-based nanocarriers for vaginal drug delivery. *Adv Drug Deliv Rev* 2015;92:53-70. doi: 10.1016/j.addr.2014.12.004

25. Lin Y-H, Chiou S-F, Lai C-H, Tsai S-C, Chou C-W, Peng S-F, et al. Formulation and evaluation of water-in-oil amoxicillin-loaded nanoemulsions using for helicobacter pylori eradication. *Process biochem* 2012;47(10):1469-78. doi: 10.1016/j.procbio.2012.05.019

26. Abbas S, Bashari M, Akhtar W, Li WW, Zhang X. Process optimization of ultrasound-assisted curcumin nanoemulsions stabilized by osa-modified starch. *Ultrason Sonochem* 2014;21(4):1265-74. doi: 10.1016/j.ultsonch.2013.12.017

27. Lai SK, O'Hanlon DE, Harrold S, Man ST, Wang YY, Cone R, et al. Rapid transport of large polymeric nanoparticles in fresh undiluted human mucus. *Proc Natl Acad Sci U S A* 2007;104(5):1482-7. doi: 10.1073/pnas.0608611104

28. Hielscher T. Ultrasonic production of nano-size dispersions and emulsions. in: Dans European Nano Systems Workshop-ENS, Paris, France; 2005.

29. Costa EM, Silva S, Pina C, Tavaria FK, Pintado M. Antimicrobial effect of chitosan against periodontal pathogens biofilms. *SOJ Microbiol Infect Dis* 2014;2(1):1-6. doi: 10.15226/sojmid.2013.00114

30. Mehta S, Verstraelen H, Peremans K, Villeirs G, Vermeire S, De Vos F, et al. Vaginal distribution and retention of a multiparticulate drug delivery system, assessed by gamma scintigraphy and magnetic resonance imaging. *Int J Pharm* 2012;426(1-2):44-53. doi: 10.1016/j.ijpharm.2012.01.006

31. Ilem-Ozdemir D, Asikoglu M, Ozkilic H, Yilmaz F, Hosgor-Limoncu M, Ayhan S. (99m) tc-doxycycline hyclate: A new radiolabeled antibiotic for bacterial infection imaging. *J Labelled Comp Radiopharm* 2014;57(1):36-41. doi: 10.1002/jlcr.3135

32. Hanson JM, McGregor JA, Hillier SL, Eschenbach DA, Kreutner AK, Galask RP, et al. Metronidazole for bacterial vaginosis. A comparison of vaginal gel vs. Oral therapy. *J Reprod Med* 2000;45(11):889-96.

33. Levine H, Watson N. Comparison of the pharmacokinetics of crinone 8% administered vaginally versus prometrium administered orally in postmenopausal women(3). *Fertil Steril* 2000;73(3):516-21. doi: 10.1016/S0015-0282(99)00553-1

34. Spencer JP, Schroeter H, Rechner AR, Rice-Evans C. Bioavailability of flavan-3-ols and procyanidins: Gastrointestinal tract influences and their relevance to bioactive forms in vivo. *Antioxid Redox Signal* 2001;3(6):1023-39. doi: 10.1089/152308601317203558

8

An Alignment-Independent 3D-QSAR Study of FGFR2 Tyrosine Kinase Inhibitors

Behzad Jafari[1,2,3], Maryam Hamzeh-Mivehroud[1,2], Ali Akbar Alizadeh[1], Mehdi Sharifi[1,2], Siavoush Dastmalchi[1,2]*

[1] *Biotechnology Research Center, Tabriz University of Medical Sciences, Tabriz, Iran.*
[2] *School of Pharmacy, Tabriz University of Medical Sciences, Tabriz, Iran.*
[3] *Students Research Committee, Tabriz University of Medical Sciences, Tabriz, Iran.*

Keywords:
· 3D-QSAR
· Docking
· GRIND descriptors
· Tyrosine kinase inhibitors
· FGFR2

Abstract

Purpose: Receptor tyrosine kinase (RTK) inhibitors are widely used pharmaceuticals in cancer therapy. Fibroblast growth factor receptors (FGFRs) are members of RTK superfamily which are highly expressed on the surface of carcinoma associate fibroblasts (CAFs). The involvement of FGFRs in different types of cancer makes them promising target in cancer therapy and hence, the identification of novel FGFR inhibitors is of great interest. In the current study we aimed to develop an alignment independent three dimensional quantitative structure-activity relationship (3D-QSAR) model for a set of 26 FGFR2 kinase inhibitors allowing the prediction of activity and identification of important structural features for these inhibitors.

Methods: Pentacle software was used to calculate grid independent descriptors (GRIND) for the active conformers generated by docking followed by the selection of significant variables using fractional factorial design (FFD). The partial least squares (PLS) model generated based on the remaining descriptors was assessed by internal and external validation methods.

Results: Six variables were identified as the most important probes-interacting descriptors with high impact on the biological activity of the compounds. Internal and external validations were lead to good statistical parameters (r^2 values of 0.93 and 0.665, respectively).

Conclusion: The results showed that the model has good predictive power and may be used for designing novel FGFR2 inhibitors.

Introduction

It is well known that the interaction between different components of tumor microenvironment play crucial role in progression and malignancy of the tumor.[1] Among the cells present in the turmeric area, fibroblasts were gained much attention due to having distinguished characteristics compared with fibroblasts in normal tissues. Such fibroblasts in turmeric area are termed carcinoma associate fibroblasts (CAFs) and are detectable in various tumors including breast, prostate, lung, colon and pancreas cancers.[2]

Fibroblast growth factor receptors (FGFRs) presented on the surface of CAFs are belong to the transmembrane receptors known as receptor tyrosine kinases (RTKs) comprised of three immunoglobulin-like domains at the extracellular region connected via a single transmembrane region to the intracellular tyrosine kinase domain.[3] FGFR family consist of four closely related receptors called FGFR1 to FGFR4. Ligand-activated FGFRs activate signaling pathways in the cell which lead to cell proliferation, growth, differentiation, migration, and survival.[4] Similar to other RTKs, deregulation of these receptors can trigger numerous diseases including cancer. FGFR2 as one of the important factors on the surface of

CAFs is overexpressed in some human cancers including stomach, pancreas, and breast. Moreover, mutations of this receptor can lead to intrinsically active form of FGFR2 reported in endometrial and lung cancers.[5] Inhibition of RTKs as a promising target in treatment of different kinds of cancers has been led to development of remarkable therapeutic agents.[6] Most of these tyrosine kinase inhibitors (TKI) at different clinical phases are the small molecules targeting ATP-binding site of the kinase domain of RTKs.[7]

In the context of developing new therapeutics, high-throughput studies combined with computational analyses are effective tools for lead compound discovery.[8] Quantitative structure-activity relationship (QSAR) is one of the most commonly *in silico* methods for the prediction of biological activity of compounds by transforming their chemical and structural properties into numerical values which can then be linked to their potencies using mathematical models.[9] There are different types of QSAR from dimensionality point of view of which 3D-QSAR method is extensively used in drug design and discovery process. In this methodology, 3D-descriptors which are representative of atomic arrangement in 3D space are

---

*Corresponding author: Siavoush Dastmalchi, Email: dastmalchi.s@tbzmed.ac.ir

employed to be used in alignment-dependent or alignment free analyses. In alignment-dependent analysis the studied compounds are required to be aligned with each other whereas in alignment free method there is no need for superpositioning of molecules prior to development of 3D models, which can be considered as an advantage. GRid-Independent Descriptors (GRIND) is one of the alignment-independent methods[10,11] in which molecular interaction fields (MIF) are used to describe the interaction energy between ligands and different types of probes.[12] Then data mining are performed on the pool of calculated descriptors according to their impact on the biological activity followed by calculating favorable and unfavorable interactions.[13]

In the current study we aimed to develop a 3D-QSAR model using GRIND algorithm for a set of FGFR2 kinase inhibitors to identify the needed structural requirements.

The results of the current study may be used for designing novel FGFR2 inhibitors.

Materials and Methods
Data set preparation
A set of 26 small molecules with inhibitory activity on FGFR2 were collected from the literature.[14-16] Inhibitory activities of the studied compounds reported in Kd (nM) were converted to pK_d values. The transformed data would be used as dependent variable in 3D-QSAR study. Table 1 presents the structures and corresponding pK_d values of FGFR2 kinase inhibitors. The 3D structures of the molecules were generated using the Built Optimum option of Hyperchem software (version 8.0.8) followed by energy minimization using MM+ force field based on Polack-Ribiere algorithm.[17] Then, the structures were fully optimized based on the semiemperical method at AM1 level of theory.[18]

Table 1. Structures and biological activities of FGFR2 inhibitors

No	Name	Structure	pK_d
1	AST-487		5.7
2	axitinib		7
3	brivanib		7
4	cediranib		7.5
5	dasatinib		5.8
6	dovitinib		6.4

No	Name	Structure	pK_d
7	federatinib		6.3
8	foretinib		6.1
9	JNJ-28312141		5.4
10	KW-2449		6.1
11	lestaurtinib		6.2
12	midostaurin		5.6
13	MLN-8054		5.8
14	NVP-TAE684		6.6

No	Name	Structure	pK$_d$
15	pazopanib		6.7
16	PD-173955		7.5
17	PHA-665752		5.3
18	PLX-4720		5.5
19	PP-242		6.7
20	sorafenib		5.6
21	staurosporine		7

No	Name	Structure	pK$_d$
22	SU-14813		6.1
23	sunitinib		6.2
24	tamatinib		7.1
25	tozasertib		6.2
26	vandetanib		6

Molecular docking study

The crystal structure of kinase domains for FGFR1 and FGFR2 (PDB IDs: 5A46 and 3RI1 respectively) were retrieved from Protein Data Bank. Docking analysis of the energy-minimized compounds was performed using AutoDock software version 4.2[19] running under LINUX operating system. The binding site was determined based on position of co-crystallized inhibitor compound. AutoGrid was used for the preparation of the grid map using a grid box. The grid size was set to 40 × 40 × 40 xyz points with grid spacing of 0.375 Å and the box was centered at point with -15.788, 23.568, and -33.739 (x, y, and z) coordinates. For docking experiment, Lamarckian genetic algorithm (LGA) was employed in a way that the number of generation,

energy evaluations, and individuals in the population were set to 27000, 2.5× 10^6, and 150, respectively. The number of docking solutions was set to 100, and the default values were accepted for the rest of parameters.

Calculation of GRIND descriptors and model building

The docking solutions for each compound were filtered based on the similarity to the reference structure (i.e. dovitinib) using Shape-it™ software.[20] The selected conformers were introduced to Pentacle program to generate GRIND-based descriptors. To do this, first MIFs were generated using GRID-based fields in which the interaction energies between atoms of molecules and different probes including hydrophobic (DRY), hydrogen bond donor, HBD (O), hydrogen bond acceptor, HBA (N1), and shape (TIP) probes at the given cutoff distance are calculated. The interaction energies (E_{xyz}) at each grid point called node were the sum of Lennard-Jones energy (E_{lj}), hydrogen bond (E_{hb}), and electrostatic interactions (E_{el}). Based on the defined cutoff, the nodes having energies lower than the cutoff were discarded. To this end, ALMOND algorithm was employed to extract the most relevant regions from MIFs according to the field intensity at a node and the mutual node-node distances between the selected nodes. Finally, MIFs were encoded by maximum autocorrelation and cross-correlation algorithm for generating correlograms in which the product of node-node energies were plotted vs the distances between the nodes.

Modeling and statistical analyses

The entire dataset was randomly divided into training and test sets containing 21 and 5, compounds, respectively. For generating 3D-QSAR model, fractional factorial design (FFD), was applied on training subset of data for obtaining the descriptors explaining the important interactions with defined probes. FFD method was carried out until no significant change in the model statistical parameters such as r^2 and q^2 was observed. The remaining descriptors were subjected to partial least squares (PLS) regression where the descriptors internally cross-validated using leave-one-out (LOO), leave-two-out (LTO), and random-group-out (RGO). The PLS model was also externally evaluated with 5 randomly selected test set compounds. To further evaluate the robustness of the generated model, y-scrambling test was carried out by ten times randomly scrambling the activity data for the train set and generating PLS models as outlined above. The generated PLS models were utilized to predict the activity of test set compounds.

Results and Discussion

Targeting carcinoma associate fibroblasts (CAFs) as one of the important components presented in the microenvironment of turmeric area was the focus of many research activities recently.[1,2,21,22] FGFR proteins as the cell surface elements of CAFs interact with their endogenous ligands and interfere with these interactions by small molecule inhibitors is one of the promising strategies which may lead to the development of new anticancer agents.[4] In general, the drug development processes require extensive experimental studies to find and improve the potency and pharmacokinetics of drug candidates via optimizing their 3D structures and physicochemical properties. Identification of novel TKIs are no exception and variety of technologies such as high-throughput screening are being employed extensively to develop druggable compounds acting as tyrosine kinase inhibitor.[23] The highly expensive and time-consuming procedure of drug development requires the utilization

of complementary in silico methods to cut-down the cost and time and increase the success rate.[11] In the current study we have used in silico QSAR approach based on alignment independent method to generate a 3D model for activity prediction of a set of FGFR2 inhibitors. One of the important issues in alignment independent 3D-QSAR calculations is the use of active conformation of the studied compounds. To consider an appropriate measure regarding this criterion, the best fitting conformers of the compounds to the reference structure dovitinib were selected after docking procedure. The experimental data showing the receptor bound form of reference compound (FGFR2- dovitinib complex) is not available, however, its crystal structure in complex with TK domain of closely homologous receptor FGFR1 has been reported previously.[24] By superpositioning the crystal structures of TK domains of FGFR1 and 2, the bound conformation of dovitinib at the TK domain of FGFR2 was identified and subsequently was used as the reference structure to filter the docking results. The filtered conformations for the TK inhibitors were submitted to Pentacle software for alignment independent 3D-QSAR analyses. FFD feature selection was applied to select important independent variables calculated by the software in relation to the dependent variable pK_d. Based on the remained variables PLS model was generated. Figure 1 represents PLS coefficients of variables which were selected by applying FFD on the GRIND descriptors using Pentacle software. The important descriptors based on their corresponding PLS coefficients were listed in Table 2. According to Table 2 two descriptors have positive impact on the biological activity of the compounds while four of them have negative impact.

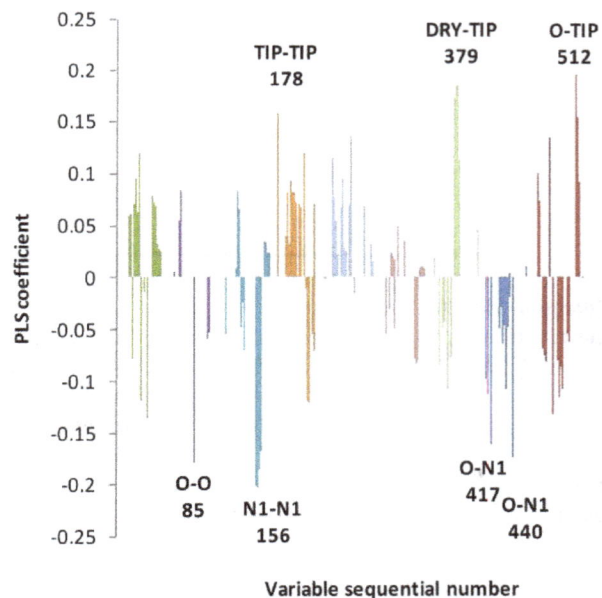

Figure 1. 2LV PLS coefficient plots for the obtained model. The most intensive variables are labeled by sequential numbers. 2LV indicates 2 latent variables; PLS, partial least squares.

Table 2. The most important structural variables in the 3D-QSAR model

Probes	Distance (Å)	Variable	Impact	Expression	Element
O-O	10.8-11.2	85	negative	about half of the compounds	NH of the amide in the ring or outside the ring and NH or its bioisoesters
O-N1	13.6-14	440	negative	almost all of the compounds	amine of indole/ piperazine/ pyrrole piperidine/ pyridine/ quinolone and hydroxyl /amine of endmost moiety or NH between two heterocyclic ring or indole ring
O-N1	4.4-4.8	417	negative	almost all of the compounds	amide carbonyl/ sulfonamide nitrogen and oh of endmost moiety/ NH of amide or NH in the indole ring
O-TIP	19.2-19.6	512	positive	one third of the compounds	NH in the ring or amide and endmost heterocyclic ring/methyl attached to the indole ring
DRY-TIP	12.2-12.8	379	positive	all of the compounds	indole/quinolone ring (or bioisoesters) and halide/alkyl in the end most moiety
N1-N1	16-16.4	156	negative	one third of the compounds	nitrogen of the heterocyclic compounds (piperazine and indole ring) and nitrogen of amide

Variable 379 belonging to DRY-TIP block with positive impact on biological activity has been observed for all of the compounds. The higher the activity of the compound is, the higher the DRY-TIP values. In this variable, DRY as a hydrophobic probe interacts with indole or quinolone rings or their corresponding bioisosteres and is connected to TIP interacting moieties such as halides or alkyl groups at the endmost part of the compounds separated with a distance ranging from 12.2 to 12.8 Å. In compounds 10, 11, and 12, with more rigid structures, the TIP interacting groups are indole or indazole groups. The quantity of DRY-TIP variable for the reference compound dovitinib (structure 6 in this study) in the receptor bound conformation is in good agreement with its potency (i.e., pK_d value), validating the statement made regarding the importance of this variable. Moreover, the inspection of experimental dovitinib-FGFR1 structure shows that the DRY-TIP interacting structural components are involved in interactions with Leu[630], Val[492], and Gly[567] residues in kinase domain of FGFR1.[24] Another important cross correlogram with positive impact on the activity is O-TIP, which relates NH of ring or amide groups with hot spot part at the far end of heterocyclic ring or methyl group attached to indole ring with a distance ranging from 19.2-19.6Å (variable 512). This is also in close agreement with the crystal structure (PDB ID: 4AGD)[25] of VEGF receptor (VEGFR) in complex with Sunitinib (structure 23). Sunitinib is able to interact via NH of its indole ring with Glu[917] of VEGFR.

Another important variable negatively influencing the activity is auto-corralogram O-O (variable 85). This variable indicates that the presence of two hydrogen bond donor groups on the compounds separated by 10.8-11.2Å is not favorable. These H-bond donor groups with the relative distances identified in variable 85 are presented by NH or OH moieties, and are shown just in less potent compounds. Thakur et al. has solved the structure of dasatinib (compound 5) bound to human protein tyrosine kinase 6 (PDB ID 5H2U) and identified a hydrogen bond interaction between its NH group positioned between two heterocyclic rings with Met[267] residue.[26] However, the second H-bond donor group is not participated in any H-

bond interaction, which may suggest an unfavorable effect for the presence of latter group at the defined distance from the former group.

Variables 440 and 417 belonging to O-N1 cross-correlogram are among the informative variables, which have negative impact on the inhibitory activity of the compounds. These variables are expressed by all compounds in the dataset. The effect of descriptor 417 is more pronounced for less potent compounds. The structure-activity relationship (SAR) study on some dovitinib analogues showed that the presence of a hydrogen bond donor-acceptor such as hydroxyl or amine group is important for FGFR1 TK inhibitory activity.[27] In dovitinib this H-bond donor-acceptor group is the NH2 moiety acting as the H-bond acceptor characteristics of the O-N1 variable, which seems to have negative effect on inhibitory activity. Apparently, this is in contrast to the results of SAR studies reported by Renhowe et al., who found this group as a necessary structural feature for having TK inhibitory activity. The source of such seemingly clear disagreement may be the huge differences in the chemical structures of the compounds used in this study with theirs all being close analogues of dovitinib. Apart from this, the compounds lacking the H-bond donor-acceptor group in Renhowe study are either inactive or very less active, while all compounds in this study are active and the unfavorable effect attributed to the N1 interacting group participating in O-N1 variable shows only its relative effect in this dataset. Moreover, the biological activity values are measured using TKs from different receptors (FGFR1 and 2), which makes comparison more difficult. In contrast to the variable 417, O-N1 variable 440 includes wide variety of structural moieties and shows less linear correlation to the activity.

At last but not least, the last selected variable 156 is of N1-N1 block with the highest negative impact on the biological activity. This descriptor is observed only in weaker compounds implying that the presence of N1-N1 interacting groups at the distance of 16-16.4 Å unfavors TK inhibition. Figure 2 represents 6 probe interaction blocks for compound 23.

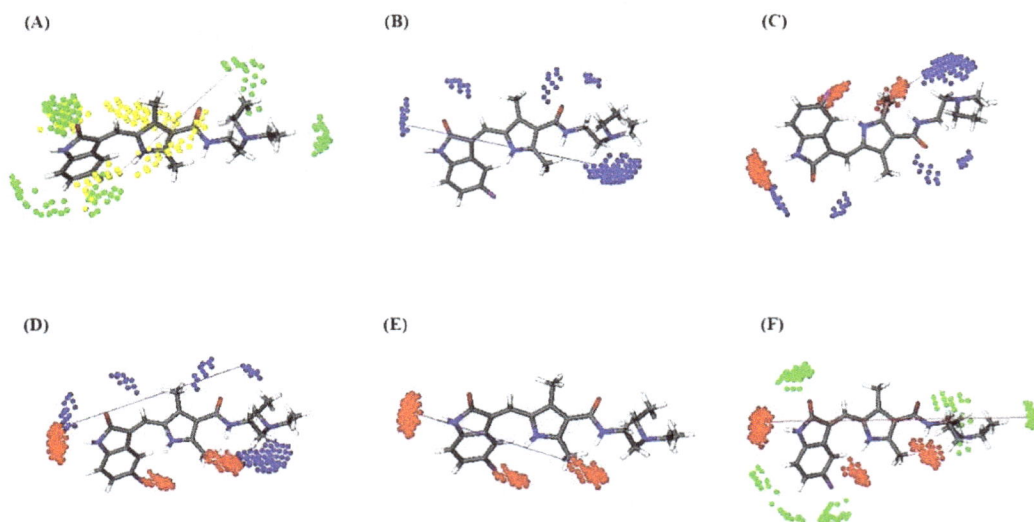

Figure 2. The most important structural elements associated with variables: (a) DRY-TIP 379; (b) N1-N1 156; (c) O-N1 417; (d) O-N1 440; (e) O-O 85; (f) O-TIP 512

Considering that the study was carried out using 26 inhibitors, only 5 compounds (20% of data set) were randomly selected as the test set and the remaining 21 compounds were used to develop the model. Using bigger test set would have adversely affected the predictivity of the model due to loss of information as the result of developing the model by fewer training set compounds. Table 3 shows the statistics for the PLS model generated using training set FGFR2 inhibitors for three latent variables (3LV). Internal validations with leave-one-out (LOO), leave-two-out (LTO), and five random-group-out (RGO) methods were performed to assess robustness of the model. The results suggested a significant correlation between PLS components and FGFR2 inhibitory activities of the compounds. In order to assess the predictive performance of the model, a subset of 5 randomly selected molecules as the test set (shown in Table 4) were used for the prediction. By monitoring the changes in the statistical indices (shown in Table 3), two latent variables (2LVs) were selected as the optimum number of PLS components for the model interpretation.

Table 3. Statistics for the PLS model for FGFR2 inhibitors

LV	SSX	SSX$_{ACC}$	SDEC	SDEP	r^2	r^2_{ACC}	$q^2_{ACC}(LOO)$	$q^2_{ACC}(LTO)$	$q^2_{ACC}(5RG)$
1	10.55	10.55	0.21	0.38	0.87	0.87	0.59	0.55	0.49
2	10.76	21.31	0.15	0.29	0.06	0.93	0.75	0.71	0.65
3	10.16	31.47	0.11	0.29	0.03	0.96	0.76	0.75	0.67

Table 4. Observed vs predicted inhibitory activities for FGFR2 inhibitors used in this work

Comp	pK$_d$ (exp)	pK$_d$ (pred)	Comp	pK$_d$ (exp)	pK$_d$ (pred)
1	5.7	5.77	14	6.6	6.48
2	7	7.06	15	6.7	6.85
3	7	7.04	16[a]	7.5	6.79
4	7.5	7.65	17	5.3	5.41
5	5.8	5.87	18	5.5	5.48
6	6.4	6.37	19[a]	6.7	6.63
7[a]	6.3	6.53	20	5.6	5.65
8	6.1	6.03	21	7	6.82
9[a]	5.4	5.95	22	6.1	6.00
10	6.1	5.95	23	6.2	6.13
11	6.2	6.29	24	7.1	6.92
12	5.6	5.82	25	6.2	6.20
13[a]	5.8	5.59	26	6	5.91

[a]Test set compounds.

Figure 3 presents experimental value of pK$_d$ against predicted activities for the training and test sets. External validation assessment showed a good predictivity for the model with r^2 of 0.665 and SDEP of 0.29 measured for the test compounds. For further validation of the model, ten *y-randomization* tests were performed by randomly scrambling the biological activities for each data point. The results showed that the average squared correlation coefficient (r^2) was -0.292 indicating that the model was not developed by chance. Another validity criterion measured for the developed model was the percentage of prediction errors. A useful rule of thumb is that a prediction error for the test set compounds smaller than or equal to 10% of the training set activity range should be considered acceptable, while an error value greater than 20% is considered a high percentage error. The calculated mean absolute error for the test set compounds was

0.35 (equal to 15% of training set activity range) which is greater than 10% of the activity range for the training set compounds. But, it is less than 20% of the range, which collectively considering the results of all validation assessments seems reasonable.[28] The applicability domain was defined according to the method developed by Roy et al, termed applicability domain using standardization approach.[29] For this purpose PLS latent variables obtained from 3D-QSAR model and pK_d values were used as X and Y variables, respectively. The result showed that there are no outliers among the dataset compounds. Hence the model can be applied for the prediction of FGFR2 tyrosine kinase inhibitory activity of compounds having structures similar to those used in this study. Taken together, working with small data set has some challenging issues concerning external validation. However, this limitation can be overcome by providing more data obtained from experimental procedures.

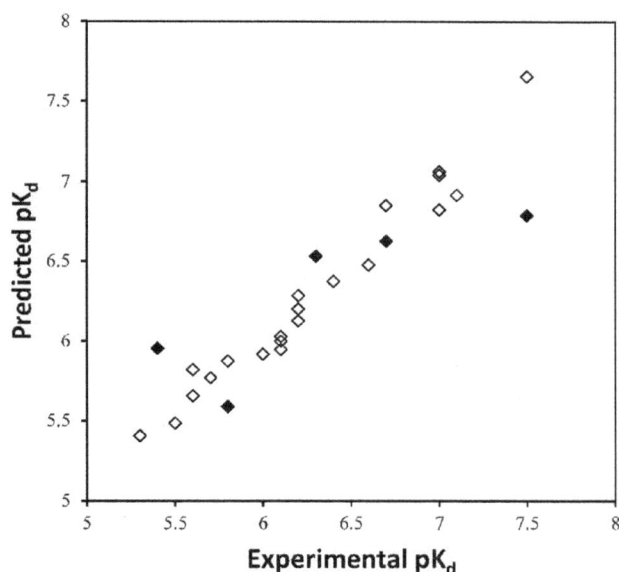

Figure 3. Experimental vs predicted pK_d for compounds. Open squares indicate training set and filled circles show the test set compounds

Conclusion
In summary, an alignment independent 3D-QSAR model was generated for a set of tyrosine kinase inhibitors (TKIs) evaluated on FGFR2. The model was verified with internal and external validation methods as well as *y-scrambling* technique. The results showed that the model has good predictive power with acceptable statistics. According to the selected correlograms, indole and quinolone rings as well as their bioisosteres are important moieties in the structures. These structural features are involved in hydrogen bond and hydrophobic interactions. Moreover, in some compounds substitution of these moieties with small heterocyclic groups helps to retain the functionality of the compounds. The result of the current investigation can be used in designing the novel FGFR2 tyrosine kinase inhibitors.

Acknowledgments
The authors would like to thank the Research Office and Biotechnology Research Center of Tabriz University of Medical Sciences for providing financial support under the Postgraduate Research Grant scheme for the PhD thesis of BJ.

Ethical Issues
Not applicable.

Conflict of Interest
The authors declare no conflict of interests.

References
1. Lin J, Liu C, Ge L, Gao Q, He X, Liu Y, et al. Carcinoma-associated fibroblasts promotes the proliferation of a lingual carcinoma cell line by secreting keratinocyte growth factor. *Tumour Biol* 2011;32(3):597-602. doi: 10.1007/s13277-011-0158-5
2. Togo S, Polanska UM, Horimoto Y, Orimo A. Carcinoma-associated fibroblasts are a promising therapeutic target. *Cancers (Basel)* 2013;5(1):149-69. doi: 10.3390/cancers5010149
3. Katoh M. Fgfr inhibitors: Effects on cancer cells, tumor microenvironment and whole-body homeostasis (review). *Int J Mol Med* 2016;38(1):3-15. doi: 10.3892/ijmm.2016.2620
4. Haugsten EM, Wiedlocha A, Olsnes S, Wesche J. Roles of fibroblast growth factor receptors in carcinogenesis. *Mol Cancer Res* 2010;8(11):1439-52. doi: 10.1158/1541-7786.MCR-10-0168
5. Powers CJ, McLeskey SW, Wellstein A. Fibroblast growth factors, their receptors and signaling. *Endocr Relat Cancer* 2000;7(3):165-97.
6. Hartmann JT, Haap M, Kopp HG, Lipp HP. Tyrosine kinase inhibitors - a review on pharmacology, metabolism and side effects. *Curr Drug Metab* 2009;10(5):470-81.
7. Madhusudan S, Ganesan TS. Tyrosine kinase inhibitors in cancer therapy. *Clin Biochem* 2004;37(7):618-35. doi: 10.1016/j.clinbiochem.2004.05.006
8. Nandi S, Bagchi MC. Qsar of aminopyrido[2,3-d]pyrimidin-7-yl derivatives: Anticancer drug design by computed descriptors. *J Enzyme Inhib Med Chem* 2009;24(4):937-48. doi: 10.1080/14756360802519327
9. John CD. The history and development of quantitative structure-activity relationships (QSARs). *Int J Quant Struct-Prop Relat (IJQSPR)* 2016;1(1):1-44. doi: 10.4018/IJQSPR.2016010101
10. Pastor M, Cruciani G, McLay I, Pickett S, Clementi S. Grid-independent descriptors (grind): A novel class of alignment-independent three-dimensional molecular descriptors. *J Med Chem* 2000;43(17):3233-43.
11. Wilkes JG, Stoyanova-Slavova IB, Buzatu DA. Alignment-independent technique for 3d qsar analysis. *J Comput Aided Mol Des* 2016;30(4):331-45. doi: 10.1007/s10822-016-9909-0
12. Goodford PJ. A computational procedure for determining energetically favorable binding sites on

biologically important macromolecules. *J Med Chem* 1985;28(7):849-57.

13. Artese A, Cross S, Costa G, Distinto S, Parrotta L, Alcaro S, et al. Molecular interaction fields in drug discovery: Recent advances and future perspectives. *Comput Molec Sci* 2013;3(6):594-613. doi: 10.1002/wcms.1150

14. Davis MI, Hunt JP, Herrgard S, Ciceri P, Wodicka LM, Pallares G, et al. Comprehensive analysis of kinase inhibitor selectivity. *Nat Biotechnol* 2011;29(11):1046-51. doi: 10.1038/nbt.1990

15. Southan C, Sharman JL, Benson HE, Faccenda E, Pawson AJ, Alexander SP, et al. The iuphar/bps guide to pharmacology in 2016: Towards curated quantitative interactions between 1300 protein targets and 6000 ligands. *Nucleic Acids Res* 2016;44(D1):D1054-68. doi: 10.1093/nar/gkv1037

16. Wodicka LM, Ciceri P, Davis MI, Hunt JP, Floyd M, Salerno S, et al. Activation state-dependent binding of small molecule kinase inhibitors: Structural insights from biochemistry. *Chem Biol* 2010;17(11):1241-9. doi: 10.1016/j.chembiol.2010.09.010

17. Allinger NL. Conformational analysis. 130. Mm2. A hydrocarbon force field utilizing v1 and v2 torsional terms. *J Am Chem Soc* 1977;99(25):8127-34. doi: 10.1021/ja00467a001

18. Stewart JJP. Optimization of parameters for semiempirical methods I. Method. *J Comput Chem* 1989;10(2):209-20. doi: 10.1002/jcc.540100208

19. Morris GM, Goodsell DS, Halliday RS, Huey R, Hart WE, Belew RK, et al. Automated docking using a lamarckian genetic algorithm and an empirical binding free energy function. *J Comput Chem* 1998;19(14):1639-62. doi: 10.1002/(SICI)1096-987X(19981115)19:14<1639::AID-JCC10>3.0.CO;2-B

20. Grant JA, Gallardo MA, Pickup BT. A fast method of molecular shape comparison: A simple application of a gaussian description of molecular shape. *J Comput Chem* 1996;17(14):1653-66. doi: 10.1002/(SICI)1096-987X(19961115)17:14<1653::AID-JCC7>3.0.CO;2-K

21. Shimoda M, Mellody KT, Orimo A. Carcinoma-associated fibroblasts are a rate-limiting determinant for tumour progression. *Semin Cell Dev Biol* 2010;21(1):19-25. doi: 10.1016/j.semcdb.2009.10.002

22. Sugihara H, Ishimoto T, Yasuda T, Izumi D, Eto K, Sawayama H, et al. Cancer-associated fibroblast-derived cxcl12 causes tumor progression in adenocarcinoma of the esophagogastric junction. *Med Oncol* 2015;32(6):618. doi: 10.1007/s12032-015-0618-7

23. Hojjat-Farsangi M. Small-molecule inhibitors of the receptor tyrosine kinases: Promising tools for targeted cancer therapies. *Int J Mol Sci* 2014;15(8):13768-801. doi: 10.3390/ijms150813768

24. Klein T, Vajpai N, Phillips JJ, Davies G, Holdgate GA, Phillips C, et al. Structural and dynamic insights into the energetics of activation loop rearrangement in fgfr1 kinase. *Nat Commun* 2015;6:7877. doi: 10.1038/ncomms8877

25. McTigue M, Murray BW, Chen JH, Deng YL, Solowiej J, Kania RS. Molecular conformations, interactions, and properties associated with drug efficiency and clinical performance among vegfr tk inhibitors. *Proc Natl Acad Sci U S A* 2012;109(45):18281-9. doi: 10.1073/pnas.1207759109

26. Thakur MK, Birudukota S, Swaminathan S, Battula SK, Vadivelu S, Tyagi R, et al. Co-crystal structures of PTK6: With dasatinib at 2.24 Å, with novel imidazo[1,2-a]pyrazin-8-amine derivative inhibitor at 1.70 Å resolution. *Biochem Biophys Res Commun* 2017;482(4):1289-95. doi: 10.1016/j.bbrc.2016.12.030

27. Renhowe PA, Pecchi S, Shafer CM, Machajewski TD, Jazan EM, Taylor C, et al. Design, structure-activity relationships and in vivo characterization of 4-amino-3-benzimidazol-2-ylhydroquinolin-2-ones: A novel class of receptor tyrosine kinase inhibitors. *J Med Chem* 2009;52(2):278-92. doi: 10.1021/jm800790t

28. Roy K, Das RN, Ambure P, Aher RB. Be aware of error measures. Further studies on validation of predictive QSAR models. *Chem Intell Lab Syst* 2016;152:18-33. doi: 10.1016/j.chemolab.2016.01.008

29. Roy K, Kar S, Ambure P. On a simple approach for determining applicability domain of QSAR models. *Chem Intell Lab Syst* 2015;145:22-9. doi: 10.1016/j.chemolab.2015.04.013

9

Effects of Ectoine on Behavior and Candidate Genes Expression in ICV-STZ Rat Model of Sporadic Alzheimer's Disease

Niloofar Bazazzadegan[1], Marzieh Dehghan Shasaltaneh[2], Kioomars Saliminejad[3], Koorosh Kamali[3], Mehdi Banan[1], Reza Nazari[2], Gholam Hossein Riazi[2], Hamid Reza Khorram Khorshid[1]*

[1] Genetics Research Center, University of Social Welfare and Rehabilitation Sciences, Tehran, Iran.

[2] Laboratory of Neuro-organic Chemistry, Institute of Biochemistry and Biophysics (IBB), University of Tehran, Tehran, Iran.

[3] Reproductive Biotechnology Research Center, Avicenna Research Institute, ACECR, Tehran, Iran.

Keywords:
· Sporadic Alzheimer disease
· Ectoine
· Gene expression
· Morris Water Maze test
· STZ- rat model

Abstract

Purpose: Alzheimer's disease (AD) is pathologically defined by the presence of amyloid plaques and tangles in the brain, therefore, any drug or compound with potential effect on lowering amyloid plaques, could be noticed for AD management especially in the primary phases of the disease. Ectoine constitutes a group of small molecule chaperones (SMCs). SMCs inhibit proteins and other changeable macromolecular structures misfolding from environmental stresses. Ectoine has been reported successfully prohibit insulin amyloid formation in vitro.

Methods: We selected eight genes, *DAXX, NFκβ, VEGF, PSEN1, MTAP2, SYP, MAPK3* and *TNFα* genes which had previously showed significant differential expression in Alzheimer human brain and STZ- rat model. We considered the neuroprotective efficacy by comparing the expression of candidate genes levels in the hippocampus of rat model of Sopradic Alzheimer's disease (SAD), using qPCR in compound-treated and control groups as well as therapeutic effects at learning and memory levels by using Morris Water Maze (MWM) test.

Results: Our results showed significant down-regulation of *Syp, Mapk3* and *Tnfα* and up-regulation of *Vegf* in rat's hippocampus after treatment with ectoine comparing to the STZ-induced group. In MWM, there was no significant change in swimming distance and time for finding the hidden platform in treated comparing to STZ-induced group. In addition, it wasn't seen significant change in compound-treated comparing to STZ-induced and control groups in memory level.

Conclusion: It seems this compound may have significant effect on expression level of some AD- related genes but not on clinical levels.

Introduction

Alzheimer's disease (AD) is the most prevalent type of dementia among aged people which is clinically bolded by continuous memory loss and a slow deterioration in cognitive function.[1] AD is neuropathologically specified by loss of neurons and synapses, especially in the hippocampus and cortex, the extracellular agglomeration of neuritic plaques, containing amyloid-β (Aβ) peptide, and the presence of intracellular neurofibrillary tangles (NFT) composed of hyperphosphorylated tau protein.[2-6] The great majority of AD cases are sporadic with aging, type 2 diabetes and apolipoprotein E4 as the essential risk factors.[7] Other mechanisms may commence before the emergence of tau and Aβ pathologies in sporadic AD pathogenesis.[8,9] These mechanisms include vascular pathology,[10] mitochondrial dysfunction,[11] oxidative stress,[12] hypoxia,[13] insulin resistance,[14] and chronic neuroinflammation.[15]

A nomination causal event in sporadic Alzheimer's disease (SAD) is distracted brain insulin metabolism.[16] Early abnormalities in brain glucose/energy metabolism are pronounced in parietotemporal and frontal areas with high glucose requirement and high insulin sensitivity which suggests damaged insulin signaling in the pathogenesis of SAD.[17,18,19] Injecting streptozotocin, a glucosaminenitrosourea toxic to pancreatic β cells, into rat brain induced the phosphorylation of the tau protein, amyloid deposits and other SAD symptoms.[19-21] The aims of management in AD patients have been to ameliorate or at least slow the loss of memory and cognition and to preserve independent function. Acetylcholinesterase suppressors are first-line factors for the remedy of mild to moderate AD.[22-25] Even though small changes in action mechanisms, these inhibitors have different detrimental effects.[26,27] The most accepted adverse effects are nausea, vomiting, and diarrhea;

cardiovascular and neurological adverse effects are comparable. The incidence of negative effects is precisely related to the dose administered.[27] Therapy with rivastigmine, donepezil or galantamine as Acetylcholinesterase inhibitors for six months to one year resulted in kind of enhanced cognitive function.[23] Improvements in daily behavior and activities also were eminent in patients cured with one of these factors; however, none of them has a major therapy efficacy and the clinical importance of these effects is ambiguous. Whenever there is no effective treatment for AD, substances with efficient inhibition of the amyloid formation have been sought as drug candidates for AD management.[28-31]

Ectoine is a heterocyclic amino acid or a partially hydrogenated pyrimidine derivative (1,4,5,6-tetrahydro-2-methyl-4-pyrimidinecarboxylic acid.[32] Ectoines are common solutes of aerobic heterotrophic bacteria and compose a class of small molecule chaperones (SMCs). SMCs stack to high intracellular concentrations, inhibiting the misfolding of proteins and other unstable macromolecular structures from environmental stresses.[33-36] SMCs have already known as eminently effective in maintaining enzymatic activities against heating, freezing and drying.[33,37] Regarding to a reporting, SMCs like ectoine, betaine, trehalose, citrulline could successfully constrain insulin amyloid formation *in vitro* (Arora, Ha et al. 2004).[38] All findings propose the effect of SMCs against amyloid formation, which may make them permanent drug candidates for medicating neurodegenerative diseases in the future. Ectoine maintains proteins and enzymes from proteolysis, thermal stress and change of the pH or the salt concentration. Studies showed its potency to maintain various proteins, nucleic acids, membranes and whole cells.[33,37,39-42] Many genes have been reported to

be related with AD which they have shown expression changes in Alzheimer model and human brain comparing to normal group.[43,44] Among them *DAXX*, *NFκβ*, *VEGF* genes with the role in apoptosis, inflammation and angiogenesis showed significant statistical diversity in Alzheimer human brain.[43] Furthermore, *Psen1*, *Mtap2*, *Syp*, *Mapk3* and *Tnf α* genes with the role in γ-secretase, cytoskeleton, synapses, kinase and inflammation showed significant statistical diversity in STZ rat model.[44]

Regarding possible mechanisms of AD like inflammation and oxidative stresses in the brain, and role of various genes in these proceedings, the neuroprotective efficacy was investigated by comparing the expression levels of the mentioned genes in the hippocampus of rat model of SAD using qPCR in treated and untreated groups. Moreover, the remedial effects were considered at learning and memory levels as well.

Materials and Methods

Thirty one mature male *Wistar* rats with 250-300 g weight were used in this research. They were kept in cage with adequate food and water, in a stable environment at 22°C and 12h light/dark cycle.[45] Animals were distributed into four groups each containing of seven to eight rats: the control group (Eight rats) received no medication and surgery; the sham group (Eight rats) had bilateral intracerebroventricular (ICV) injection of aCSF as the vehicle of STZ; the Alzheimer group (Seven rats) which received bilateral ICV infusion of STZ, and the treated STZ group (Eight rats) which received the compound for fifteen days after modeling as intrapritoneal injection (6 mg/day).[38] All groups except the control one had five recovery days after surgery and before treatment with aCSF, STZ and compound-treated. All procedures were shown in details in Figure 1.

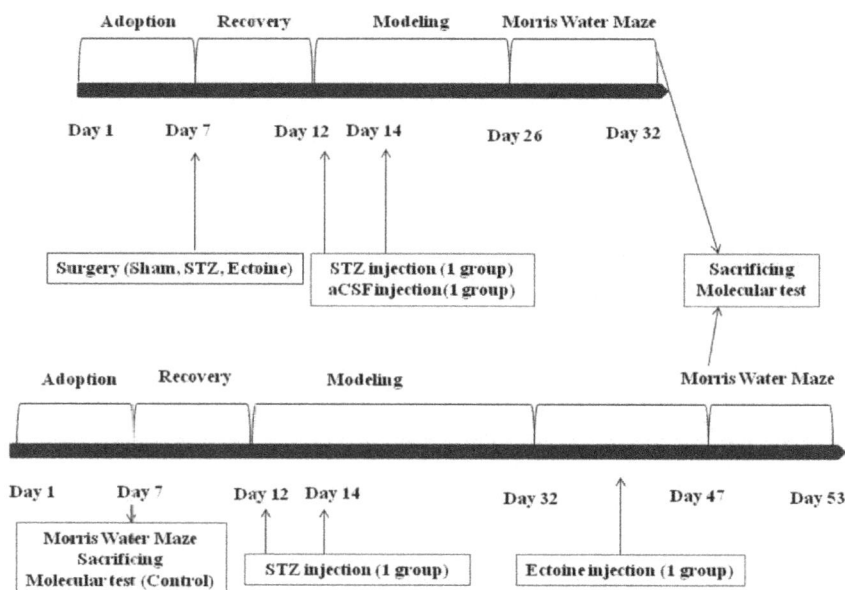

Figure 1. The schematic figure is representative of all procedures. Four rat groups were grouped as control, sham, STZ and Ectoine-treated after adoption days and recruited in treatments and tests

Learning and memory examined for all group of rats using Morris Water Maze (MWM) test after treatment.[46] The maze was a round black pool with 150 cm diameter, 60 cm height. Maze was filled with water to a depth of 40 cm with temperature of about 23°C. Four identical spaced places at the circumference of the pool divided the pool into four quadrants, and were used as beginning parts. An escape platform of 10 cm diameter was located 2 cm beneath the surface of the water at a fixed position in the center of one of the quadrants. All rats were participated to a daily session of four training trials for five consecutive days. Each rat was permitted to find the latent platform within sixty seconds. The time spent to detect the platform (Escape latency), the distance each rat swam to find the platform (Path Length) and the swimming speed (Velocity) were recorded. One day after acquisition, a probe test was performed to evaluate memory level by removing platform.[47]

After MWM test, they were immolated and all hippocampi were dissected and reserved in RNA protector solution at -20°C.[48] All processes were performed according to the National Institute of Health Guide for the care and use of laboratory animals.[49]

Total RNAs were extracted from hippocampus tissues using UP100H ultrasonic processor (Germany) and RNeasy Plus Mini Kit (Qiagen, Hilden, Germany) conferring to the manufacturer's protocol. Purity and integrity of RNAs were specified using Nano-drop spectrophotometer and gel electrophoresis. cDNA synthesis was performed using RevertAid™ First Strand cDNA Synthesis Kit (Fermentas, Thermo Fisher Scientific) according to the manufacturer's protocol.

The relative expression levels of the eight genes *Daxx, Nfkb, Vegf, Psen1, Mtap2, Syp, Mapk3* and *Tnf α* in rat hippocampus of each group were detected using SYBR green Real Time PCR (Takara SYBR Master Mix (Shiga, Japan) in ABI 7500 Real-time PCR system (Applied Biosystem, Foster city, CA, USA) and). All genes expression normalizations were done by *Actb* endogenous control.[50,51] Cycle threshold (Ct) values were used to calculate fold changes in gene expression between groups using REST 2009 software. P-values less than 0.0125 for analysis by REST and in other analysis less than 0.05 were considered statistically significant. MWM test data were analyzed by GraphPad Prism 6 software; Kruskal Wallis (Dunn's multiple comparisons test) test was used for three recorded factors (escape latency, path length and the swimming speed) in all treated and untreated groups separately during five days.

Results
MWM Test Results
After evaluating the learning and memory level changes using MWM test, our results represented a remarkable gradual decrease in swimming distance and time for finding the hidden platform during five days in all groups, despite of no significant change in these two criteria in -treated comparing to the STZ-induced group

during five days, Figure 2a, b and c are representative of MWM test analyses among treated and untreated groups. The swimming speed did not show significant change during five trial days among groups except in STZ group. Probe test results showed no significant memory change in - treated comparing to STZ-induced and control groups (Figure 3).

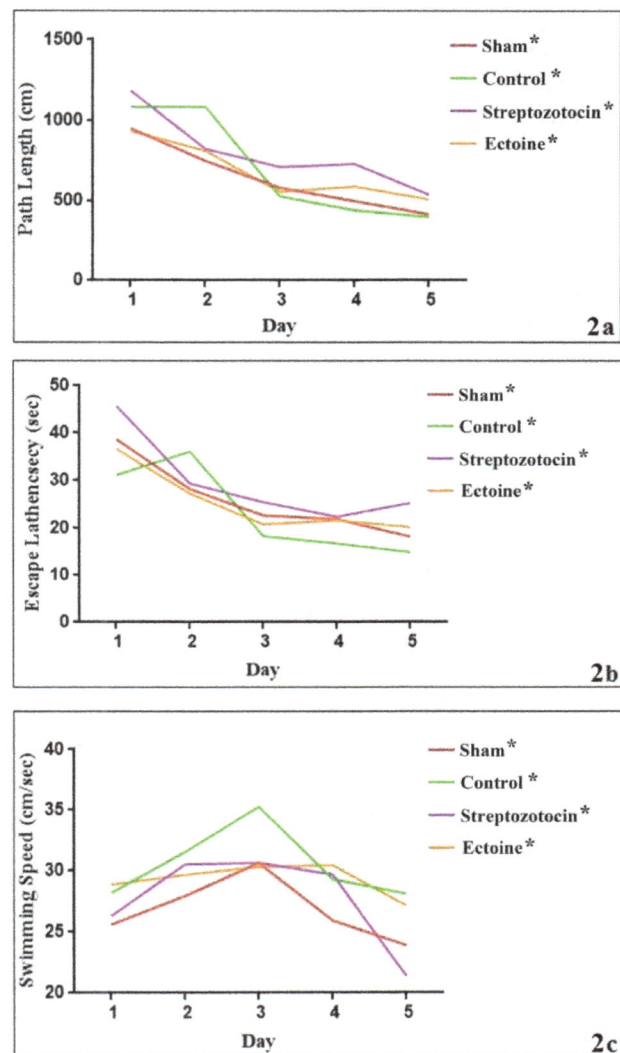

Figure 2. The mean value of path length (swimming distance), escape latency (time for finding hidden platform) and swimming speed (velocity) during five continuous days in all treated and control groups were represented in 1a, 1b and 1c respectively. (*) is representative of significant difference in swimming distance and time for finding hidden platform throughout trial days in all groups. Kruskal Wallis (Dunn's multiple comparisons test) test was used for three recorded factors (escape latency, path length and the swimming speed) in all treated and untreated groups separately during five days

Expression of Candidate Genes
Syp, Mapk3 and *Tnf α* genes were down-regulated and *Vegf* gene was upregulated in rat's hippocampus after two weeks treatment with comparing to STZ-induced group (Table 1). Statistically significant change (p-value ≤ 0.01) was observed in expression level of *Syp, Mapk3, Tnf α* and *Vegf* with decreasing ~ 3, 4.5 and 2- fold in the

Syp, Mapk3 and *Tnf α* also increasing 2- fold in *Vegf* (Figure 4). As it is obvious in Figure 4b, *Syp* showed no significant up-regulation in the STZ-induced comparing to the control group also, in the -treated comparing to the STZ- induced group there was a significant down-regulation (P-value= 0.002). Also in Figure 4c no significant down-regulation of *Mapk3* gene was observed in the STZ-induced comparing to the control group, whereas significant 4.5-fold down-regulation was seen in the -treated comparing to the STZ-induced group (P-value=0.000). As it is obvious in Figure 4d, *Tnfα* showed significant down-regulation in STZ-induced comparing to control group (P-value= 0.008) the same in -treated versus STZ-induced group with about 2- fold reduction (P-value= 0.01). Figure 4a is representative of the expression of *Vegf which* was remarkably decreased in the STZ-induced comparing with the control group (P-value= 0), but its expression showed about 2-fold significant up-regulation in the -treated comparing to the STZ-induced group (P-value= 0.001).

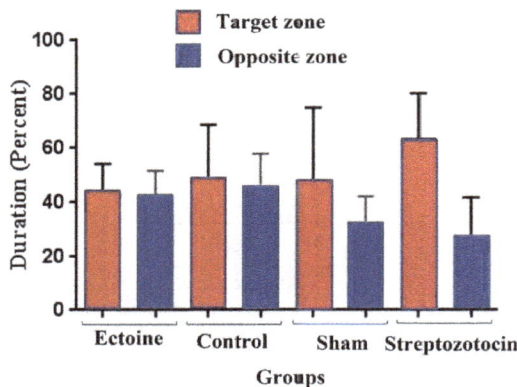

Figure 3. Inability of rats to find the hidden platform was assessed by probe test. The median with interquartile range of percentage of time spending in target (The zone in which hidden platform located) and opposite zone (The opposite zone of target zone) in the sixth day (four trials) of the test in all treated and control groups. Data were analyzed by GraphPad Prism 6 software

Table 1. The table is representative of the eight gene expression levels in Ectoine-treated comparing to the Alzheimer (STZ) group. Asterisk shows significant p-value

Gene	Ectoine-treated/STZ	p-value	Up or down regulation
Daxx	1.9	0.117	Up-regulation
Nfκb	0.7	0.238	Down- regulation
Vegf	2.2	0.001*	Up-regulation
Syp	0.36	0.002*	Down-regulation
Psen1	1.05	0.823	Up-regulation
Mapk3	0.2	0.000*	Down-regulation
Mtap2	0.6	0.095	Down-regulation
Tnfα	0.45	0.017*	Down-regulation

Discussion

In this study, we evaluated expression of eight candidate genes (*Daxx, Nfkb, Vegf Psen1, Mtap2, Syp, Mapk3* and *Tnf α*) for Alzheimr's disease in RNA level in AD rat model. Our results showed that three genes, *Syp, Mapk3* and *Tnf α* were significantly down-regulated in the treated compared to the STZ-induced group as same as up-regulation of *Vegf*.

Synaptic loss and dysfunction are reported to be the molecular basis of cognitive defect in AD.[52,53] Chen et al. (2012) reported their finding as notably reduced expression of synaptophysin (*Syp*) in the hippocampus of icv-STZ mice. Also other Synapse-related genes were found not to be significantly reduced in STZ- induced model even some of them were up-regulated.[44] In the present study, as it is obvious in Figure 4b, *Syp* showed no significant up-regulation in the STZ-induced comparing to the control group also, in the -treated comparing to the STZ- induced group there was a significant down-regulation.

Mitogen-activated protein kinase 3 (*Mapk3*) is an anti-apoptosis gene which is also involved in neuron plasticity .[44] Protein phosphorylation regulates neuronal plasticity, APP processing and tau aggregation.[54] Regarding studies, several protein kinases disorder in AD brain or play many roles in the disease. In the study by chen et al. (2012), gene expressions of some AD-related protein kinases showed down-regulation in STZ-induced mice, but only *Mapk3* expression change was significant. In our study no significant down-regulation of this gene was observed in the STZ-induced comparing to the control group, whereas significant 4.5-fold down-regulation was seen in the -treated comparing to the STZ-induced group.

Many evidences indicate that neuroinflammation can act as an independent factor at very early stage of AD, where the immune-related genes and cytokines are the important factors. It was reported that proinflammatory cytokines such as TNFα are elevated in the CSF and plasma of AD patients.[55] Several biologic medications against TNFα have decreased Aβ deposition, behavioral impairments and inflammation in AD animal models,[56-59] which suggest that TNFα is a deleterious agent in AD term and can serve as a reliable AD target. It has been reported that persistent neuronal TNFα expression in 3xTg AD mice led to large amount of neuronal loss.[60] In present study, *Tnfα* showed significant down-regulation in STZ-induced comparing to control group the same in -treated versus STZ-induced group with about 2- fold reduction.

VEGF levels in AD patient have been controversial. According to the available data, it is postulated that reduced *VEGF* expression might be proved in AD.[61] Increased levels of this gene in the hippocampal cortex of AD patients comparing to normal brain were reported.[62] Some genetic studies have described that *VEGF* levels cause neurodegeneration in part by harming neural tissue perfusion.[63] Gene array analysis has shown up-regulation of angiogenesis relevant genes in the AD brain.[64] In our study, the expression of *Vegf* was significantly decreased in the STZ-induced compared to the control group, but its expression showed about 2-fold significant up-regulation in the -treated comparing to the STZ-induced group.

MWM test results represented a significant gradual decrease in swimming distance and time for finding the hidden platform during five training days in all groups, but not significant change was seen in the -treated comparing to the STZ-induced group. Probe test results showed no significant memory change in the compound-

treated comparing to the STZ-induced and control groups.

According to the previous studies that were reported in the treatment of mild to moderate atopic dermatitis also, ectoine ameliorates ischemia reperfusion injury after intestinal transplantation in rats. Moreover, it causes recovery of neutrophil apoptosis in lung inflammation. Therefore, it can be effective systemically in different diseases.[65-67] Regarding previous report, it could successfully prohibit insulin amyloid formation *in vitro*.[38]

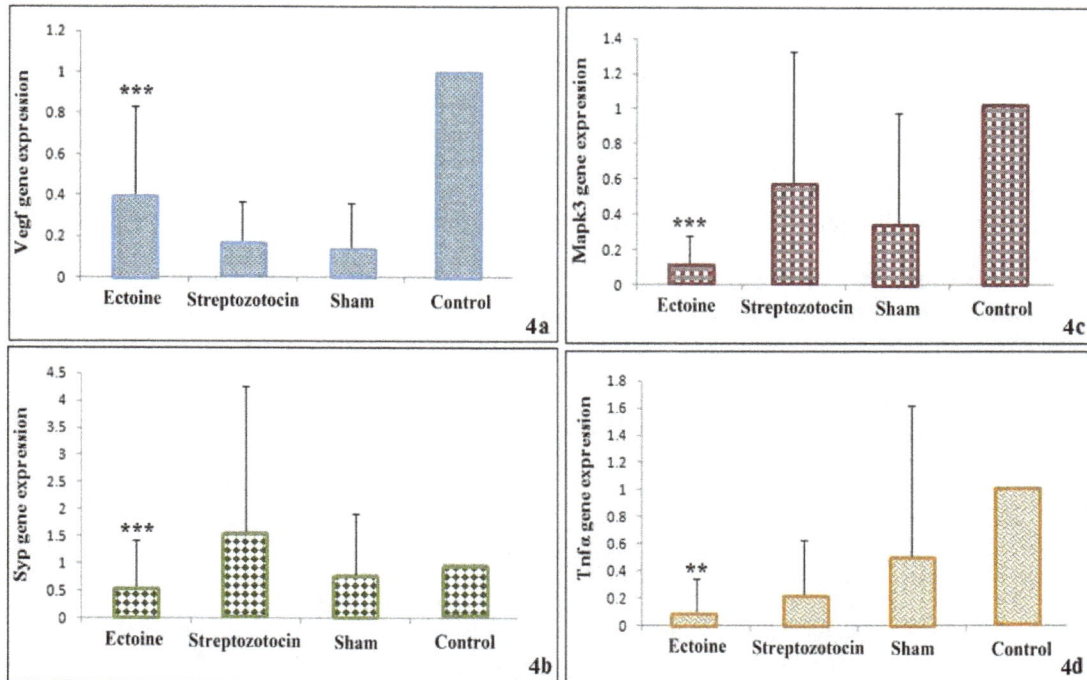

Figure 4. The expression level of *Vegf, Syp, Mapk3* and *Tnf-α* genes in all treated and control groups are shown in this figure. Significant expression changes of Ectoine-treated group comparing to Alzheimer group were labeled out with asterisk

Conclusion

Finally, regarding to both behavioral and gene expression results, it could be concluded that ectoine may have significant effects on expression level of genes related to angiogenesis, synapsis, kinases and inflammation but, not on clinical level. It is recommended to use transgenic animals that could be very helpful to study gene expression levels in Alzheimer's disease. Using transgenic animals could be used to study the effects of our compound in prevention of amyloid beta protein and fibrillary tangles formation. Moreover, using different doses of the ectoine maybe have more effective results on Alzheimer disease. Another study that could be helpful is to use the ectoine before construction of Alzheimer models to observe its effects in prevention of the disease. Duration of ectoine administration is another important factor which might be more efficient on Alzheimer treatment and at last route of administration, for instance intravenous (IV) instead of intraperitoneal could be resulted in better management of Alzheimer's disease.

Acknowledgments

We would like to thank all colleagues specially Dr. Saeed Talebi who helped us in gene expression analysis and Dr. Parvaneh Daneshmand for useful comments. The study was supported by the University of Social Welfare and Rehabilitation Sciences, Tehran, Iran.

Ethical Issues

Not applicable.

Conflict of Interest

Authors declare no conflict of interest in this study.

References

1. Querfurth HW, LaFerla FM. Alzheimer's disease. *N Engl J Med* 2010;362(4):329-44. doi: 10.1056/NEJMra0909142
2. Selkoe DJ. Alzheimer's disease results from the cerebral accumulation and cytotoxicity of amyloid beta-protein. *J Alzheimers Dis* 2001;3(1):75-80. doi: 10.3233/jad-2001-3111

3. Goedert M, Spillantini MG. A century of Alzheimer's disease. *Science* 2006;314(5800):777-81. doi: 10.1126/science.1132814

4. Moreira PI, Honda K, Zhu X, Nunomura A, Casadesus G, Smith MA, et al. Brain and brawn: Parallels in oxidative strength. *Neurology* 2006;66(2 Suppl 1):S97-101. doi: 10.1212/01.wnl.0000192307.15103.83

5. Moreira PI, Santos MS, Seica R, Oliveira CR. Brain mitochondrial dysfunction as a link between Alzheimer's disease and diabetes. *J Neurol Sci* 2007;257(1-2):206-14. doi: 10.1016/j.jns.2007.01.017

6. Moreira PI, Duarte AI, Santos MS, Rego AC, Oliveira CR. An integrative view of the role of oxidative stress, mitochondria and insulin in Alzheimer's disease. *J Alzheimers Dis* 2009;16(4):741-61. doi: 10.3233/JAD-2009-0972

7. Hoyer S. Causes and consequences of disturbances of cerebral glucose metabolism in sporadic alzheimer disease: Therapeutic implications. *Adv Exp Med Biol* 2004;541:135-52.

8. Krstic D, Madhusudan A, Doehner J, Vogel P, Notter T, Imhof C, et al. Systemic immune challenges trigger and drive Alzheimer-like neuropathology in mice. *J Neuroinflammation* 2012;9:151. doi: 10.1186/1742-2094-9-151

9. Chételat G. Alzheimer disease: Aβ-independent processes-rethinking preclinical AD. *Nat Rev Neurol* 2013;9(3):123-4. doi: 10.1038/nrneurol.2013.21

10. Zlokovic BV. Neurovascular pathways to neurodegeneration in Alzheimer's disease and other disorders. *Nat Rev Neurosci* 2011;12(12):723-38. doi: 10.1038/nrn3114

11. Ankarcrona M, Mangialasche F, Winblad B. Rethinking Alzheimer's disease therapy: are mitochondria the key? *J Alzheimers Dis* 2010;20(S2):579-90. doi: 10.3233/JAD-2010-100327

12. Castellani RJ, Perry G. Pathogenesis and disease-modifying therapy in Alzheimer's disease: the flat line of progress. *Arch Med Res* 2012;43(8):694-8. doi: 10.1016/j.arcmed.2012.09.009

13. Orešič M, Hyötyläinen T, Herukka S, Sysi-Aho M, Mattila I, Seppänan-Laakso T, et al. Metabolome in progression to Alzheimer's disease. *Transl Psychiatry* 2011;1:e57. doi: 10.1038/tp.2011.55

14. Kuusisto J, Koivisto K, Mykkänen L, Helkala EL, Vanhanen M, Hänninen T, et al. Association between features of the insulin resistance syndrome and Alzheimer's disease independently of apolipoprotein E4 phenotype: cross sectional population based study. *BMJ* 1997;315(7115):1045-9. doi: 10.1136/bmj.315.7115.1045

15. Krstic D, Knuesel I. Deciphering the mechanism underlying late-onset Alzheimer disease. *Nat Rev Neurol* 2013;9(1):25-34. doi: 10.1038/nrneurol.2012.236

16. Cardoso S, Correia S, Santos RX, Carvalho C, Santos MS, Oliveira CR, et al. Insulin is a two-edged knife on the brain. *J Alzheimers Dis* 2009;18(3):483-507. doi: 10.3233/JAD-2009-1155

17. Henneberg N, Hoyer S. Desensitization of the neuronal insulin receptor: a new approach in the etiopathogenesis of late-onset sporadic dementia of the Alzheimer type (SDAT)? *Arch Gerontol Geriatr* 1995;21(1):63-74. doi: 10.1016/0167-4943(95)00646-3

18. Hoyer S. The brain insulin signal transduction system and sporadic (type II) Alzheimer disease: an update. *J Neural Transm (Vienna)* 2002;109(3):341-60. doi: 10.1007/s007020200028

19. Hoyer S. Glucose metabolism and insulin receptor signal transduction in Alzheimer disease. *Eur J Pharmacol* 2004;490(1-3):115-25. doi: 10.1016/j.ejphar.2004.02.049

20. Grünblatt E, Hoyer S, Riederer P. Gene expression profile in streptozotocin rat model for sporadic Alzheimer's disease. *J Neural Transm (Vienna)* 2004;111(3):367-86. doi: 10.1007/s00702-003-0030-x

21. de la Monte SM, Tong M. Mechanisms of nitrosamine-mediated neurodegeneration: potential relevance to sporadic Alzheimer's disease. *J Alzheimers Dis* 2009;17(4):817-25. doi: 10.3233/JAD-2009-1098

22. American Psychiatric Association Practice Guidelines for the treatment of psychiatric disorders: compendium 2006. Arlington, Virginia: American Psychiatric Association; 2006.

23. Birks J. Cholinesterase inhibitors for alzheimer's disease. *Cochrane Database Syst Rev* 2006(1):CD005593. doi: 10.1002/14651858.CD005593

24. Dementia: A NICE-SCIE guideline on supporting people with dementia and their carers in health and social care. Leicester (UK): British Psychological Society; 2007.

25. Qaseem A, Snow V, Cross JT Jr, Forciea MA, Hopkins R Jr, Shekelle P, et al. Current pharmacologic treatment of dementia: a clinical practice guideline from the American College of Physicians and the American Academy of Family Physicians. *Ann Intern Med* 2008;148(5):370-8. doi: 10.7326/0003-4819-148-5-200803040-00008

26. Raina P, Santaguida P, Ismaila A, Patterson C, Cowan D, Levine M, et al. Effectiveness of cholinesterase inhibitors and memantine for treating dementia: evidence review for a clinical practice guideline. *Ann Intern Med* 2008;148(5):379-97. doi: 10.7326/0003-4819-148-5-200803040-00009

27. Lockhart IA, Mitchell SA, Kelly S. Safety and tolerability of donepezil, rivastigmine and galantamine for patients with Alzheimer's disease: Systematic review of the 'real-world' evidence. *Dement Geriatr Cogn Disord* 2009;28(5):389-403. doi: 10.1159/000255578

28. Tjernberg LO, Näslund J, Lindqvist F, Johansson J, Karlström AR, Thyberg J, et al. Arrest of beta-

amyloid fibril formation by a pentapeptide ligand. *J Biol Chem* 1996;271(15):8545-8. doi: 10.1074/jbc.271.15.8545

29. McLaurin J, Cecal R, Kierstead ME, Tian X, Phinney AL, Manea M, et al. Therapeutically effective antibodies against amyloid-β peptide target amyloid-β residues 4-10 and inhibit cytotoxicity and fibrillogenesis. *Nat Med* 2002;8(11):1263-9. doi: 10.1038/nm790

30. Gestwicki JE, Crabtree GR, Graef IA. Harnessing chaperones to generate small-molecule inhibitors of amyloid ß aggregation. *Science* 2004;306(5697):865-9. doi: 10.1126/science.1101262

31. Liu R, Yuan B, Emadi S, Zameer A, Schulz P, McAllister C, et al. Single chain variable fragments against β-amyloid (Aβ) can inhibit Aβ aggregation and prevent Aβ-induced neurotoxicity. *Biochemistry* 2004;43(22):6959-67. doi: 10.1021/bi049933o

32. Galinski EA, Pfeiffer HP, Truper HG. 1,4,5,6-tetrahydro-2-methyl-4-pyrimidinecarboxylic acid. A novel cyclic amino acid from halophilic phototrophic bacteria of the genus ectothiorhodospira. *Eur J Biochem* 1985;149(1):135-9. doi: 10.1111/j.1432-1033.1985.tb08903.x

33. Lippert K, Galinski EA. Enzyme stabilization be ectoine-type compatible solutes: protection against heating, freezing and drying. *Appl Microbiol Biotechnol* 1992;37(1):61-5. doi: 10.1007/bf00174204

34. Nunes OC, Manaia CM, Da Costa MS, Santos H. Compatible Solutes in the Thermophilic Bacteria Rhodothermus marinus and "Thermus thermophilus". *Appl Environ Microbiol* 1995;61(6):2351-7.

35. Santos H, da Costa MS. Organic solutes from thermophiles and hyperthermophiles. *Methods Enzymol* 2001;334:302-15. doi: 10.1016/s0076-6879(01)34478-6

36. Vorob'eva LI. Stressors, stress reactions, and survival of bacteria: a review. *Prikl Biokhim Mikrobiol* 2004;40(3):261-9.

37. Göller K, Galinski EA. Protection of a model enzyme (lactate dehydrogenase) against heat, urea and freeze-thaw treatment by compatible solute additives. *J Mol Catal B Enzym* 1999;7(1-4):37-45. doi: 10.1016/s1381-1177(99)00043-0

38. Arora A, Ha C, Park CB. Inhibition of insulin amyloid formation by small stress molecules. *FEBS Lett* 2004;564(1-2):121-5. doi: 10.1016/S0014-5793(04)00326-6

39. Knapp S, Ladenstein R, Galinski EA. Extrinsic protein stabilization by the naturally occurring osmolytes β-hydroxyectoine and betaine. *Extremophiles* 1999;3(3):191-8. doi: 10.1007/s007920050116

40. Andersson MM, Breccia JD, Hatti-Kaul R. Stabilizing effect of chemical additives against oxidation of lactate dehydrogenase. *Biotechnol Appl Biochem* 2000;32(3):145-53. doi: 10.1042/ba20000014

41. Barth S, Huhn M, Matthey B, Klimka A, Galinski EA, Engert A. Compatible-solute-supported periplasmic expression of functional recombinant proteins under stress conditions. *Appl Environ Microbiol* 2000;66(4):1572-9. doi: 10.1128/aem.66.4.1572-1579.2000

42. Borges N, Ramos A, Raven ND, Sharp RJ, Santos H. Comparative study of the thermostabilizing properties of mannosylglycerate and other compatible solutes on model enzymes. *Extremophiles* 2002;6(3):209-16. doi: 10.1007/s007920100236

43. Lukiw WJ. Gene expression profiling in fetal, aged, and Alzheimer hippocampus: a continuum of stress-related signaling. *Neurochem Res* 2004;29(6):1287-97. doi: 10.1023/b:nere.0000023615.89699.63

44. Chen Y, Tian Z, Liang Z, Sun S, Dai Cl, Lee MH, et al. Brain gene expression of a sporadic (icv-STZ Mouse) and a familial mouse model (3xTg-AD mouse) of Alzheimer's disease. *PLoS One* 2012;7(12):e51432. doi: 10.1371/journal.pone.0051432

45. Daneshmand P, Saliminejad K, Dehghan Shasaltaneh M, Kamali K, Riazi GH, Nazari R, et al. Neuroprotective Effects of Herbal Extract (Rosa canina, Tanacetum vulgare and Urtica dioica) on Rat Model of Sporadic Alzheimer's Disease. *Avicenna J Med Biotechnol* 2016;8(3):120-5.

46. Morris RG. Morris water maze. *Scholarpedia* 2008;3(8):6315. doi: 10.4249/scholarpedia.6315

47. Zhou S, Yu G, Chi L, Zhu J, Zhang W, Zhang Y, et al. Neuroprotective effects of edaravone on cognitive deficit, oxidative stress and tau hyperphosphorylation induced by intracerebroventricular streptozotocin in rats. *Neurotoxicology* 2013;38:136-45. doi: 10.1016/j.neuro.2013.07.007

48. Paxinos G, Watson C. The Rat Nervous Coordinates: The New Coronal Set. New York: Elsevier; 2004.

49. Guide for the care and use of laboratory animals. Washington, DC: National Academies; 1985.

50. Silver N, Cotroneo E, Proctor G, Osailan S, Paterson KL, Carpenter GH. Selection of housekeeping genes for gene expression studies in the adult rat submandibular gland under normal, inflamed, atrophic and regenerative states. *BMC Mol Biol* 2008;9:64. doi: 10.1186/1471-2199-9-64

51. Moura AC, Lazzari VM, Agnes G, Almeida S, Giovenardi M, Veiga AB. Transcriptional expression study in the central nervous system of rats: what gene should be used as internal control? *Einstein (Sao Paulo)* 2014;12(3):336-41. doi: 10.1590/s1679-45082014ao3042

52. Terry RD, Masliah E, Salmon DP, Butters N, DeTeresa R, Hill R, et al. Physical basis of cognitive alterations in Alzheimer's disease: synapse loss is the major correlate of cognitive impairment. *Ann Neurol* 1991;30(4):572-80. doi: 10.1002/ana.410300410

53. Arendt T. Synaptic degeneration in Alzheimer's disease. *Acta Neuropathol* 2009;118(1):167-79. doi: 10.1007/s00401-009-0536-x

54. Iqbal K, Liu F, Gong CX, Alonso Adel C, Grundke-Iqbal I. Mechanisms of tau-induced neurodegeneration. *Acta Neuropathol* 2009;118(1):53-69. doi: 10.1007/s00401-009-0486-3

55. Brosseron F, Krauthausen M, Kummer M, Heneka MT. Body fluid cytokine levels in mild cognitive impairment and Alzheimer's disease: a comparative overview. *Mol Neurobiol* 2014;50(2):534-44. doi: 10.1007/s12035-014-8657-1

56. Russo I, Caracciolo L, Tweedie D, Choi SH, Greig NH, Barlati S, et al. 3,6'-Dithiothalidomide, a new TNF-α synthesis inhibitor, attenuates the effect of Aβ1-42 intracerebroventricular injection on hippocampal neurogenesis and memory deficit. *J Neurochem* 2012;122(6):1181-92. doi: 10.1111/j.1471-4159.2012.07846.x

57. Tweedie D, Ferguson RA, Fishman K, Frankola KA, Van Praag H, Holloway HW, et al. Tumor necrosis factor-α synthesis inhibitor 3,6'-dithiothalidomide attenuates markers of inflammation, Alzheimer pathology and behavioral deficits in animal models of neuroinflammation and Alzheimer's disease. *J Neuroinflammation* 2012;9:106. doi: 10.1186/1742-2094-9-106

58. Detrait ER, Danis B, Lamberty Y, Foerch P. Peripheral administration of an anti-TNF-α receptor fusion protein counteracts the amyloid induced elevation of hippocampal TNF-α levels and memory deficits in mice. *Neurochem Int* 2014;72:10-3. doi: 10.1016/j.neuint.2014.04.001

59. Gabbita SP, Johnson MF, Kobritz N, Eslami P, Poteshkina A, Varadarajan S, et al. Oral TNFα Modulation Alters Neutrophil Infiltration, Improves Cognition and Diminishes Tau and Amyloid Pathology in the 3xTgAD Mouse Model. *PloS One* 2015;10(10):e0137305. doi: 10.1371/journal.pone.0137305

60. Janelsins MC, Mastrangelo MA, Park KM, Sudol KL, Narrow WC, Oddo S, et al. Chronic neuron-specific tumor necrosis factor-alpha expression enhances the local inflammatory environment ultimately leading to neuronal death in 3xTg-AD mice. *Am J Pathol* 2008;173(6):1768-82. doi: 10.2353/ajpath.2008.080528

61. Mateo I, Llorca J, Infante J, Rodríguez-Rodríguez E, Fernández-Viadero C, Pena N, et al. Low serum VEGF levels are associated with Alzheimer's disease. *Acta Neurol Scand* 2007;116(1):56-8. doi: 10.1111/j.1600-0404.2006.00775.x

62. Tang H, Mao X, Xie L, Greenberg DA, Jin K. Expression level of vascular endothelial growth factor in hippocampus is associated with cognitive impairment in patients with Alzheimer's disease. *Neurobiol Aging* 2013;34(5):1412-5. doi: 10.1016/j.neurobiolaging.2012.10.029

63. Oosthuyse B, Moons L, Storkebaum E, Beck H, Nuyens D, Brusselmans K, et al. Deletion of the hypoxia-response element in the vascular endothelial growth factor promoter causes motor neuron degeneration. *Nat Genet* 2001;28(2):131-8. doi: 10.1038/88842

64. Pogue AI, Lukiw WJ. Angiogenic signaling in Alzheimer's disease. *NeuroReport* 2004;15(9):1507-10. doi: 10.1097/01.wnr.0000130539.39937.1d

65. Pech T, Ohsawa I, Praktiknjo M, Overhaus M, Wehner S, Von Websky M, et al. A natural tetrahydropyrimidine, ectoine, ameliorates ischemia reperfusion injury after intestinal transplantation in rats. *Pathobiology* 2013;80(2):102-10. doi: 10.1159/000342792

66. Marini A, Reinelt K, Krutmann J, Bilstein A. Ectoine-containing cream in the treatment of mild to moderate atopic dermatitis: a randomised, comparator-controlled, intra-individual double-blind, multi-center trial. *Skin Pharmacol Physiol* 2014;27(2):57-65. doi: 10.1159/000351381

67. Sydlik U, Peuschel H, Paunel-Görgülü A, Keymel S, Krämer U, Weissenberg A, et al. Recovery of neutrophil apoptosis by ectoine: a new strategy against lung inflammation. *Eur Respir J* 2013;41(2):433-42. doi: 10.1183/09031936.00132211

10

Development and Optimization of a New Chemoenzymatic Approach for the Synthesis of Peracetylated Lactosamine (Intermediate for the Synthesis of Pharmacologically Active Compounds) Monitored by RP-HPLC Method

Qais Ibrahim Abualassal[1,2][*][δ], Khaldun Mohammad Al Azzam[3][*][δ], Zead Helmi Abudayeh[1], and Loay Khaled Hassouneh[1]

[1] Faculty of Pharmacy, Isra University, Amman, Jordan.
[2] Department of Drug Sciences, University of Pavia, Italy.
[3] Preparatory Year Department, Al-Ghad International Colleges for Applied Medical Sciences, 11451 Riyadh, Kingdom of Saudi Arabia.

Keywords:
· Glycosylation reaction
· Chemo-enzymatic synthesis
· Regioselectivity
· High performance liquid chromatography
· Flash column chromatography
· *Candida rugosa*

Abstract

Purpose: To describe a chemoenzymatic approach joining an enzymatic regioselective hydrolysis of peracetylated *N*-acetyl-α-D-glucosamine (**A**) with a mild controlled acyl relocation which resulted 2-acetamido-2 deoxy-1,3,6-tri-O-acetyl-α-D-glucopyranose (**1B**).

Methods: Immobilization of lipase on decaoctyl (DSEOD) and octyl-agarose (OSCL) was carried out as reported by the work of Bastida *et al*. The newly developed RP-HPLC method for examining the enzymatic hydrolysis was carried out isocratically utilizing a HPLC system.

Results: The new approach resulted the target compound (**B**) in 95% yield after purification utilizing flash column chromatography. *Candida rugosa*-lipase immobilized ondecaoctyl-sepabeads was the best catalyst in terms of activity and region-selectivity in the hydrolysis of substrate (**A**), delivering the deacetylation at C6 position (98% general yield).

Also, a reversed-phase high-performance liquid-chromatographic (RP-HPLC) method for controlling the region-selective hydrolysis of peracetylated *N*-acetyl-α-D-glucosamine (**A**) with a mild monitored acyl movement which led to 2-acetamido-2-deoxy-1,3,6-tri-O-acetyl-α-D-glucopyranose (**1B**) has additionally been developed. The developed RP-HPLC method was utilized as fingerprints to follow the hydrolysis of substrate (**A**) and to determine its purity and additionally yield. Furthermore, the acquired compound (**B**) was further purified by flash chromatography. Compound (**B**) was further characterized utilizing ^{1}HNMR and mass spectrometry.

Conclusion: An efficient chemoenzymatic procedure to optimize the preparation of peracetylated lactosamine **B** containing acetyl ester as extraordinary protecting group is presented. Compound **B** is a significant intermediate for the synthesis of pharmacologically active compound (e.g. complex oligosaccharides for biochemical, biophysical, or biological examinations). Besides, reaction monitoring utilizing HPLC proposes more exact information than spectroscopic methods.

Introduction

Carbohydrates are viewed as a key part in various biological processes. Given their differing difficulty in all cells, it is not surprising that glycans have various assorted part in different physiological processes. The physiological processes are made out of sophisticated multi-cell living organism form. Honestly, a generous number of bioactive compounds are glycosylated and the sugar moiety is considered as a key for their bioactivity.[1] Of them, glycoproteins found in cell–cell recognition of various pathologies are of remarkable interest.[2] Actually, oligosaccharides found in glycoproteins are recognized by lectin receptors, the key part for carbohydrate-mediated recognition actions.[3] For example, lacto oligosaccharides series are incorporated into a couple of structures with high biological concern (e.g., glycolipids and glycoproteins) (Figure1).[4-6]

The destiny of carbohydrate science will be great by the use of its products. The access to oligosaccharides by separation from natural sources is believed tedious and subsequently it gives simply little material that consistently needs the targeted level of purity. The synthesis of high purity oligosaccharides is considered a challenge. Additionally, it is critical for improvement of glycobiology branch.[7] The absence of fruitful and successful methods for synthesis decreased the usage and the examination of oligosaccharides for therapeutic and diagnostic applications. The preparation of monodeprotected sugar is one of the basic building stones in accomplishing complex oligosaccharides.[8,9]

Due to the complexity of structure as well as variability of oligosaccharides, it has been highlighted more than in case of proteins or DNA. Moreover, they are not

*Corresponding authors: Qais Ibrahim Abualassal and Khaldun Mohammad Al Azzam, Email:

controlled by genes and complex polymer, thus they are not valid techniques. For example, PCR for the nucleic acids or recombinant DNA procedure for proteins, found in bacteria, is profitable for the manufacturing on a quantitative scale.[10] Therefore; the preparation of large amounts of carbohydrates starting from natural sources is

suitable to conduct studies or even utilize them as pharmacological substances. Additionally, the advances in glycobiology are constrained because of the absence of efficient techniques to characterize and sequence polysaccharides.[7]

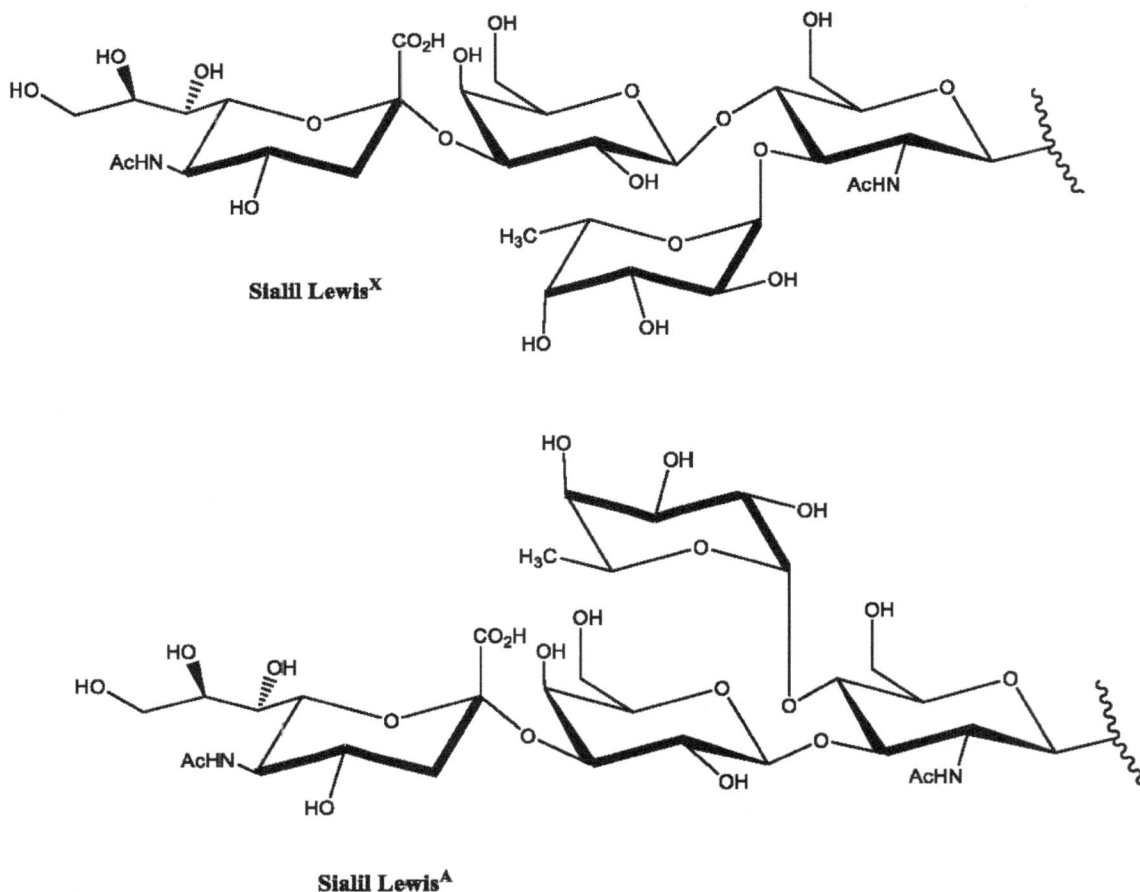

Sialil Lewis^X

Sialil Lewis^A

Figure 1. Oligosaccharides as a key component for carbohydrate determinates highly expressed on the surface of malignant cells.

The advances in chemical synthesis of carbohydrates to find more successful, effective and automated techniques is crucial for the development in glycobiology. It is vital to be used in oligosaccharides in therapeutic and diagnostic area. Herein, it should be highlighted that the synthesis of large amounts of oligosaccharides can improve the production of medication more effectively than the relating natural products.[11-13]

The online/inline evaluation is viewed as a capable tool for controlling and monitoring organic reactions through scale-up step. In addition, the kinetic data obtained from these reviews not just permits control of reactions in routine production but also encourages the design of robust methods and subsequently better idea of the reaction mechanisms.[14] Also, it decreases the tedious work prior reaction controlling through expelling the requirement for manual sampling. This methodology is valuable in conditions where a percentage rate of the reaction compositions are labile or even where the reaction mixture may be dangerous to operator.[15,16]

Flash chromatography technique offers a quick and efficient strategy for separation of mixtures requiring rational resolution.[17] Furthermore, it can be applied for both modes namely; normal phase and reversed phase sepration.[18] Other advantages such as high flow rate with low pressure, thus good separation in a short time and under a reasonable chromatographic conditions could be achieved.[17]

Since long time, our potential research group has been focusing on the mono-protective approach which is necessary for the synthesis of oligosaccharides.[19] In this work, we investigated, optimized and developed another chemoenzymatic approach for the synthesis of oligosaccharides. The last is considered a key intermediate in the regioselective enzymatic hydrolysis of peracetylated pyranoses that catalyzed by the immobilized lipases. Literature review reveals that no reports have been reported for the chemoenzymatic approach for the synthesis or optimization of peracetylated lactosamine (PL) or even using reversed-phase high performance liquid chromatography (RP-HPLC) and flash chromatography methods as monitoring tools for the hydrolysis and purifying, respectively.

In the present work, we concentrated on the development and optimization of another chemoenzymatic approach for the synthesis of PL. In addition, the subsequent acyl movement of the hydrolyzed product to obtain the particularly monodeprotected acyl-pyranose holding a free hydroxyl group at C4 position has additionally been examined. These synthons were successfully and effectively used as an important part in the synthesis of oligosaccharides. The immobilized acetyl xylan esterase (ACEXE) has also been used as another approach for the hydrolysis of substrate **A**. Also, sensitive and direct method is considered important to screen the hydrolysis of substrate **A** and to purify the obtained product **B**. Along these, RP-HPLC and flash chromatographic methods have also been developed in this work.

Materials and Methods
Reagents and chemicals
The octyl-sepharose CL-4B (OSCL) and decaoctyl Sepabeads ECOD/S (DSEOD) were purchased from Amersham Pharmacia Biotech Co. (Uppsala, Sweden). N-acetyl-D-glucosamine ($C_8H_{15}NO_6$), β-D-galactose pentaacetate ($C_{16}H_{22}O_{11}$), lipase from *Candida rugosa lipase* (CRGL), HPLC grade acetnitrile (CH_3CN) and methanol (CH_3OH), ethyl acetate $CDCl_3$-d, sulfuric acid (H_2SO_4), dichloromethane (CH_2Cl_2), ethanol (CH_3CH_2OH), anhydrous sodium sulfate (Na_2SO_4), tetramethylsilane (TMS) ($Si(CH_3)_4$), triethylamine (($C_2H_5)_3N$), sodium chloride (NaCl), boron trifluoride diethyl etherate ($BF_3 \cdot O(C_2H_5)_2$), sodium azide (NaN_3), toluene ($C_6H_5CH_3$), and sodium hydroxide (NaOH), were obtained from Sigma-Aldrich (Milan, Italy). Immobilized acetylxylan esterase (ACEXE) (*Bacillus pumilus*) was a kind gift from ACS Dobfar SPA. All other reagents were of high analytical grade. Substrates that were not commercially available were synthesized in our lab utilizing reported protocols.

Immobilization of CRGL on DSEOD and OSCL
Immobilization of lipase on DSEOD and OSCL was done based on the protocol described by Bastida *et al.*[20] In brief, an exact amount of enzymatic extract was diluted with the aid of phosphate buffer solution (25 mM, pH 7) and then kept under continuous mixing for 30 min. An exact amount of DSEOD and OSCL, (conditioned previously with the same buffer solution and then dried on glass funnel for 1 min) was added to the enzymatic solution in a ratio of (1:10, v/v). After that, the suspension was kept under gentle mixing at room temperature for 3 h. The route of immobilization was tested through Bradford assay method.

Once finished, the enzymatic preparation was isolated using filter paper on glass funnel, washed out using distilled water and with a solution of sodium azide of concentration 0.02% w/v. The yield was assessed through the determination of the weight in mg of protein found in the supernatant. The activity of the enzymatic solution was assessed using ethyl-butyrate test (section 2.3).

Estimation of lipase activity using ethyl butyrate assay test
A 16 mL solution of phosphate buffer of concentration 100 mM, pH 7 was mixed with 4 mL of ethyl butyrate. Then, 100 μL of free enzyme or 50 mg of the enzymatic solution was poured to the solution prepared under vigorous mixing. Throughout the assay (15-20 min), the pH was controlled and kept constant during the addition of NaOH solution (50 or 100 mM) with the aid of programmed titration pH-meter (Metrohm 718 STAT Titrino, Herisau, Switzerland). In light of the consumed amount of NaOH solution, the activity was estimated and expressed in U/g or U/mL.

Procedure for enzymatic hydrolysis in aqueous medium
The enzymatic hydrolysis of **A** was achieved in 50 mM phosphate buffer and with the aid of 20% acetonitrile (pH 4, and 5) to assure full solubilization through mechanical blending. The reaction began at ambient temperature after addition of the immobilized enzyme solution. The pH was kept constant, during the reaction, via programmed titration. The reason of keeping pH constant is to avoid the chemical acyl movement that may happen in the per-*O*-acetylated carbohydrates hydrolysis.[21]

The course of the hydrolysis was controlled by HPLC. The products were evaluated using the synthetic standards isolated. After the whole usage of the substrate, the reaction was stopped utilizing biocatalyst and the generated products were isolated by extraction with the aid of ethyl acetate. The organic layer was dried over anhydrous sodium sulfate, then filtered, and dried under vacuum. The residue was further purified by flash chromatography, and after that it has been subjected to NMR spectroscopy and mass spectrometry for characterization.

Chemical acyl migration/movement
The immobilized biocatalyst was separated by normal filtration. The solution that contains 6-OH derivative **1A** was incubated at pH 9 and 4°C to facilitate the acyl migration from position C4 to C6. RP-HPLC was used, as mentoring tool, to control obtaining the targeted substrate **1B**. At that point, the solution was saturated utilizing sodium chloride and subsequently separated by ethyl acetate. Anhydrous sodium sulfate was used as drying agent to dry the organic layer, then separated and afterward dried under vacuum. The crude products (unrefined) was purified utilizing flash chromatography.

Synthesis of 1A
Enzymatic hydrolysis method was followed for the synthesis of this compound as prescribed by the earlier protocol. Moreover, silica gel flash chromatography was applied for purification of the crude product. A mixture of methanol/dichloromethane using the following ration 5:95,v/v was used for successful elution. The obtained

yield (98%) was determined after purification by flash chromatography. Retention factor (R_f) was 0.32. HPLC chromatographic conditions applied were 20% acetonitrile in phosphate buffer, 10 mM, pH 4, and at flow rate of 1.0 mL/min. Retention time (t_R) was 5.70 min.

Synthesis of 1B

The method of acyl migration/movement mentioned above was adopted for the synthesis of this compound. Moreover, silica gel flash chromatography was applied for the purification of the crude product using a mixture of methanol/dichloromethane (5:95, v/v) to provide the desired glassy white solid product. The yield obtained was 90% after purification by flash chromatography. HPLC chromatographic conditions applied were 15% acetonitrile in phosphate buffer, 10 mM, pH 4, and at flow rate of 1.0 mL/min. t_R was 7.50 min.

Synthesis of product B

A 1.77 g or 3.597 mmol of 2,3,4,6-tetra-O-acetyl-α-D-galactopyranosyltrichloro acetimidate (2) and 0.5 g or 1.44 mmol of **1B** were dissolved in 10 mL CH_2Cl_2. After that, boron trifluoride diethyletherate (0.346 mL or 2.769 mmol) was added in the presence of activated molecular sieves (4Å). Then, mixing at room temperature and under nitrogen was done. After mixing for 5 h, the reaction was quenched by adding 0.39 mL of triethylamine. After that the residue was further purified utilizing flash column chromatography using a mixture of methanol/toluene/ethyl acetate, 1:6:8, v/v to give the requested product. The yield was 95% and R_f 0.24.

Biocatalysts recycling

To look at the reusability or reusing of the immobilized enzymes specified before, the hydrolysis of **A** was examined under comparable conditions. As the highest conversion was accomplished, the reaction mixture was filtered under reduced pressure, washed and after that the immobilized biocatalyst was reused for the following reaction.

^{1}H NMR and mass spectrometry

The ^{1}H NMR spectra were conducted in deuterated chloroform ($CDCl_3$) for **B**. The analysis was achieved at 298 K, 400.1 and 100.6 MHz using a Bruker Avance 400 MHz Spectrometer (Bruker, Karlsruhe, Germany). The Bruker Avance instrument was equipped with a 5 mm BBI inverse gradient probe. Also, the spectrometer used was equipped with a Topspin Programming Package on a workstation running Windows Operating System. Chemical shifts were recorded based on the internal reference TMS. The purified **B** was dissolved in $CDCl_3$. The products obtained by enzymatic hydrolysis were characterized by 2D-Cozy (Correlated Spectroscopy), HSQC (Heteronuclear Single Quantum Correlation) and HMBC (Heteronuclear Multiple Bond Correlation). In addition, 2D NMR was carried out to allocate the correct position of the hydrolysis.

TLC

TLC was carried out on a 0.2 mm layer silica gel pre-coated aluminum sheets purchased from Merck, Darmstadt, Germany. The mobile phases used in TLC analysis comprise of methanol/ethyl acetate/toluene of ratio 16:8, v/v/v and methanol/dichloromethane of ratio 5:95, v/v were utilized to track the preparation of **1B** and **B**, respectively. The spots on TLC were identified by spraying the plates with a mixture consisting of 5% H_2SO_4 solution in ethanol, then by warming to 150 °C. Silica gel 60 of 40–63 μm, was purchased from Merck and utilized for flash chromatography. R_f values were 0.24 and 0.30 for the **1B** and **B**, respectively.

RP-HPLC for monitoring the enzymatic hydrolysis

A new RP-HPLC method was applied for controlling/monitoring the enzymatic hydrolysis process. It was carried out using isocratic elution. The HPLC system (model L-7100) used (Merck-Hitachi, Darmstad, Germany) equipped with a pump (model, L-7100), an interface (model, L-7000), a diode array detector (model, L-7400), an auto sampler (model, L-7200) with a 20 μL sample loop, a degasser (model, L-7612) and a high pressure gradient mixer. LaChrom Software (version 3.2.1) was used to record the data analysis. Separation was achieved utilizing a Phenomenex C-18 column (250 x 4.6 mm, i.d., 5 μm) (Chemtek Analitica, Anzola Emilia, Italy). Other chromatographic conditions such as column oven at 25°C and at a detection wavelength of 220 nm were applied. The flow rate was 1.0 mL/min using a mixture of 20 and 15% acetonitrile in 10 mM phosphate buffer, adjusted to pH 4 as a mobile phase for **1A** and **1B**, respectively. t_R were 5.70, and 7.50 min for **1A** and **1B**, respectively (chromatograms are not shown).

Flash chromatography

The selection of column dimension to be used in flash chromatography was done based on the sample size to be purified. In this work 30 cm × 1.5 cm or larger column was chosen. It was manually packed with silica gel 60 of an average particle size ranged between 40-63 μm, (60 g silica per 1 g of product). In the beginning, the sample was dissolved in a minimum amount of mobile phase. Then it was loaded onto the column. After that, the isocratic elution started using mixtures of methanol-dichloromethane with a ratio of 5:95, v/v (**1A** and **1B**), or toluene-ethyl acetate-methanol with a ratio of 8:6:1, v/v (**B**) as mobile phases. The flash chromatography was run at 10 cm min^{-1}. The detection wavelength was 220 nm. The effluents from the column were collected into test tubes of 10 mL each. Fractions with same peak purity were combined, concentrated and then dried under reduced pressure. The collected extracts were determined by HPLC (chromatograms are not shown).

Results and Discussion
Enzymatic hydrolysis

The enzymatic hydrolysis of alpha PL (1) utilizing two unique enzymes (Scheme 1) was investigated. Keeping in mind the end goal is to optimize the yield of the product where the deprotection took place at the position of C6. Moreover, the enzymatic hydrolysis of 2-acetamido-2-deoxy-1,3,4,6-tetra-O-acetyl α-D-glucopyranose (**1**), was carried out in a phosphate buffer solution, containing 10 or 20% acetonitrile. The later was done to guarantee full solubilization of the starting materials. The reactions took place at acidic pH to avoid any possibility for acyl group migration/movement from one -OH⁻ to the next that could generate undesired *by-products*.[22] Hydrolysis reactions were followed by TLC as well as HPLC.

For better screening of **A**, two different enzymes were used. The first one is called lipase obtained from CRGL immobilized on two different hydrophobic supports namely; DSEOD and OSCL. The second is ACEXE obtained from *Bacillus pumilus* which immobilized on acrylic resin and epoxy groups as functional groups.

The reaction continued with a high regioselectivity at carbon 6 position as indicated in Table 1. The results of

the previous reaction was in agreement with the results reported for the hydrolysis of **A** that catalyzed by CRGL and immobilized at pH 4.[21,22] CRGL immobilized on DSEOD showed a higher regioselectivity as well as activity in 24 h (98%) in comparison with the hydrolysis which catalyzed by CRGL immobilized on OSCL within 48h (27%) once the hydrolysis took place at pH 5. Actually, CRGL immobilized on these two hydrophobic matrixes revealed diverse region-selectivities and rate of biotransformation at the previous pH for **1A**.

In order to explore the reaction catalyzed by the biocatalyst CRGL which immobilized on DSEOD, an increasing concentration of **A**, to attain a preparative amount of **1A**, was used. Surprisingly, we noticed that the performance of CRGL was inversely proportional to substrate concentration in the range 64-98% yield. Precisely when the biocatalyst ACEXE was used, the hydrolysis of **A** proceeded with unexpected results (13% yield of **1A**, Table 1).

Table 1. Hydrolysis of substrate **A** catalyzed by different immobilized enzymes.

Substrate	Conc. (mM)	Enzyme[a]	pH	Time[b] (h)	Conv.[c] (%)	Products (%)[d] 6OH	(others)	Rate[e]
					Scheme 1. Regioselective enzymatic hydrolysis of substrate **A**.			

Scheme 1. Regioselective enzymatic hydrolysis of substrate **A**.

Substrate	Conc. (mM)	Enzyme[a]	pH	Time[b] (h)	Conv.[c] (%)	6OH	(others)	Rate[e]
		ACEXE	5	3	91	13 (**1A**)	77	0.47
	5	CRGL-OSCL	4	48	52	46 (**1A**)	6	0.04
			5	48	75	27 (**1A**)	48	0.04
1		CRGL-DSEOD	5	24	100	98 (**1A**)	2	0.18
	10	CRGL-DSEOD	5	7	98	75 (**1A**)	23	0.37
	50	CRGL-DSEOD	5	24	94	64 (**1A**)	30	0.54

Key to abbreviations:

[a]: Reaction conditions: 5-10 mM of substrate in 15 mL of KH_2PO_4, 50 mM buffered solution, containing 10% CH_3CN; Temperature, 25°C.

[b]: ACEXE (97 U/gr): 58U; CRGL-OSCL (170 U/gr): 100 U; CRGL-DSEOD (116 U/gr): 100 U.

[c]: 20-50 mM of substrate in 25-30 mL of KH_2PO_4, 50 mM buffered solution, containing 20% CH_3CN; Temperature, 25°C.

[d]: ACEXE(97U/gr): 145U – 233U; CRGL -DSEOD(190U/gr): 150 U.

[e]: [a]ACEXE = Acetyl xylan esterase from *Bacillus pumilus*; CRGL-OSCL = Lipase from *Candida rugosa* immobilized on octyl-agarose (Octyl SepharoseR CL-4B); CRGL-DSEOD = Lipase da *Candida rugosa* on decaoctyl-sepabeads (Sepabeads DSEOD/S); [b] Reaction time; [c] % of substrate converted; [d] Yield of the monodeprotected products (APs-6OH) at the maximum of conversion; [e] Initial rate in μ mol min-1 x Ul, calculated at 20% conversion. Results reported were calculated without considering conversion factor.

HPLC method development

Chromatographic methods are considered fundamental for monitoring the hydrolysis of drug substances or even synthesis of any new compound. This includes the analysis of intermediates and the synthesized reaction mixtures at particular intervals of time. It helps also in checking the purity, yield of reaction products generated

and particular impurities which affect reaction. The current HPLC method has been adopted to follow/monitor the progress of reaction during the route of the hydrolysis of **A**, its conversion to **1A** and purity and yield of the **1A**.

A few chromatographic conditions have been investigated while developing the current HPLC method.

For instance solvents, mobile phase, stationary phase, and detection wavelength. The chromatographic separation was accomplished using C18 column as it gave a base-line separation between the two substrates under examination (A and 1A) and from *by-products* (chromatograms are not shown). The common challenge faced while screening the formation of 1A, once the A subjected to hydrolysis, was to achieve complete base-line separation between the two substrates upon hydrolysis by ACEXE or CRGL. The cause of such challenge was attributed to similarity in structures as prescribed in Table 1 and from other *by-products* accordingly. After that, the reaction mixture was chromatographed on a reversed phase column and analyzed at 220 nm. Isocratic elution mode was applied which comprised of 15 and 20 % acetonitrile in phosphate buffer (10 mM, pH 4) as mobile phase for the hydrolysis of 1A and 1B, respectively.

After checking the reactions by RP-HPLC method, we noticed diverse *by-products* produced. These *by-products* were entitled by shorter retention times. This was attributed to the nature of the hydrophilic compounds (hydrolyzed monosaccharides in many positions). Specifically, the deprotection at C6 position. Indeed, after 24 h, the substrate was converted at 98% of the targeted monosaccharide 1A and only 2% of *by-products* generated. As known, the absence of other peaks indicates the good purity of the isolated compounds. Then again, the hydrolysis of A catalyzed by ACEXE was very unspecific, producing only 13% of 1A and 77% of other products (Table 1).

Next, the mild acyl migration/movement was investigated to get the tetraacetylated glycopyranoses containing a free hydroxyl group at the C4 position. The last compound is considered useful being as a building block in the synthesis of PL 3. In this manner, the 6-hydroxy derivative 1A (aqueous solution, pH 9 and 4°C) was converted to product 1B and then isolated in a yield of 90% (scheme 1).

Starting from A using CRGL immobilized on DSEOD, the hydrolysis was performed at pH 5 and 25 °C. It helps in obtaining 1A in a good yield. After that, separation of the immobilized enzyme by filtration was carried out. Next, the reaction conditions were altered by lowering the temperature to 4 °C and at the same time increasing pH to 9. Under these conditions used, a controlled acetyl group movement/migration from 4 to 6 position gave 1B with 90% yield after isolation as indicated in Scheme 1. In order to quench the reaction, acidification at pH ranged between 4-5 was conducted. After that, extraction of 4-hydroxy 1B in organic solvent was done. Then, flash chromatography was applied to purify the desired compound 1B. The purified compound was isolated and characterized by RP-HPLC. Synthetic standards were used for identification purposes.

In addition, we described herein the optimization of a new method for the synthesis of PL. It represents a basic element in the structure of glycosidic antitumor carbohydrate. The 4-hydroxy derivative of the PL 2

(acceptor), once prepared using the chemoenzymatic process, was used as starting material in the glycosilation reaction for the synthesis of B. It was obtained through the reaction with 2,3,4 tetra-O-acetyl-α-D-galactopyranosyl trichloroacetimidate 2 prepared as in the protocol reported (donor).[23]

In glycosylation reaction, it is necessary for the reaction to take place that the donor molecule possesses in the anomeric position a good leaving group. Moreover, in the presence of promoting agent, it allows the formation of carbocationic intermediate that is able to react with the hydroxyl group of desired acceptor. The glycocidic bond must be in β configuration in order to get the desired B. Thus, it is deemed necessary to control bond configuration during the bond formation. This could be achieved through the neighboring group participation due to the presence of acetyl group at position 2 (C). This occurs through the formation of a cyclic structure called dioxolium ring which provides a steric shield for the face α of the molecule. The importance of such formation of this intermediate permits the nucleophile (acceptor) to determine the nucleophilic attack from the β face of the electrophile (donor). Also, it allows the achievement of the chemical bond in the desired configuration.

To improve the yield of synthesis of B, it was analyzed under various reaction conditions. It was performed by coupling reaction between the two building blocks namely; 1B and 2,3,4,6-tetra-O-acetyl-α-D-galactopyranosyl trichloroacetimidate 2 which prepared based on the protocol reported.[23] Parameters such as the molar ratio (between donor 2 and acceptor 1B), and temperature have been investigated. The results of the current study revealed that the yield of B was enhanced up to 95%. This is indicated in Table 2 and ascertained after the product of interest subjected to purification using flash chromatography utilizing the molar proportion of 2.5:1 (2:1B) and borontrifluoride diethyl etherate as promoting agent at room temperature (Table 2).

Table 2. Optimization of glycosylation reaction conditions.

Acceptor (eq)	Donor (eq)	Time (h)	T (°C)	Products	Yield(%)
1[1B]	1.5	6	-20	B	28
1[1B]	1.5	5	0	B	52
1[1B]	1.5	5	RT	B	55
1[1B]	2	5	RT	B	88
1[1B]	2.5	5	RT	B	95

Key to abbreviations:
1B: 2-Acetamido-1,3,6-tri-O-acetyl- 2-deoxy-α-D-glucopyranose.
Donor: 2,3,4,6-Tetra-O-acetyl-α-D-galactopyranosyl trichloroacetimidate (2).
[a] Compound 1B, BF₃·OEt₂, CH₂Cl₂, MS 4 Å.

Flash chromatography method development (purification procedure)

As known, TLC is considered a straight approach for selecting of mobile phase to be used in silica gel flash chromatography.[14,24] Furthermore, to start chromatographic purification, it is recommended to refer to protocols in literature as a guidance in selecting a versatile mobile phase and a column suitable to the solubility, molecular weight, and hydrophobic character of the analyte to be analyzed.[14,25,26] In the current work, no reports have been published for flash purification of substrates **1B** and **B**. Therefore, development and determination of a suitable procedure is a challenging step of this work. Several mixtures of mobile phases were examined such as methanol/ ethyl acetate/toluene (1:6:8, v/v/v) and methanol/dichloromethane (5:95, v/v) to accomplish the purification of **1B** and **B**, respectively.

The best organic solvent ratio to be used was determined by trial and error.

On the other hand, several of solvent systems were examined in TLC separation of the two substrates. For example, methanol/dichloromethane, ethyl acetate/chloroform, acetone/hexane, methanol/chloroform, methanol/ethyl acetate, acetone/chloroform, and methanol/toluene/ethyl acetate). The best separation achieved among the systems examined on TLC was accomplished as mentioned earlier.

NMR spectroscopy

The final step is to verify the structure of **B** after purification using flash chromatography. Characterization has been done by ^{1}HNMR spectra (spectra are not shown) while Figure 2 shows the mass spectrometry.

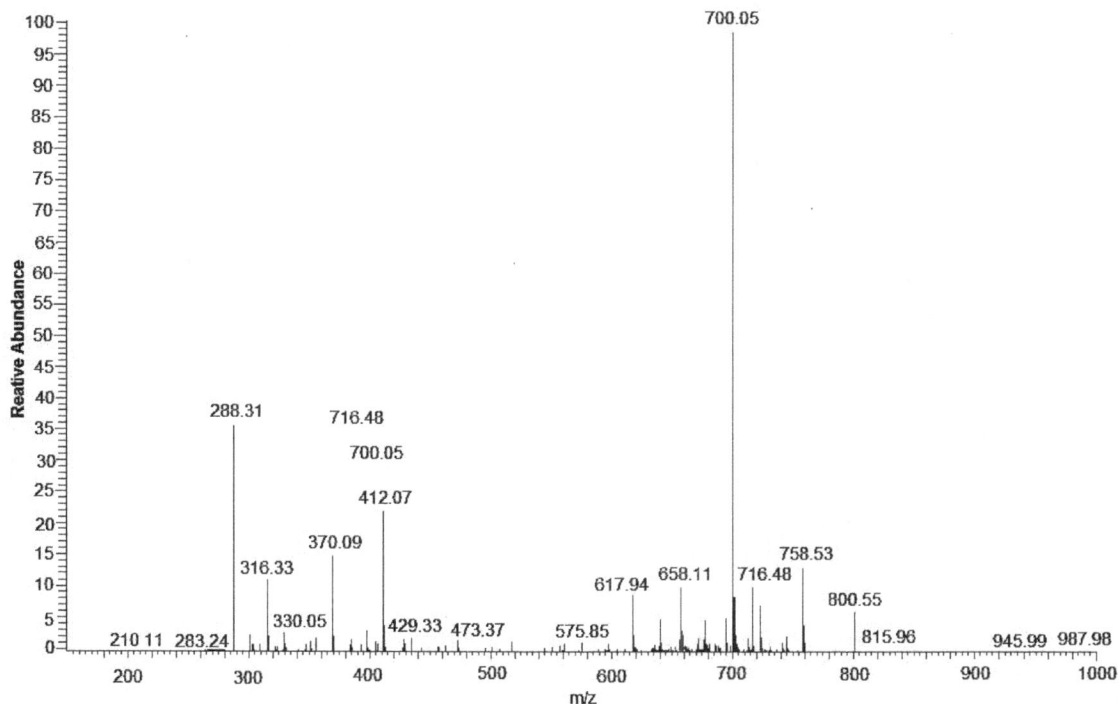

Figure 2. Mass spectrometry of the targeted compound (**B**).

^{1}H-NMR (400 MHz, CDCl$_3$): δ = 1.94-2.19 (8s, 24H, Ac), 3.85-3.92 (m, 3H, H-4, H-5 and H-5'), 4.06-4.16 (m, 3H, H-6a',H-6b' and H-6a), 4.38-4.44 (m, 2H, H-2, H-6b), 4.53 (d,1H, *J* = 8 Hz, H-1'), 4.98 (dd, 1H, H-3'), 5.15 (dd, 1H, H-2'), 5.25 (dd,1H, H-3), 5.39 (dd,1H, H-4'), 5.72 (d, 1H, *J* = 8.8 Hz, NH), 6.1 (d, 1H, *J* = 3.2, H-1).
MS (ESI)+ m/z: calcd for C$_{28}$H$_{39}$NO$_{18}$: 677.21, found: 700.20 [M+Na]$^+$

1D and 2D NMR study of B

The values of the ^{1}H NMR chemical shifts for **B** in CDCl$_3$ solution are reported in the previous section 3.4. Referring to the ^{1}H NMR chemical shifts for **B** illustrated eight signals appeared as singlet in the most high-field region of δ = 1.94 ppm, δ = 1.98 ppm, δ = 2.06 ppm, δ =

2.08 , δ = 2.11, δ = 2.13, δ = 2.16, δ = 2.19, for 8s, 24H, and COCH$_3$, respectively. This is due to the protons in CH$_3$ presents in COCH$_3$ groups (8s, 24H, COCH$_3$). Additionally, a multiplet which appeared in the high-field region at δ = 3.85-3.92 ppm was assigned to the three protons namely; m, 3H, H-4, H-5 and H-5'. A resonating, which appeared as multiplet at the range of δ = 4.06 - 416 ppm were assigned for protons (m, 3H, H-6a', H-6b' and H-6a). On the other hand, the multiplet at the range of δ = 4.38 - 4.44 ppm was assigned to the protons namely; m, 2H, H-2, H-6b. Moreover, proton H-1'was assigned for the doublet which appeared at the range of δ = 4.53 ppm (d, 1H, *J* = 8 Hz, H-1'). The doublet of doublet at δ = 4.98 dd ppm, was assigned to the proton (dd, 1H, H-3'). Also, the ^{1}H NMR data showed that the signals of the protons due to 1H, H-2' was assigned as doublet of doublet at δ = 5.15 ppm (dd, 1H, H-2'). The signal of proton due to 1H, H-3 appeared at δ = 5.25 ppm (dd, 1H, H-3). The signal of proton due to 1H, H-4' appeared at δ = 5.39 ppm (dd, 1H, H-4'). Additionally, the signal of proton due to 1H, NH appeared at δ = 5.72 ppm (d, 1H, J = 8.8 Hz, NH) and the signal of H-1 appeared as a doublet at δ = 6.1 ppm (d, J = 3.2 Hz, 1H, H-1).

Conclusion

An efficient chemoenzymatic procedure in order to optimize the preparation of PL 3 containing acetyl ester as extraordinary protecting group is presented herein. Compound **B** is a significant intermediate for the synthesis of pharmacologically active compound (e.g., complex oligosaccharides for biochemical, biophysical, or biological examinations and so on).[27] Immobilized lipase from CRGL has been contrasted and the immobilized ACEXE from *Bacillus pumilus*, with regard to their exploitation in biotransformation of PL 1. CRGL was immobilized on two diverse solid supports, to be specific; OSCL, and DSEOD including hydrophobic adsorption. While ACEXE was covalently linked to the matrix by means of oxirane-groups sepabeads. The hydrolysis of **A** which catalyzed by CRGL affirmed that the performance of the immobilized enzyme is strongly affected by the kind of support. Lipase immobilized on DSEOD was more active and regioselective than the lipase immobilized on OSCL, producing **1A** in 98% at 100% of conversion, and 27% at 75% of conversion of **A**, respectively.

Besides, reaction monitoring utilizing HPLC proposes more exact information than spectroscopic methods. For instance, it gives the content of starting material, product and the impurities during the course of the reaction. Besides, these outcomes help researchers and scientist to optimize and enhance the reaction conditions, improve the quality and quantity of the product. Moreover, we conclude that HPLC is considered as an effective and important tool for *in-process* analysis. It aids to increase the quality, quantity of the products and reduce the manufacturing cost. In this work, an isocratic HPLC method for controlling the hydrolysis of **A** to **1A** with the guide of ACEXE and CRGL-OSCL was developed. The newly developed method was observed to be simple, and able of separating the two substrates in addition to all *by-products* connected with the process of hydrolysis. In this way, this method can be valuable for *in-process* control and additionally quality affirmation in the pharmaceutical industry.

Acknowledgments

This work was funded by Drug Sciences Department, Pavia University, Italy.

Ethical Issues

Not applicable.

Conflict of Interest

The authors declare no conflict of interests.

References

1. Varki A, Cummings RD, Esko JD, Freeze HH, Stanley P, Bertozzi CR, et al. Essential of Glycobiology. New York: Cold Spring Harbor Laboratory Press; 2009.
2. Bertozzi CR, Kiessling LL. Chemical glycobiology. *Science* 2001;291(5512):2357-64.
3. Lis H, Sharon N. Lectins: carbohydrate-specific proteins that mediate cellular recognition. *Chem Rev* 1998;98(2):637-74.
4. Broder W, Kunz H. A new method of anomeric protection and activation based on the conversion of glycosyl azides into glycosyl fluorides. *Carbohydr Res* 1993;249(1):221-41.
5. Broder W, Kunz H. Glycosyl azides as building blocks in convergent syntheses of oligomeric lactosamine and lewis(x) saccharides. *Bioorg Med Chem* 1997;5(1):1-19.
6. Chuang HY, Ren CT, Chao CA, Wu CY, Shivatare SS, Cheng TJ, et al. Synthesis and vaccine evaluation of the tumor-associated carbohydrate antigen rm2 from prostate cancer. *J Am Chem Soc* 2013;135(30):11140-50. doi: 10.1021/ja403609x
7. Seeberger PH, Werz DB. Synthesis and medical applications of oligosaccharides. *Nature* 2007;446(7139):1046-51. doi: 10.1038/nature05819
8. Schmidt RR. New methods for the synthesis of glycosides and oligosaccharide are there alternative to the koenigs-knorr method? *Angew Chem Int Edit* 1986;25(3):212-35. doi: 10.1002/anie.198602121
9. Kocienski PJ. Protecting Groups. 3 rd ed. New York: Georg Thieme Verlag: Stuttgart; 2005.
10. Gamblin DP, Scanlan EM, Davis BG. Glycoprotein synthesis: An update. *Chem Rev* 2009;109(1):131-63. doi: 10.1021/cr078291i
11. Boltje TJ, Buskas T, Boons GJ. Opportunities and challenges in synthetic oligosaccharide and glycoconjugate research. *Nat Chem* 2009;1(8):611-22. doi: 10.1038/nchem.399
12. Davis BG. Synthesis of glycoproteins. *Chem Rev* 2002;102(2):579-602.
13. Stallforth P, Lepenies B, Adibekian A, Seeberger PH. 2009 claude s. Hudson award in carbohydrate chemistry. Carbohydrates: A frontier in medicinal chemistry. *J Med Chem* 2009;52(18):5561-77. doi: 10.1021/jm900819p
14. Abualassal Q, Al Azzam KM, Jilani JA. Regioselective deprotection of the monosaccharide-bearing thiocyanomethyl group at the anomeric position monitored by reversed-phase hplc method. *Biomed Chromatogr* 2016;30(9):1416-22. doi: 10.1002/bmc.3699
15. Wartewig S, Neubert RH. Pharmaceutical applications of mid-ir and raman spectroscopy. *Adv Drug Deliv Rev* 2005;57(8):1144-70. doi: 10.1016/j.addr.2005.01.022

16. Schafer WA, Hobbs S, Rehm J, Rakestraw ADA, Orella C, McLaughlin M, et al. Mobile tool for HPLC reaction monitoring. *J Org Process Res Dev* 2007;11(5):870-6. doi: 10.1021/op7000854

17. Yu XX, Wang QW, Xu XJ, Lv WJ, Zhao MQ, Liang ZK. Preparative isolation of Heteroclitin D from Kadsurae Caulis using normal-phase flash chromatography. *J Pharm Anal* 2013;3(6):456-9. doi: 10.1016/j.jpha.2013.07.004

18. Weber P, Hamburger M, Schafroth N, Potterat O. Flash chromatography on cartridges for the separation of plant extracts: Rules for the selection of chromatographic conditions and comparison with medium pressure liquid chromatography. *Fitoterapia* 2011;82(2):155-61. doi: 10.1016/j.fitote.2010.08.013

19. Bavaro T, Filice M, Bonomi P, Abu Alassal Q, Speranza G, Guisan JM, et al. Regioselective deprotection of peracetylated disaccharides at the primary position catalyzed by immobilized acetyl xylan esterase from Bacillus pumilus. *Eur J Org Chem* 2011; 31: 6181-5. doi: 10.1002/ejoc.201100944

20. Bastida A, Sabuquillo P, Armisen P, Fernandez-Lafuente R, Huguet J, Guisan JM. A single step purification, immobilization, and hyperactivation of lipases via interfacial adsorption on strongly hydrophobic supports. *Biotechnol Bioeng* 1998;58(5):486-93.

21. Terreni M, Salvetti R, Linati L, Fernandez-Lafuente R, Fernandez-Lorente G, Bastida A, et al. Regioselective enzymatic hydrolysis of acetylated pyranoses and pyranosides using immobilised lipases. An easy chemoenzymatic synthesis of alpha- and beta-d-glucopyranose acetates bearing a free secondary c-4 hydroxyl group. *Carbohydr Res* 2002;337(18):1615-21.

22. Filice M, Bavaro T, Fernandez-Lafuente R, Pregnolato M, Guisan JM, Palomo JM, et al. Chemo-biocatalytic regioselective one-pot synthesis of different deprotected monosaccharides. *Catal Today* 2009;140:11-8. doi: 10.1016/j.cattod.2008.07.016

23. Cheng H, Cao X, Xian M, Fang L, Cai TB, Ji JJ, et al. Synthesis and enzyme-specific activation of carbohydrate-geldanamycin conjugates with potent anticancer activity. *J Med Chem* 2005;48(2):645-52. doi: 10.1021/jm049693a

24. Wei Z, Luo M, Zhao C, Wang W, Zhang L, Zu Y, et al. An efficient preparative procedure for main flavone aglycones from Equisetum palustre L. using macroporous resin followed by gel resin flash chromatography. *Sep Purif Technol* 2013;118:680-9. doi: 10.1016/j.seppur.2013.07.045

25. Snyder LR, Kirkland JJ, Glajch JL. Practical HPLC Method Development. 2nd ed. New York: John Wiley & Sons; 1997.

26. Patsavas MC, Byrne RH, Liu X. Purification of meta-cresol purple and cresol red by flash chromatography: Procedures for ensuring accurate spectrophotometric seawater pH measurements. *Mar Chem* 2013;150:19-24. doi: 10.1016/j.marchem.2013.01.004

27. Filice M, Palomo JM. Monosaccharide derivatives as central scaffolds in the synthesis of glycosylated drugs. *RSC Adv* 2012;2:1729-42. doi: 10.1039/C2RA00515H

11

Cord Blood Cells Responses to IL2, IL7 and IL15 Cytokines for mTOR Expression

Anahita Mohammadian[§], Elahe Naderali[§], Seyedeh Momeneh Mohammadi, Aliakbar Movasaghpour, Behnaz Valipour, Mohammad Nouri, Hojjatollah Nozad Charoudeh*

Stem Cell Research Center, Tabriz university of Medical Sciences, Tabriz, Iran.

Keywords:
· Cord blood
· mTOR
· Cytokines

Abstract

Purpose: Mammalian target of rapamycin (mTOR)is important in hematopoiesis and affect cell growth,differentiation and survival. Although previous studies were identified the effect of cytokines on the mononuclear cells development however the cytokines effect on mTOR in cord blood mononuclear cells was unclear. The aim of this study was to evaluate mTOR expression in cord blood mononuclear and cord blood stem cells (CD34+ cells) in culture conditions for lymphoid cell development.

Methods: Isolation of The mononuclear cells (MNCs) from umbilical cord blood were done with use of Ficollpaque density gradient. We evaluated cultured cord blood mononuclear and CD34+ cells in presece of IL2, IL7 and IL15 at distinct time points during 21 days by using flow cytometry. In this study, we presented the role of IL2, IL7 and IL15 on the expression of mTOR in cord blood cells.

Results: mTOR expression were increased in peresence of IL2, IL7 and IL15 in day 14 and afterword reduced. However in persence of IL2 and IL15 expression of mTOR significantly reduced. mTOR expression in CD34+ cells decreased significantly from day7 to day 21 in culture.

Conclusion: cytokines play important role in mTOR expression during hematopoiesis and development of cord blood mononuclear cells.

Introduction

Mammalian target of rapamycin (mTOR), a serine/threonine kinase has important role in cell growth, differentiation and survival in hematopoiesis.[1-3] both extracellular and intracellular signals can activate mTOR complex includs mTOR complex 1(mTORC1) and mTOR complex 2(mTORC2). Every changes in cells and microenvironment of cells for example cell nutrient ,stress, cytokine , hormone receptors and immuneregulatory signals are able to activate mTOR signaling pathway.[4-6] It has shown that mTOR pathway is clearly important in regulation of adaptive immune cells activation.[7,8] Recently studies suggested that mTOR controls the activity of B, T and natural killer cells[4] antigen receptors and vis versa cytokine receptors (for example IL-2 receptor)can activate mTOR signaling.[8,9] Morever mTOR have a critical role in the decisions between effector and regulatory T cell lineage commitment,[10] and influences on the migratory properties of murine CD8+ T lymphocytes.[8.11] Despite of limited studies about mTOR role in B cells activity, it was shown that inhibition of mTOR by rapamycin reduce B cell proliferation and differentiation of plasma cell.[4,12,13] Cell cycle progression from G1 into S phase was controlled by mTOR in NK cells,[14] however mTOR couldnot affect on NK cell cytotoxicity and cytokine production.[14,15] IL-2 plays important role in T cell growth, proliferation of activated B cells and on NK cells differentiation.[16] Also IL15 has important role in NK and CD8 T cell devlopment.[17,18] It has shown that IL-7 is a key cytokine in B, T cell proliferation and thymic NK cell development.[16]

It is clearly known that cord blood cells are an important source for stem cell transplantation and immune cell therapy. It is well to underestand mTOR expression during development of B, T and NK cells from cord blood cells.

Herein, we evaluated mTOR expression in mononuclear and CD34+ umbilical cord blood cells and wethere IL-2, IL-7 and IL-15 could alter mTOR expression during in vitro culture.

Materials and Methods

Mononuclear cord blood isolation and CD34+ cells enrichment

Cord blood sampling has been done as reported in previous studies[16,19-21] Umbilical cord blood samples of full-term normal deliveries assembled and diluted 1:2 with phosphate buffered saline (PBS) plus 10% fetal bovine serum (FBS). Separating of mononuclear cells were done with use of Ficollpaque (GE healthcare -1.078

---

*Corresponding author: Hojjatollah Nozad Charoudeh, Email: nozadh@tbzmed.ac.ir, §: Equal contribution in first author

g/ml), by centrifuge. Isolated MNCs collected and washed twice in RPMI 1640(Gibco) plus 5% fetal bovine serum (FBS; Gibco). Cord blood mononuclear cells (MNCs) were incubated with 100 μl of CD34+ micro beads (Miltenyi Biotec, Germany Cat no: 130100453) for 30 minutes, cells were passed through LS MACS column (Miltenyi Biotec, Germany) and enriched CD34+ cells were collected in 15 ml tubes by flushing the column. Purity of CD34+ cells evaluated by flow cytometry in FACSCalibur (BD Bioscience) and data analyzed by Flow software version X.0.7.

Culture condition

Seeding of the 10^5 MNCs and isolated CD34+ cells were accomplished in 96-well plates in 250 μL of RPMI1640 supplemented with 20% FBS, 1% penicillin/streptomycin (Gibco), plus cytokines with final concentrations of: SCF (40 ng/ml), Flt3 ligand (FL, 40 ng/mL), interleukin-7 (IL-7, 40 ng/mL), IL-15 (40 ng/mL), and IL-2 (40 ng/mL) (all cytokines were purchased from PeproTech, USA). All cultures have done for 21 days at 37°C with replacing of half of the culture medium every week. Cultured cells were collected in indicated days and analyzed by flow cytometry for mTOR positive cells.

Flow cytometry

Harvested cells were incubated with monoclonal mTOR Antibody (Novus Biologicals USA, Cat no: IC1537P) for 20 minutes in 4 degrees. Stained cells were evaluated by BD caliber (BDebioscience). Between 10,000 to 30,000 events were collected and analyzed using BD flowjo.

Result

mTOR expression in umbilical cord blood mononuclear cells during culture with by existence of Cytokines

Mammalian target of rapamycin (mTOR) has important role in cell growth, differentiation and survival in hematopoiesis.[1-3]

We cultured 1x 10^5 cord blood mononuclear cells and evaluated the relation between IL2, IL7 and IL15 cytokines and expresssion of mTOR in vitro by FACS at indicated time points (Figure 1-A).

mTOR expression in presence of all cytokines increased in day14 (59.7%) and decreased in day 21 (19.7) in compaire with day 7 (26.4%). The highest mTOR expression was seen in day 14 and There was significant decline of mTOR expression in day 21 (Figure 1-B).

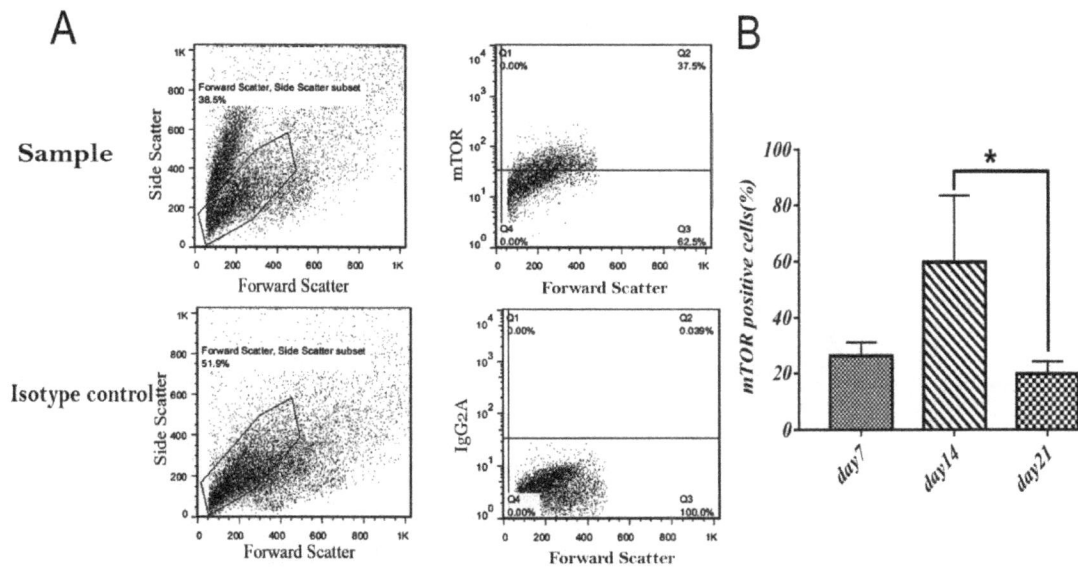

Figure 1. Expression of mTOR in cord blood mononuclear cells. (A) Representative FACS plots for mTOR expression. (B) Mean(SD) proportion of mTOR expression was evaluated in harvested cord blood mononuclear cells in indicated time points.in presence of SCF+FLt3+IL2+IL7+IL15. Values shown are mean ± SD from 3 independent experiments with 20-30 wells analyzed (*p <0.05).

Rlationship between mTOR expression and immune cell cytokines

To evaluate the effect of IL2, IL7 and IL15 on mTOR expression, cord blood mononuclear cells were culcured with IL2, IL7 and IL15 for 21 days. The SCF and Flt3 were suplemented in to all groups. mTOR expression was significantly lower in presence of IL15 (8.2%). Also mTOR expression reduced after co-culture with IL2 (22%) but did not altered in presence

of IL7 (32.4 %) in comparison with SCF and Flt3 (31%) (Figure 2).

mTOR expression in CD34$^+$ cells

We cultured 1x10^5 CD34+ cells for 21 days without cytokines and observed expression of mTOR by flow cytometry in vitro conditions at distinct days (Figure 3-A). the percentage of mTOR positive cells decreased from day 0 to day 21 significantly from 96% to 26%. mTOR expression was lowest in day 14 (20 %) (Figure 3-B).

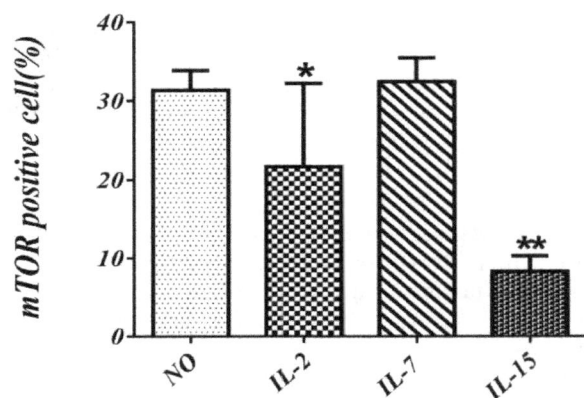

Figure 2. Evaluation of mTOR expression in cord blood mononuclear cells in vitro in presence of different cytokines at day 21. SCF and Flt3L have been included in all groups. Values shown are mean ± SD from 3 independent experiments with 10-12 wells analyezed in each groups (**p <0.01).

Discution

mTOR signaling is necessary during immune cell development, particularly in activated cells that are proliferative (for example activated T and B lymphocytes) and illustrated that mTOR activation in immune cells is higher than most of the other non-immune cells during development.[8,19,20] mTOR is involve in sensing of the immune microenvironment and dictating immune function and differentiation.[6] In this study we showed that mTOR expression in cord blood mononuclear as well as in $CD34^+$ cells decreased during development which was affected by cytokinese. IL2 and IL15 had dominant role,in particular mTOR expression was influenced by IL15 more than IL2. Cytokines are soluble mediators of intercellular signals and regulate and activate the adaptive and innate immunity.[21,22] Immune cell cytokines(IL-2, IL-7 and IL-15) control development of Natural killer cell, T and B lymphocyte and regulate hematopoiesis, proliferation, self-renewal, differentiation and senescence of HSCs (Hematopoietic stem cells).[23,24] mTOR is sensitive to the various environmental or cellular signals and the fate of immune cells was affected by interaction of these signals on each other.[5,25-27] mTOR plays essential role in lymphocytes.[8] mTOR via effect on T-bet expression and IL-7 and IL-15 receptors can control STAT5 signaling indirectly,[5] also mTOR is activated in response to IL-2 signaling. IL-2 maintains the tolerance between effector and regulatory T cells.[10] mTOR controls proper migration of $CD8^+$ T lymphocytes, although its not completely demonstrated in vivo and require more evidence. However mTOR implicate in controlling intraction between actin and microtubule cytoskeletons in T cells. Progression of cell cycle from G1 into S phase controlled by mTOR pathway in IL-2-stimulated T lymphocytes. deletion of the Cdk inhibitor protein p27Kip1 by IL-2 is able activate Cdk that rapamycin prevente this process in T cells.[28] Also cell cycle progression was controlled by mTOR in (NK) cells.[15]

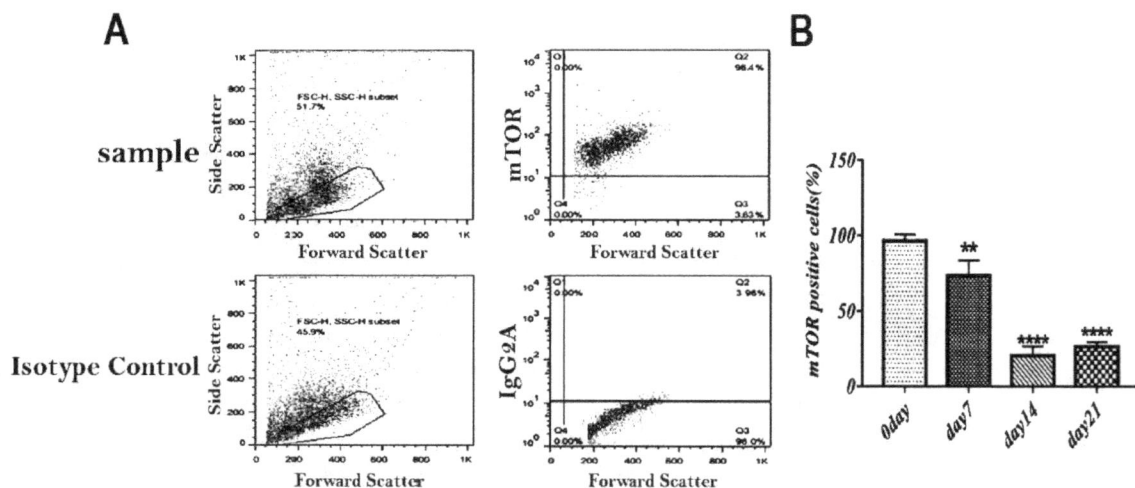

Figure 3. Expression of mTOR in cord blood CD34+ cells in vitro in indicated time points. (A) Representative FACS plots, (B) Mean(SD) percentage of mTOR expression in harvrested cells in different time points. Mean value preseanted from 12-18 wells were analyzed. Pvalue between day 7 and 14 and 21 (**p <0.01, and ****p<0.0001).

Conclusion

Taken together, mTOR expreseed in cord blood cells cells during culture with IL2, IL7 and IL15 and it is important factor in Immune cell development in particular in cord blood derived B, T and NK cell in response to key immune cell cytokines. It is important to investigate mTOR behaveier in furture study.

Acknowledgments

This work has been approved by Novin School of Advanced Medical Sciences and financially supported by Research Council of Tabriz University of Medical Sciences with Grant code: 5.104.1209.

Ethical Issues

This study was approved by ethical committee of Tabriz University of Medical Sciences with ethical number: 5.4.10696.

Conflict of Interest

The authors report no conflicts of interest.

References

1. Drayer AL, Olthof SG, Vellenga E. Mammalian Target of Rapamycin Is Required for Thrombopoietin-Induced Proliferation of Megakaryocyte Progenitors. *Stem Cells* 2006;24(1):105-14. doi: 10.1634/stemcells.2005-0062
2. Cruz R, Hedden L, Boyer D, Kharas MG, Fruman DA, Lee-Fruman KK. S6 kinase 2 potentiates interleukin-3-driven cell proliferation. *J Leukoc Biol* 2005;78(6):1378-85. doi: 10.1189/jlb.0405225
3. Rohrabaugh SL, Campbell TB, Hangoc G, Broxmeyer HE. Ex vivo rapamycin treatment of human cord blood CD34+ cells enhances their engraftment of NSG mice. *Blood Cells Mol Dis* 2011;46(4):318-20. doi: 10.1016/j.bcmd.2011.02.006
4. Xu X, Ye L, Araki K, Ahmed R. mTOR, linking metabolism and immunity. *Semin Immunol* 2012;24(6):429-35. doi: 10.1016/j.smim.2012.12.005
5. Saleiro D, Platanias LC. Intersection of mTOR and STAT signaling in immunity. *Trends Immunol* 2015;36(1):21-9. doi: 10.1016/j.it.2014.10.006
6. Delgoffe GM, Pollizzi KN, Waickman AT, Heikamp E, Meyers DJ, Horton MR, et al. The kinase mTOR regulates the differentiation of helper T cells through the selective activation of signaling by mTORC1 and mTORC2. *Nat Immunol* 2011;12(4):295-303. doi: 10.1038/ni.2005
7. Hay N, Sonenberg N. Upstream and downstream of mTOR. *Genes Dev* 2004;18(16):1926-45. doi: 10.1101/gad.1212704
8. Weichhart T, Säemann MD. The multiple facets of mTOR in immunity. *Trends Immunol* 2009;30(5):218-26. doi: 10.1016/j.it.2009.02.002
9. Fruman DA. Towards an understanding of isoform specificity in phosphoinositide 3-kinase signalling in lymphocytes. *Biochem Soc Trans* 2004;32(Pt 2):315-9. doi: 10.1042/bst0320315
10. Delgoffe GM, Kole TP, Zheng Y, Zarek PE, Matthews KL, Xiao B, et al. The mTOR kinase differentially regulates effector and regulatory T cell lineage commitment. *Immunity* 2009;30(6):832-44. doi: 10.1016/j.immuni.2009.04.014
11. Sinclair LV, Finlay D, Feijoo C, Cornish GH, Gray A, Ager A, et al. Phosphatidylinositol-3-OH kinase and nutrient-sensing mTOR pathways control T lymphocyte trafficking. *Nat Immunol* 2008;9(5):513-21. doi: 10.1038/ni.1603
12. Wicker LS, Boltz RC Jr, Matt V, Nichols EA, Peterson LB, Sigal NH. Suppression of B cell activation by cyclosporin A, FK506 and rapamycin. *Eur J Immunol* 1990;20(10):2277-83. doi: 10.1002/eji.1830201017
13. Donahue AC, Fruman DA. Distinct signaling mechanisms activate the target of rapamycin in response to different B-cell stimuli. *Eur J Immunol* 2007;37(10):2923-36. doi: 10.1002/eji.200737281
14. Säemann MD, Haidinger M, Hecking M, Hörl WH, Weichhart T. The multifunctional role of mTOR in innate immunity: implications for transplant immunity. *Am J Transplant* 2009;9(12):2655-61. doi: 10.1111/j.1600-6143.2009.02832.x
15. Thomson AW, Turnquist HR, Raimondi G. Immunoregulatory functions of mTOR inhibition. *Nat Rev Immunol* 2009;9(5):324-37. doi: 10.1038/nri2546
16. Aliyari Z, Alemi F, Brazvan B, Tayefi Nasrabadi H, Nozad Charoudeh H. CD26+ Cord Blood Mononuclear Cells Significantly Produce B, T, and NK Cells. *Iran J Immunol* 2015;12(1):16-26.
17. Kobayashi H, Dubois S, Sato N, Sabzevari H, Sakai Y, Waldmann TA, et al. Role of trans-cellular IL-15 presentation in the activation of NK cell-mediated killing, which leads to enhanced tumor immunosurveillance. *Blood* 2005;105(2):721-7. doi: 10.1182/blood-2003-12-4187
18. Cooper MA, Fehniger TA, Turner SC, Chen KS, Ghaheri BA, Ghayur T, et al. Human natural killer cells: a unique innate immunoregulatory role for the CD56(bright) subset. *Blood* 2001;97(10):3146-51. doi: 10.1182/blood.V97.10.3146
19. Shillingford JM, Murcia NS, Larson CH, Low SH, Hedgepeth R, Brown N, et al. The mTOR pathway is regulated by polycystin-1, and its inhibition reverses renal cystogenesis in polycystic kidney disease. *Proc Natl Acad Sci U S A* 2006;103(14):5466-71. doi: 10.1073/pnas.0509694103
20. Weimbs T. Polycystic kidney disease and renal injury repair: common pathways, fluid flow, and the function of polycystin-1. *Am J Physiol Renal Physiol* 2007;293(5):F1423-32. doi: 10.1152/ajprenal.00275.2007
21. Khaziri N, Mohammadi M, Aliyari Z, Soleimani Rad J, Tayefi Nasrabadi H, Nozad Charoudeh H. Cord Blood Mononuclear Cells Have a Potential to Produce NK Cells Using IL2Rg Cytokines. *Adv Pharm Bull* 2016;6(1):5-8.
22. Rochman Y, Spolski R, Leonard WJ. New insights into the regulation of T cells by γc family cytokines. *Nat Rev Immunol* 2009;9(7):480-90. doi: 10.1038/nri2580
23. Copley MR, Beer PA, Eaves CJ. Hematopoietic stem cell heterogeneity takes center stage. *Cell Stem Cell* 2012;10(6):690-7. doi: 10.1016/j.stem.2012.05.006
24. Brazvan B, Farahzadi R, Mohammadi SM, Montazer Saheb S, Shanehbandi D, Schmied L, et al. Key Immune Cell Cytokines Affects the Telomere Activity of Cord Blood Cells In vitro. *Adv Pharm Bull* 2016;6(2):153-61. doi: 10.15171/apb.2016.022
25. Powell JD, Pollizzi KN, Heikamp EB, Horton MR. Regulation of immune responses by mTOR. *Annu*

Rev Immunol 2012;30:39-68. doi: 10.1146/annurev-immunol-020711-075024

26. Yang H, Wang X, Zhang Y, Liu H, Liao J, Shao K, et al. Modulation of TSC-mTOR signaling on immune cells in immunity and autoimmunity. *J Cell Physiol* 2014;229(1):17-26. doi: 10.1002/jcp.24426

27. Contreras AG, Dormond O, Edelbauer M, Calzadilla K, Hoerning A, Pal S, et al. mTOR-understanding the clinical effects. *Transplant Proc* 2008;40(10 Suppl):S9-S12. doi: 10.1016/j.transproceed.2008.10.011

28. Nourse J, Firpo E, Flanagan WM, Coats S, Polyak K, Lee MH, et al. Interleukin-2-mediated elimination of the p27Kip1 cyclin-dependent kinase inhibitor prevented by rapamycin. *Nature* 1994;372(6506):570-3. doi: 10.1038/372570a0

siRNA-Mediated Silencing of CIP2A Enhances Docetaxel Activity Against PC-3 Prostate Cancer Cells

Saiedeh Razi Soofiyani[1,2], **Akbar Mohammad Hoseini**[1], **Ali Mohammadi**[1], **Vahid Khaze Shahgoli**[1], **Behzad Baradaran**[1][*][δ], **Mohammad Saeid Hejazi**[3,2][*][δ]

[1] *Immunology Research Center, Tabriz University of Medical Sciences, Tabriz, Iran.*
[2] *Department of Molecular Medicine, Faculty of Advanced Biomedical Sciences, Tabriz University of Medical Sciences, Tabriz, Iran.*
[3] *Molecular Medicine Research Center, Tabriz University of Medical Sciences, Tabriz, Iran.*

Keywords:
· CIP2A
· Docetaxel
· Prostate cancer
· siRNA

Abstract

Purpose: Cancerous inhibitor of protein phosphatase 2A (CIP2A) is an identified human oncoprotein which modulates malignant cell growth. It is overexpressed in human prostate cancer and in most of the human malignancies. The aim of this study was to investigate the effects of CIP2A silencing on the sensitivity of PC-3 prostate cancer cells to docetaxel chemotherapy.

Methods: PC-3 cells were transfected using CIP2A siRNA. CIP2A mRNA and protein expression were assessed after CIP2A gene silencing using q-RT PCR and Western blotting. Proliferation and apoptosis were analyzed after treatment with docetaxol using MTT assay, DAPI staining, and flow cytometry, respectively.

Results: Silencing of CIP2A enhanced the sensitivity of PC-3 cells to docetaxel by strengthening docetaxel induced cell growth inhibition and apoptosis against PC-3 cells.

Conclusion: Silencing of CIP2A may potentiate the cytotoxic effects of docetaxel and this might be a promising therapeutic approach in prostate cancer treatment.

Introduction

Prostate cancer is the common malignancy among men and it accounts for the second cause of cancer-related death in men.[1,2] In spite of significant efforts in the treatment of prostate cancer, conventional therapies could not successfully treat the tumors. Therefore, most of the patients will develop castration resistant prostate cancer (CRPC) for the duration of 18-24 months and this is associated with poor prognosis.[3,4] Chemotherapy, using docetaxel as a taxan family member, is the first choice for the treatment of CRPC.[5,6] The anti-tumor effects of docetaxel depend on its ability to promote microtubules polymerization and stabilization, which leads to cell cycle arrest and apoptosis.[7,8] The toxicity and undesirable events in docetaxel based treatment reduce the therapeutic efficacy and limit its tolerated dose.[9] Lack of efficient treatments shows the importance of additional means to develop effective therapeutic approaches in the treatment of prostate cancer. One of the feasible approaches consists of combining a chemotherapy agent with silencing specific proteins involved in proliferation and survival of the cancer cells using RNA interference technology due to RNAi's high specificity, noticeable efficacy, and low toxicity when compared with the other reverse genetic technologies.[10-12] Cancerous inhibitor of protein phosphatase 2A (CIP2A), a human oncoprotein, is generally overexpressed in most human malignancies and its overexpression is closely associated with poor outcome in patients.[13,14] It promotes malignant cell growth and tumor progression.[15] It is overexpressed in prostate cancer samples and cell lines.[16,17]

Since, the effect of CIP2A suppression on docetaxel induced cytotoxicity against prostate cancer cells has not been reported, this study investigated the effects of CIP2A silencing on the sensitivity of PC-3 cells to docetaxel chemotherapy.

Materials and Methods

Cell culture and drug

PC-3, human prostate cancer cells (Pasteur Institute, Iran), were cultured in RPMI-1640 medium (GIBCO, Carlsbad, CA, USA) supplemented with 10% FBS (Invitrogen Life Technologies), containing 100 U/mL penicillin and 100 µg/mL streptomycin (Sigma-Aldrich, St. Louis, MO, USA) in a humidified atmosphere of 5% CO_2 at 37°C. Docetaxel, 10 mg/ml (Hospira UK Co., Ltd) was used at the concentrations of 0.39 to 50 nM.

siRNA transfection

CIP2A siRNA, negative control siRNA (not homologous to any gene), and siRNA transfection reagent were purchased from Santa Cruz Biotechnology, USA. CIP2A siRNA (human) is a pool of 3 different siRNA duplexes (Table 1). To knock down the CIP2A expression with

Corresponding authors: Behzad Baradaran, Mohammad saeid Hejazi, Email: baradaranb@tbzmed.ac.ir,
Email: msaeidhejazi@yahoo.com δ: These authors were equally contributed in this work.

CIP2A siRNA, the cells at 2×10^5/well density were seeded in 6-well plate and cultured overnight before transfection using CIP2A siRNA according to the manufacturer's instruction. Briefly, siRNA transfection medium was used to dilute siRNAs and siRNA transfection reagent. The diluted solutions were mixed gently and incubated at room temperature for 15 to 30 min. Then, the complexes were added to each well and were incubated in a humidified CO_2 incubator at 37°C for 6 h. 1 ml of RPMI-1640 medium containing 20% FBS was added to each well. After 24, 48, and 72 h, down-regulation of CIP2A was monitored using quantitative RT-PCR (qRT-PCR) and Western blotting.

Table 1. Three different siRNA duplexes.

siRNA duplexs pool	Sense	Antisense
sc-77964A	5′ CUAGCAGUAGACAUUGAAAtt 3′	5′ UUUCAAUGUCUACUGCUAGtt 3′
sc-77964B	5′ GUACCACUCUUAUAGAACAtt 3′	5′ UGUUCUAUAAGAGUGGUACtt 3′
sc-77964C	5′ GGAAGUAAGCUUCUACAAAtt 3′	5′ UUUGUAGAAGCUUACUUCCtt 3′

Quantitative RT-PCR
Total RNA was extracted from the cells using the RiboEx total RNA extraction kit (GeneAll Biotechnology CO, LTD, Korea). cDNA was synthesized using random Hexamer (rH) primer and Moloney murine leukemia virus (M-MuLV) reverse transcriptase (Fermentas Life Sciences, Vilnius, Lithuania). The primer sequences were as follows: GAPDH, forward 5′ CAAGATCATCACCAATGCCT 3′; reverse: 5′ CCCATCACGCCACAGTTTCC 3′; CIP2A, forward 5′GATTATTGGCAAATCTTTGTCGG 3′; reverse 5′CTGATGAATGTTTCGAGCATGG 3′. qPCR was done using SYBR Green Master Mix (Ampliqon III, VWR-Bie Berntsen, Denmark) on LightCycler® 96 System (Roche Diagnostics, Mannheim, Germany) as follows: 95°C for 10 min, followed by 40 cycles at 94°C for 10 s, 60°C for 30 s, and 72°C for 20 s, using GAPDH as an endogenous control for sample normalization. The relative expression level of mRNAs was calculated using the $2^{(-\Delta\Delta Ct)}$ method (Livak and Schmittgen, 2001).

Western blotting analysis
The cells lysate was prepared using RIPA Lysis Buffer System (Santa Cruz Biotechnology, USA) according to the manufacturer's instruction and was quantified using NanoDrop (Thermo Scientific, Wilmington, USA). 50 μL of protein was separated using 10% SDS-PAGE gel electrophoresis and transferred to polyvinyl difluoride membranes (Roche Diagnostics GmbH). After blocking using blocking buffer containing 0.5% Tween-20 for 2 h at 25°C, the membranes were incubated with primary antibodies against CIP2A (1:200; Santa Cruz Biotechnology, USA) and monoclonal antibody against β-actin (1:5000, Abcam) overnight at 4°C. After washing, the membranes were incubated using the secondary antibodies conjugated to horseradish peroxidase (1:3000, Razi Biotech Co, Tehran, Iran) for 2 h at room temperature. Protein bands were visualized using enhanced BM chemiluminescence blotting substrate POD (Roche Diagnostics GmbH, Mannheim, Germany) and Western blot imaging system (Sabz BIOMEDICALS, Iran). To quantify the bands intensity,

ImageJ software version 1.44 software (National Institutes of Health, Bethesda, USA) was used.

Cytotoxicity assay
PC-3 cells (7×10^3) were seeded into 96-well plates. The cells were transfected using CIP2A siRNA. 48 h after CIP2A-siRNA transfection, the cells were treated using different concentrations of the docetaxol (0.39-50 nM) for 24 h. Then, 50 μL of MTT solution (2 mg/mL) was added to each well and was incubated in the humidified incubator containing 5% CO_2 at 37°C for 4 h. Then, 200 μl of DMSO and 25 μl Sorenson buffer were added to each well. The optical density (OD) of each well was measured using a microplate reader (Awareness Technology, Palm City, FL, USA) at a wavelength of 570 nm. IC_{50}, the concentration which induced 50% cytotoxicity, was calculated using GraphPad Prism 6.01 software (GraphPad Software Inc., San Diego, CA, USA).

Treatment and control groups
PC-3 cells were subdivided into 5 groups: (A) Control group, un-treated PC-3 cells; (B) Negative control (NC) siRNA treated group, scrambled siRNA-transfected PC-3 cells; (C) CIP2A siRNA treated group, PC-3 cells were transfected using 80 pmol CIP2A siRNA; (D) DTX group, PC-3 cells were exposed to IC_{50} docetaxel treatment (3.6 nM); and (E) CIP2A siRNA + DTX group, PC-3 cells were pre-treated using CIP2A siRNA and exposed to IC_{50} docetaxel (3.6 nM).

Combination effect analysis
To study the interaction between CIP2A siRNA and docetaxel, combination effect analysis was performed based on Chou and Talalay principles.[18] CDI, the coefficient of drug interaction value, was determined using the formula:

$$CDI = SAB / (SA \times SB).$$

Where SAB is the survival rate of the combination group relative to the control group, SA and SB are the survival rate of docetaxel and CIP2A siRNA relative to the control group, respectively. CDI<1, CDI=1 and CDI>1 indicate synergistic, additive, and antagonistic effects, respectively.

DAPI staining

PC-3 cells were seeded at 7×10^3 cells/well density in 96-well plates. Following the aforementioned treatments, the cells were fixed with 4% paraformaldehyde for 60 min at 37°C, washed three times with PBS, permeablized with 0.1% Triton-X-100 for 10 min, washed with PBS, and incubated with 50 μL of DAPI solution (1/2000 dilution, in 1x TBST buffer; Sigma, St. Louis, MO, USA) for 10 min in the dark. After washing with PBS, the DAPI signals were measured using Cytation 5 (Biotk) at the wavelength of 377 to 477 nm. The apoptotic cells were characterized by condensed chromatin and fragmented nuclei.

Apoptosis assay by Annexin-V FITC/PI staining

Forty eight hours after CIP2A siRNA transfection, the cells were exposed to 3.6 nM of docetaxel for 24 h. After the exposure, the cells were harvested and resuspended in cold PBS for analysis. Annexin-V FITC/PI staining kit (Roche Diagnostics, Germany) was used to stain the cells for additional analysis of cell death according to the manufacturer's instructions. Data were collected using a BD FACS Calibur flow cytometer (San Jose, CA, USA) and were analyzed with Flowing software.

Statistical analysis

All data were presented as mean ± standard deviation (SD). Statistical differences between groups were analyzed using T test and Two-way analysis of variance (ANOVA) followed by Dunnett's multiple comparisons

with GraphPad Prism software, La Jolla California USA, http://www.graphpad.com. P value less than 0.05 was considered statistically significant.

Results and Discussion

CIP2A siRNA down-regulated CIP2A expression in PC-3 cells

To investigate the effect of CIP2A siRNA on CIP2A expression in PC-3 cells, the CIP2A expression in PC-3 cells was knocked down by specific CIP2A siRNA for 24, 48, and 72 h with 60 pmol of CIP2A siRNA. The CIP2A expression level was analyzed using qRT-PCR. The relative expression of CIP2A mRNA for 24, 48 and 72 h after transfection were 0.71, 0.52 and 0.34, respectively (Figure 1A). Then, to setup the optimum dose of CIP2A siRNA, the cells were transfected using 40, 60, and 80 pmol of siRNA for 72 h. qRT-PCR and Western blot analysis were used to determine the expression of CIP2A at mRNA and protein levels following transfection using different doses. The relative CIP2A mRNA expression level for doses 40, 60, and 80 pmol of CIP2A siRNA was 0.50, 0.35, and 0.01, while the relative CIP2A protein expression levels were %73, %42, and 5% of the control, respectively. The results showed that CIP2A expression was remarkably reduced in cells transfected using 80 pmol of CIP2A siRNA as compared to the control. The optimum knockdown dose and time were achieved on 80 pmol of siRNA, 72 h post transfection (Figure 1B, 1C and 1D). Accordingly, the following tests were performed using the same condition.

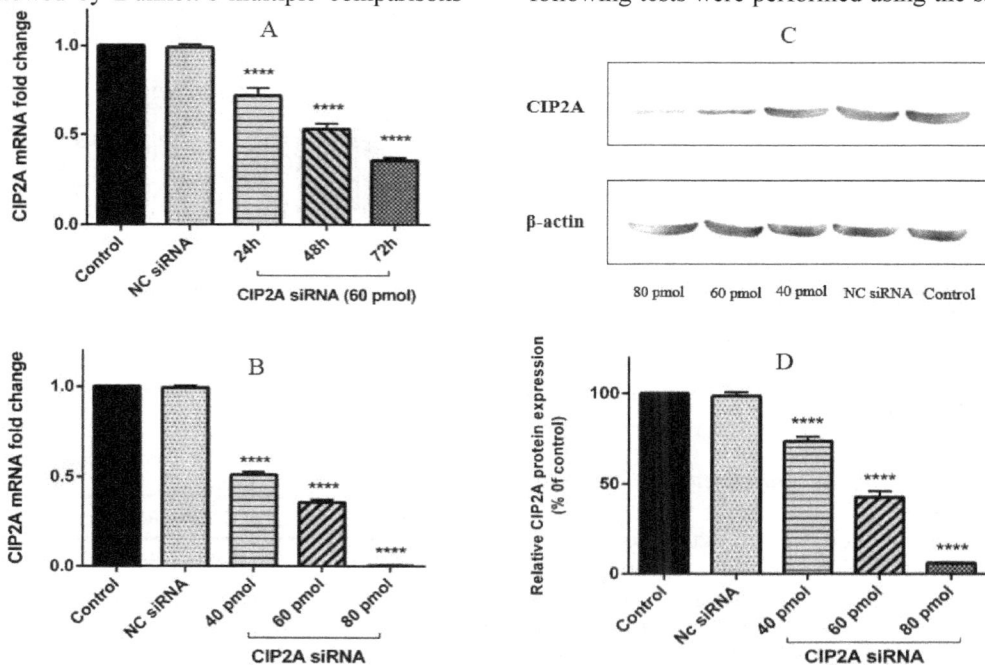

Figure 1. Suppression of CIP2A expression at mRNA and protein levels by CIP2A siRNA in PC-3 Cells. (A) q-RT PCR analysis of CIP2A expression levels in PC-3 cells following transfection with 60 mol of CIP2A specific siRNA or NC siRNA for 24, 48, and 72 h. (B) CIP2A mRNA expression levels in PC-3 cells transfected with 40, 60, and 80 pmol of specific siRNA for 72 h (1B). CIP2A expression was down regulated in time and dose dependent manner in the cells treated with CIP2A siRNA. (C) The CIP2A protein expression was determined by western blotting following transfection of cells with 40, 60 and 80 pmol of CIP2A siRNA or NC siRNA. The results showed a remarkable reduction in CIP2A expression after CIP2A transfection with 80 pmol of CIP2A siRNA, when compared with the protein level in the control group. (D) The intensity of bands was quantified and normalized to the β-actin (as an internal control) relative to CIP2A expression in the control group. The results were shown as mean±SD (n=3); ****P < 0.0001 versus control.

No significant differences were found in CIP2A mRNA and protein levels in the control groups (un-treated cells and negative siRNA group; p > 0.05).

Therefore, the results showed that silencing CIP2A with specific siRNA significantly reduced the expression of CIP2A in a time and dose dependent manner.

siRNA mediated CIP2A down-regulation inhibited the proliferation of PC-3 cells

In order to analyze the effect of CIP2A down-regulation on the proliferation and viability of PC-3 cells, MTT assay was used at different time points after CIP2A siRNA transfection. As shown in Figure 2, compared to the control group, CIP2A siRNA significantly decreased the proliferation and cell viability of P-C3 cells at 24, 48 and 72 h after transfection in a time dependent manner (p<0.0001). 24 h after CIP2A siRNA transfection, the cell viability was reduced to 81% and later dropped to 70% at 72 h. Also, no significant differences in cell viability were observed between the NC siRNA transfected cells and the un-treated control group (p>0.05). Therefore, CIP2A plays a key role in the proliferation of prostate cancer cells.

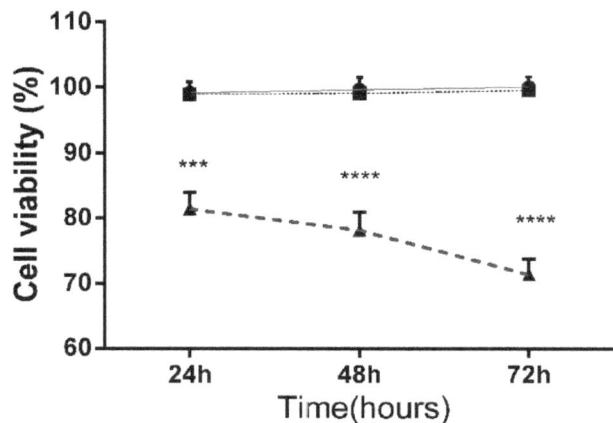

Figure 2. Effect of CIP2A silencing on PC-3 cells viability. PC-3 cells transfected with CIP2A siRNA or NC siRNA for 24, 48 and 72 h, then the effect of treatment on cell viability was determined by MTT assay. The results were shown as mean±SD (n=3); **P<0.01, ***P<0.001, ****P<0.0001 versus control. ●,■ and ▲ indicated to control group, NC siRNA treated group and CIP2A siRNA treated group , respectively.

CIP2A siRNA synergistically enhanced the cytotoxic effects of docetaxel

Sequential treatment regime was designed to explore whether CIP2A silencing could enhance the chemosensitivity of PC-3 cells to docetaxel. PC-3 cells were pre-treated with CIP2A siRNA for 48 h followed by 0.39 to 50 nM of docetaxel for 24 h and the effects of the mentioned treatment were evaluated using MTT assay. As shown in Figure 3, CIP2A siRNA significantly decreased the cell survival rate to 70% and the combination of docetaxel and CIP2A siRNA significantly decreased the cell survival rate to 45% as compared to the control. The IC$_{50}$ value of docetaxel was reduced from 3.59 to 1.97 nM after CIP2A siRNA

transfection (Figures 3 and 4). Also, the CDI values were less than 1 in all the concentrations of docetaxel which pointed to the synergistic effect between CIP2A siRNA and docetaxel (Table 2). Thus, it is suggested that CIP2A down-regulation could sensitize PC-3 cells to docetaxel.

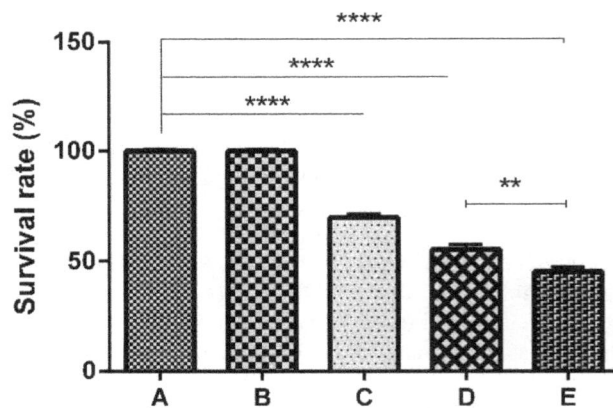

Figure 3. Effect of CIP2A siRNA on docetaxel induced cytotoxicity against PC-3 cells. PC-3 cells were transfected with CIP2A siRNA or exposed to 3.6 nM of docetaxel alone and a combination of them as shown in the methods section. The survival rate was analyzed using MTT assay. The results were shown as mean±SD (n=3); ****P<0.0001. A, B, C, D, and E indicated in the studied groups were as stated in the methods section.

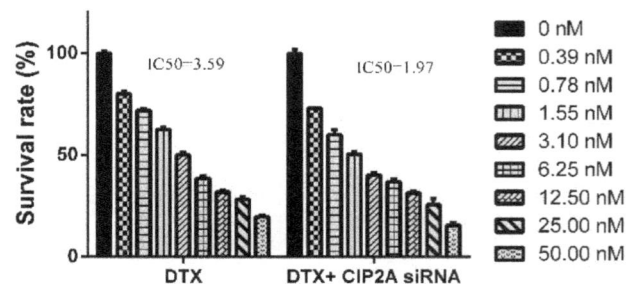

Figure 4. Effect of CIP2A silencing on the chemosensitivity of the PC-3 cells to docetaxel. 48 h after transfection with CIP2A siRNA, the cells were exposed to 0.39 to 50 nM of docetaxel for 24 h. Then, the treatments cytotoxicity was determined using MTT assay. The results were shown as mean±SD (n=3); **P<0.01 versus docetaxel treated alone cells.

Table 2. The CDI value for combination of CIP2A siRNA and 0.39 to 50 nM of docetaxel.

Concentration of CIP2A siRNA and docetaxel	CDI
80 pmol+0.39 nM	0.73
80 pmol+0.78 nM	0.68
80 pmol+1.55 nM	0.65
80 pmol+3.1 nM	0.68
80 pmol+6.25 nM	0.77
80 pmol+12.5 nM	0.86
80 pmol+25 nM	0.71
80 pmol+50 nM	0.70

Silencing of CIP2A increased apoptosis induced by docetaxel

To determine whether CIP2A suppression could enhance docetaxel induced apoptosis, DAPI and Annexin-V FITC/PI staining were used. Distinctive apoptosis-related morphological changes such as nuclear condensation were observed and nuclear fragmentation in the cells was treated using CIP2A siRNA, docetaxel, and both of them on the florescence micrographs when compared with NC siRNA treated and un-treated control groups (Figure 5). These changes, such as nuclear condensation and fragmentation, are in line with the apoptosis. The apoptotic effect of CIP2A siRNA and docetaxel on PC-3 cells was further confirmed by Annexin-V/PI staining.

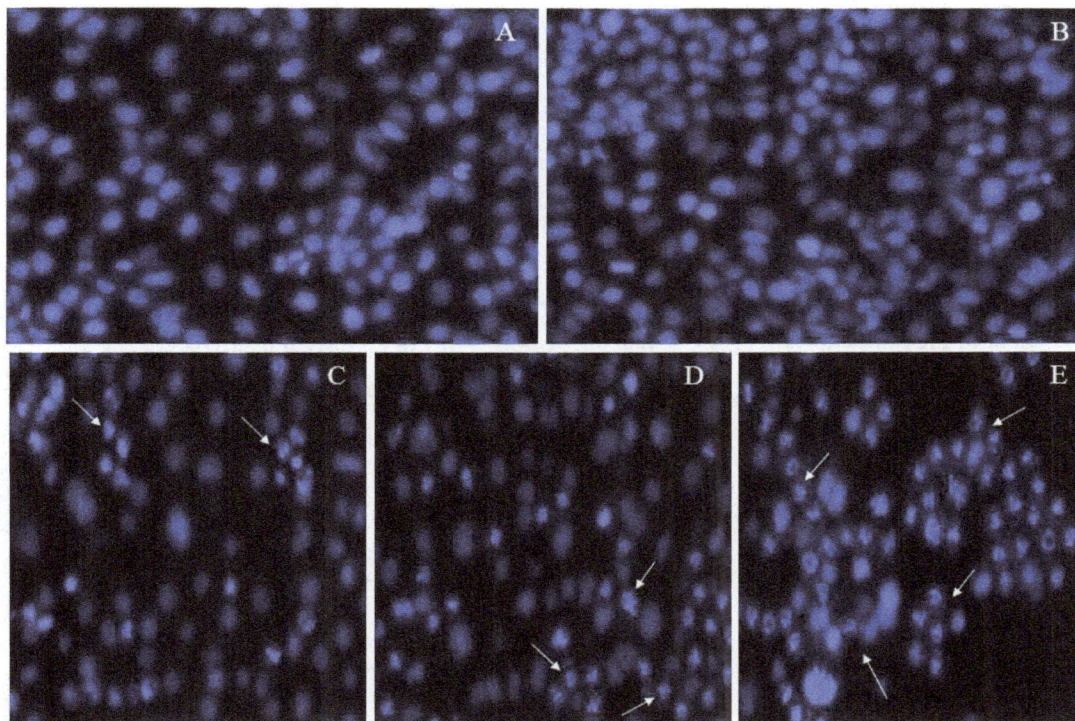

Figure 5. Nuclear morphological changes of PC-3 cells by DAPI staining. The white arrow marks indicate condensed and damaged nuclear material. A, B, C, D, and E indicated in the studied groups were as mentioned in the methods section.

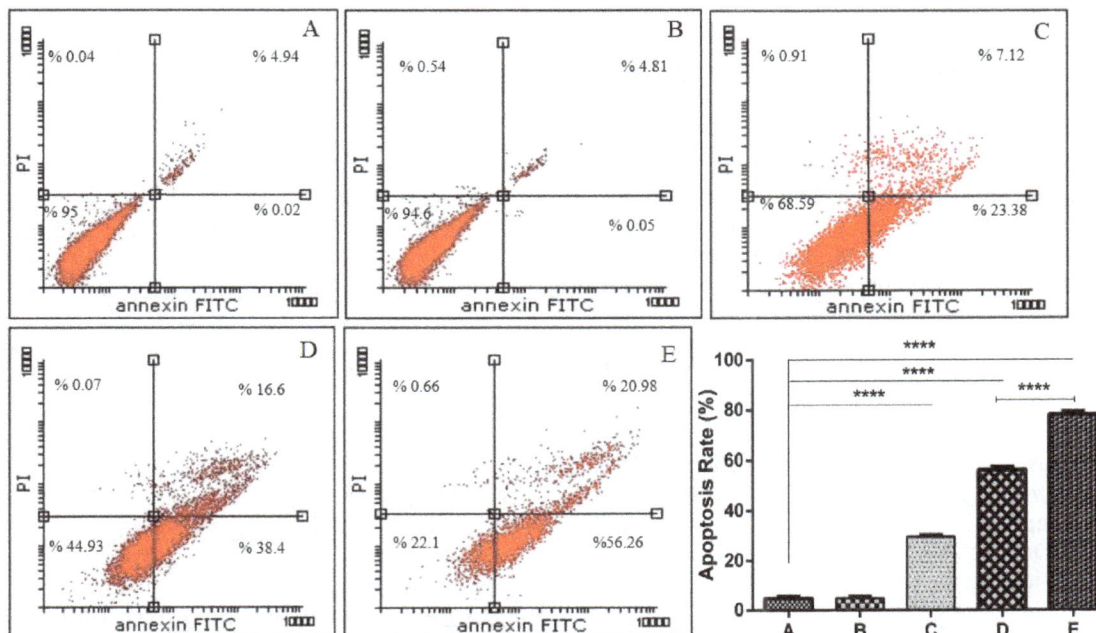

Figure 6. Effect of CIP2A silencing on docetaxel induced apoptosis. PC-3 cells were treated with CIP2A siRNA and docetaxel alone or in combination as mentioned in methods section. The apoptosis was analyzed using AnnexinV/PI staining. The results are expressed as mean±SD (n=3); ****P<0.0001 versus control. A, B, C, D, and E indicated in the studied groups were as mentioned in the methods section.

Figure 6 shows that *the apoptosis percentage* in PC-3 cells treated with CIP2A siRNA + 3.6 nM docetaxel was significantly higher than CIP2A siRNA treated cells and docetaxel treated cells alone (p<0.0001). However, no significant change was observed for NC siRNA treated group in the apoptosis rate when compared with the untreated cells. Therefore, the knockdown of CIP2A enhanced the apoptosis induction effect by docetaxel on PC-3 cells. Fang et al. showed that down-regulation of CIP2A enhanced the paclitaxel induced apoptosis in human ovarian cancer cells.[19] Also, Zhang et al. showed that the depletion of CIP2A sensitized ovarian cancer cells to cisplatin.[20] These findings are fully in agreement with the results of similar studies, which further verify the important role of CIP2A in the survival and proliferation of cancer cells.

Conclusion
Conclusively, the present study showed that silencing of CIP2A could enhance the antitumor effects of docetaxel against PC-3 cells. Therefore, targeting of CIP2A can be considered as a novel strategy for targeted prostate cancer synergy therapy.

Acknowledgments
The authors would like to thank the Immunology Research Center (IRC), Tabriz University of Medical Sciences, for the financial support of this project (No. 94/59).

Ethical Issues
Not applicable

Conflict of Interest
The authors declare no conflict of interests.

References
1. Asadi H, Orangi M, Shanehbandi D, Babaloo Z, Delazar A, Mohammadnejad L, et al. Methanolic fractions of ornithogalum cuspidatum induce apoptosis in pc-3 prostate cancer cell line and wehi-164 fibrosarcoma cancer cell line. *Adv Pharm Bull* 2014;4(Suppl 1):455-8. doi: 10.5681/apb.2014.067
2. Heidarian E, Keloushadi M, Ghatreh-Samani K, Valipour P. The reduction of il-6 gene expression, pakt, perk1/2, pstat3 signaling pathways and invasion activity by gallic acid in prostate cancer pc3 cells. *Biomed Pharmacother* 2016;84:264-9. doi: 10.1016/j.biopha.2016.09.046
3. Schurko B, Oh WK. Docetaxel chemotherapy remains the standard of care in castration-resistant prostate cancer. *Nat Clin Pract Oncol* 2008;5(9):506-7. doi: 10.1038/ncponc1201
4. Seruga B, Ocana A, Tannock IF. Drug resistance in metastatic castration-resistant prostate cancer. *Nat Rev Clin Oncol* 2011;8(1):12-23. doi: 10.1038/nrclinonc.2010.136
5. Chang AJ, Autio KA, Roach III M, Scher HI. High-risk prostate cancer [mdash] classification and therapy. *Nat Rev Clin Oncol* 2014;11(6):308-23. doi: 10.1038/nrclinonc.2014.68
6. Sasaki H, Klotz LH, Sugar LM, Kiss A, Venkateswaran V. A combination of desmopressin and docetaxel inhibit cell proliferation and invasion mediated by urokinase-type plasminogen activator (upa) in human prostate cancer cells. *Biochem Biophys Res Commun* 2015;464(3):848-54. doi: 10.1016/j.bbrc.2015.07.050
7. Perez-Martinez FC, Carrion B, Lucio MI, Rubio N, Herrero MA, Vazquez E, et al. Enhanced docetaxel-mediated cytotoxicity in human prostate cancer cells through knockdown of cofilin-1 by carbon nanohorn delivered sirna. *Biomaterials* 2012;33(32):8152-9. doi: 10.1016/j.biomaterials.2012.07.038
8. Chen X, Wang L, Zhao Y, Yuan S, Wu Q, Zhu X, et al. St6gal-i modulates docetaxel sensitivity in human hepatocarcinoma cells via the p38 mapk/caspase pathway. *Oncotarget* 2016;7(32):51955-64. doi: 10.18632/oncotarget.10192
9. Wu W, Kong Z, Duan X, Zhu H, Li S, Zeng S, et al. Inhibition of parp1 by small interfering rna enhances docetaxel activity against human prostate cancer pc3 cells. *Biochem Biophys Res Commun* 2013;442(1-2):127-32. doi: 10.1016/j.bbrc.2013.11.027
10. Mansoori B, Mohammadi A, Goldar S, Shanehbandi D, Mohammadnejad L, Baghbani E, et al. Silencing of high mobility group isoform ic (hmgi-c) enhances paclitaxel chemosensitivity in breast adenocarcinoma cells (MDA-MB-468). *Adv Pharm Bull* 2016;6(2):171-77. doi: 10.15171/apb.2016.024
11. Karami H, Baradaran B, Esfahani A, Sakhinia M, Sakhinia E. Therapeutic effects of myeloid cell leukemia-1 sirna on human acute myeloid leukemia cells. *Adv Pharm Bull* 2014;4(3):243-8. doi: 10.5681/apb.2014.035
12. Mahon KL, Henshall SM, Sutherland RL, Horvath LG. Pathways of chemotherapy resistance in castration-resistant prostate cancer. *Endocr Relat Cancer* 2011;18(4):R103-23. doi: 10.1530/erc-10-0343
13. Soofiyani SR, Hejazi MS, Baradaran B. The role of cip2a in cancer: A review and update. *Biomed Pharmacother* 2017;96:626-33. doi: 10.1016/j.biopha.2017.08.146
14. De P, Carlson J, Leyland-Jones B, Dey N. Oncogenic nexus of cancerous inhibitor of protein phosphatase 2a (cip2a): An oncoprotein with many hands. *Oncotarget* 2014;5(13):4581-602. doi: 10.18632/oncotarget.2127
15. Khanna A, Pimanda JE, Westermarck J. Cancerous inhibitor of protein phosphatase 2a, an emerging human oncoprotein and a potential cancer therapy target. *Cancer Res* 2013;73(22):6548-53. doi: 10.1158/0008-5472.can-13-1994
16. Vaarala MH, Vaisanen MR, Ristimaki A. Cip2a expression is increased in prostate cancer. *J Exp Clin Cancer Res* 2010;29:136. doi: 10.1186/1756-9966-29-136

17. Pallai R, Bhaskar A, Barnett-Bernodat N, Gallo-Ebert C, Pusey M, Nickels JT, Jr., et al. Leucine-rich repeat-containing protein 59 mediates nuclear import of cancerous inhibitor of pp2a in prostate cancer cells. *Tumour Biol* 2015;36(8):6383-90. doi: 10.1007/s13277-015-3326-1

18. Chou TC, Talalay P. Quantitative analysis of dose-effect relationships: The combined effects of multiple drugs or enzyme inhibitors. *Adv Enzyme Regul* 1984;22:27-55.

19. Fang Y, Li Z, Wang X, Zhang S. Cip2a is overexpressed in human ovarian cancer and regulates cell proliferation and apoptosis. *Tumour Biol* 2012;33(6):2299-306. doi: 10.1007/s13277-012-0492-2

20. Zhang X, Xu B, Sun C, Wang L, Miao X. Knockdown of cip2a sensitizes ovarian cancer cells to cisplatin: An in vitro study. *Int J Clin Exp Med* 2015;8(9):16941-7.

13

Modafinil Improves Catalepsy in a Rat 6-Hydroxydopamine Model of Parkinson's Disease; Possible Involvement of Dopaminergic Neurotransmission

Reza Vajdi-Hokmabad[1], Mojtaba Ziaee[2], Saeed Sadigh-Eteghad[3], Siamak Sandoghchian Shotorbani[4], Javad Mahmoudi[3]*

[1] Department of veterinary, Miyaneh branch, Islamic Azad University, Miyaneh, Iran.
[2] Medicinal Plant Research Center, Institute of Medicinal Plants, ACECR, Karaj, Iran.
[3] Neurosciences Research Center (NSRC), Tabriz University of Medical Sciences, Tabriz, Iran.
[4] Department of Immunology, Tabriz Branch, Islamic Azad University, Tabriz, Iran.

Keywords:
· 6-hydroxydopamine
· Dopaminergic neurotransmission
· Modafinil
· Parkinson's disease
· Rat

Abstract

Purpose: Modafinil is a vigilance-enhancing drug licensed for narcolepsy. The use of modafinil leads to various neuromodulatory effects with very low abuse potential. A body of evidence suggested that modafinil may have anti-parkinsonian effects. This study was designed to evaluate whether modafinil could improve motor dysfunction in the 6-hydroxydopamine (6-OHDA)-induced rat model of Parkinson's disease.

Methods: Male Wistar rats (180-220 g, n= 98) were used in this study. Parkinsonism was induced by injection of 6-hydroxydopamine (10 µg/2µl in 0.2 % ascorbic acid-saline) into the right striatum. Parkinsonian rats received intraperitoneal (ip) injections of modafinil (50, 75, and 100 mg/kg) and catalepsy-like immobility was assessed by the bar test (BT). Furthermore, involvement of dopamine D_1 and D_2 receptors in modafinil's anti-parkinsonian effects was studied. For this purpose, parkinsonian animals were pretreated with SCH23390 and raclopride (the dopamine D_1 and D_2 receptor anatgonists, respectively) or SCH23390 + raclopride, and then assessed by the BT.

Results: Modafinil (100 mg/kg) showed anti-cataleptic effects in the BT. Notably, the effect of modafinil in the BT was reversed in parkinsonian rats pretreated with raclopride (1.25 mg/kg) and/or SCH23390 + raclopride (0.75 and 1.25 mg/kg, respectively), but not in those pretreated with SCH23390 (0.75 mg/kg).

Conclusion: Acute administration of modafinil improves 6-OHDA-induced motor impairment possibly through activation of dopamine D_2 receptors.

Introduction

Parkinson's disease (PD) is the second most common neurodegenerative condition characterizing with motor symptoms including akinesia, bradykinesia, tremor at rest, rigidity[1] and leads to extensive biochemical and molecular alterations in cerebral structures that are involved in motor function.[2,3] Dopamine (DA) regulates normal motor activity through D_1 and D_2 receptors that are found postsynaptically on the dopaminergic (DAergic) neurons[4] in the striatum.[5] Studies showed that degeneration of the nigrostriatal pathway alters the brain's D_1 and D_2 receptor densities.[6,7] Such changes play a compensatory role and may consider as a promising therapeutic target in PD.[8]

L-DOPA (3,4-dihydroxyphenylalanine) restores DA level to normal value, but responses to this regimen decline over the time and the patients experience some motor abnormalities.[9] Hence, development of effective therapies to manage PD complications is of great interest.

Modafinil is a vigilance-enhancing compound[10] first approved by the Food and Drug Administration for treatment of sleep disorders such as narcolepsy, shift-work sleep disorder and obstructive-sleep apnea syndrome.[11,12] Because of its complex and wide spectrum pharmacologic profiles, there are efforts for its application in conditions such as nicotine and cocaine addiction,[11] schizophrenia, memory impairments, depression[13] and PD.[10,14] Results of positron-emission tomography (PET)[15] and micro-dialysis[16] studies have shown that modafinil has the ability to increase cerebral DA levels. Given the above, modafinil appears to provide anti-PD effects via modulation of DAergic neurotransmission. Therefore, the present study was set out to evaluate modafinil's anti-parkinsonian effects in a rat model of PD and the involvement of D_1 and D_2 DAergic receptors in this effect.

***Corresponding author:** Javad Mahmoudi, Email: mahmoudij@tbzmed.ac.ir*

Materials and Methods

Animals

Ninety eight male Wistar rats weighing 180-220 g were used for the experiment. Animals were kept under controlled conditions (12/12 h light /dark cycle: lights on at 07: 00 hours, ambient temperature $21\pm1°C$, humidity $55\pm5\%$) with unrestricted access to food and water.

Drugs and treatments

All chemicals were purchased from Sigma-Aldrich Chemical Co. (USA). For systemic administration, modafinil was suspended in saline with 0.4% sodium carboxymethyl cellulose. SCH23390 (the DA D_1 receptor antagonist) and raclopride (the DA D_2 receptor antagonist) were dissolved in distilled water. 6-OHDA was dissolved in a 0.9% normal saline solution containing 0.2% (w/v) ascorbic acid. Drugs were freshly prepared and injected intraperitoneally (ip) in a volume of 1 ml/kg body weight, except for 6-OHDA which was injected into the right striatum. Desipramine (25 mg/kg, ip) was injected 30 min before intra-striatal injection of 6-OHDA, in order to prevent the destruction of noradrenergic neurons.[17]

Two sets of experiments were performed in this study. The first experiment was conducted to assess modafinil's ability to reduce the immobility time in parkinsonian animals. In this phase, rats with 6-OHDA lesion received different doses of modafinil (50, 75, and 100 mg/kg) or its vehicle and then, after 30 minutes, were subjected to the bar test (BT).

The second set was carried out to evaluate the possible involvement of the DAergic system on the anti-immobility effect of modafinil in the BT. In this phase, individual groups of parkinsonian animals were pretreated with SCH23390 (0.75 mg/kg, ip), raclopride (1.25 mg/kg, ip) and/or both of these (or their vehicles) at the same doses in combination, and after 30 minutes, received modafinil (100 mg/kg) or the its vehicle. The doses of antagonists used in this study was approximately the same as that reported by Hauber et al.[18]

Intra-striatal injection of 6-OHDA

For stereotaxic surgery, animals were anesthetized with a combination of ketamine and xylazine (80 and 5 mg/kg, ip; respectively) and placed in a stoelting stereotaxic apparatus (stoelting, USA) in the flat skull position. The small central incision was made to make the skull appear. A 23 gauge sterile cannula was inserted into the injection site as a guide cannula for subsequent insertion of the injection tube into the striatum. The coordinates for this position, with reference to the atlas of Paxinos &Watson,[19] were: anteroposterior from bregma (AP)= 0.4 mm, mediolateral from the midline (ML)= 2.8 mm and dorsoventral from the skull (DV)= -5 mm. Subsequently, 6-OHDA (10 µg/ rat in 2 µl saline containing 0.2% ascorbic acid) was infused by an infusion pump at the flow rate of 0.2 µl/min into the right striatum. Lesioned rats were subjected to the designed protocols after a 3-week recovery period. All of these procedures were performed for sham-operated animals, but they only received intra-striatal of 2 µl vehicle of 6-OHDA (0.9% saline containing 0.2% (w/v) ascorbic acid).

Assessment of catalepsy-like immobility

Catalepsy-like immobility was assessed by using BT. As described previously, both forelegs of a rat were gently placed over a 9-cm-high horizontal bar (diameter, 0.7 cm) and the retention time in this imposed posture was considered to define catalepsy time. The end point of catalepsy was designated to occur when both front paws were removed from the bar or the animal moved its head in an exploratory fashion. The cut-off time of the test was 180 seconds.[17,20]

Verification of infusion site

To verify the infusion site, all rats were sacrificed by a high dose of ether at the end of behavioral assessments. Afterwards, the brains were removed and stored in 10% formaldehyde solution for one week prior to embedding and sectioning. Serial coronal sections (6 µm) were taken with a microtome (Leitz, Germany) and stained with haematoxylin-eosin; the scar tract made by the infusion tube was controlled with a light microscope. Whenever the emplacement of the infusion tube in striatum was incorrect, the representative data were excluded.

Statistical analysis

Statistical analysis of each data set was done by SPSS 21 software. The data were expressed as the mean ± SEM and were analyzed by two-and/or one-way ANOVA and post hoc Tukey's test. P values < 0.05 were considered to be statistically significant.

Results

Effect of 6-OHDA on the BT

One-way ANOVA revealed a significant effect of intra-striatal injection of 6-OHDA [$F(3,28)=375.27$ $p<0.001$] on the catalepsy time in comparison with control and sham-operated groups. Post hoc analysis showed that 6-OHDA (10 µg/ rat) increased catalepsy time in the BT, which indicates that this neurotoxin is able to produce marked catalepsy. Also, there was no significant difference between the sham-operated group and control rats (Figure 1).

Effect of modafinil on the BT

One-way ANOVA showed that modafinil could attenuate catalepsy time in 6-OHDA-lesioned rats [$F(3,28) = 375.27$ $p<0.001$]. Post hoc analysis indicated that modafinil only at the dose of 100 mg/kg is able to decrease the immobility time in the BT when compared with vehicle-treated 6-OHDA-lesioned rats. At lower doses (50 and 75 mg/kg), modafinil has not significant effect on the catalepsy time (Figure 1).

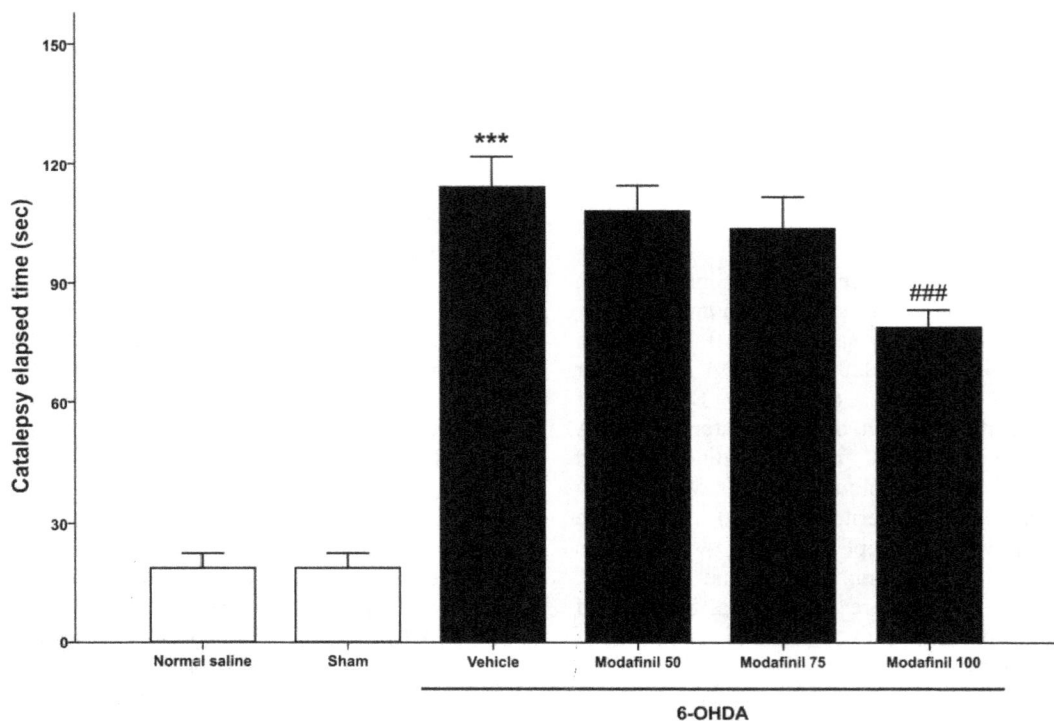

Figure 1. Effect of intraperitoneal (ip) injection of vehicle and/or different doses of modafinil (50, 75 and 100 mg/kg) on the 6-OHDA (10 µg/2 µl/rat)-induced catalepsy. Each bar represents the mean ± SEM. (n = 8) $^{***}p<0.001$ and $^{###}p<0.001$ as compared with the normal saline and vehicle received groups, respectively.

Effect of raclopride and SCH23390 pretreatment on the anti-cataleptic effect of modafinil

Modafinil (100 mg/kg, ip) reduced catalepsy ($p<0.001$) and the involvement of the DAergic neurotransmission on this effect was studied in separate groups of 6-OHDA-lesioned rats.

A two-way ANOVA revealed significant differences of modafinil treatment [$F(1,28) = 55.3$ $p<0.001$] but not SCH23390 pretreatment [$F(1,28) = 0.8$ $p>0.05$]. Also, there was significant differences of modafinil treatment interaction with SCH23390 pretreatment [$F(1,28) = 18$ $p<0.001$].

The results presented in in Figure 2A, show that pretreatment of lesioned rats with SCH23390 (0.75 mg/kg, ip) did not alter the anti-cataleptic effect of modafinil in the BT.

A two-way ANOVA showed significant differences of modafinil treatment [$F (1, 28) = 143.7$ $p< 0.001$], raclopride pretreatment [$F (1, 28) = 91.2$ $p<0.001$] and modafinil treatment interaction with raclopride pretreatment [$F (1, 28) = 6.92$ $p<0.05$].

The results presented in Figure 2B show that pretreatment of lesioned rats with raclopride (1.25 mg/kg, ip) reversed the anti-cataleptic effect of modafinil in the BT.

A two-ANOVA revealed significant differences of modafinil treatment [$(1, 28) = 169.8$ $p<0.001$], SCH23390 + raclopride pretreatment [$F (1, 28) = 218.9$ $p<0.001$] and modafinil treatment interaction with SCH23390 + raclopride pretreatment [$F (1, 28) = 8.94$ $p< 0.01$]. The results depicted in Figure 2C show that

pretreatment of lesioned rats with SCH23390 + raclopride (0.75 and 1.25 mg/kg, respectively, ip) blocked anti-cataleptic effect of modafinil in the BT.

Discussion

Our data showed that modafinil displays an anti-parkinsonian effect on the 6-OHDA lesioned rats, and this effect in part is mediated through DAergic neurotransmission.

Catalepsy or tonic immobility is a complex motor inhibition[21] in which rodents are unable to correct externally imposed abnormal posture[21,22] and revert to a normal position for initiation of exploratory behavior.[23] This behavior not only is able to mimic the state of akinesia and rigidity occurring in PD[24] but also is used to evaluate nigrostriatal function and its regulation by different neurotransmitter systems.[25] 6-OHDA is frequently used for chemical denervation of DAergic neurons[26] and those rats with DAergic lesion show marked catalepsy;[27] as a result, this neurotoxin provides simple and a reliable model for studying the anti-parkinsonian potential of drugs.[20]

In this study, a single dose of modafinil (100 mg/kg) resulted in decreased catalepsy time and normalized motor behavior in parkinsonian rats 30 min after ip injection. Pharmacokinetic findings suggest that modafinil reaches a peak concentration in brain 30 to 60 min by single systemic administration[28] and produces a rapid and significant elevation in brain DA content in dose dependent fashion.[29]

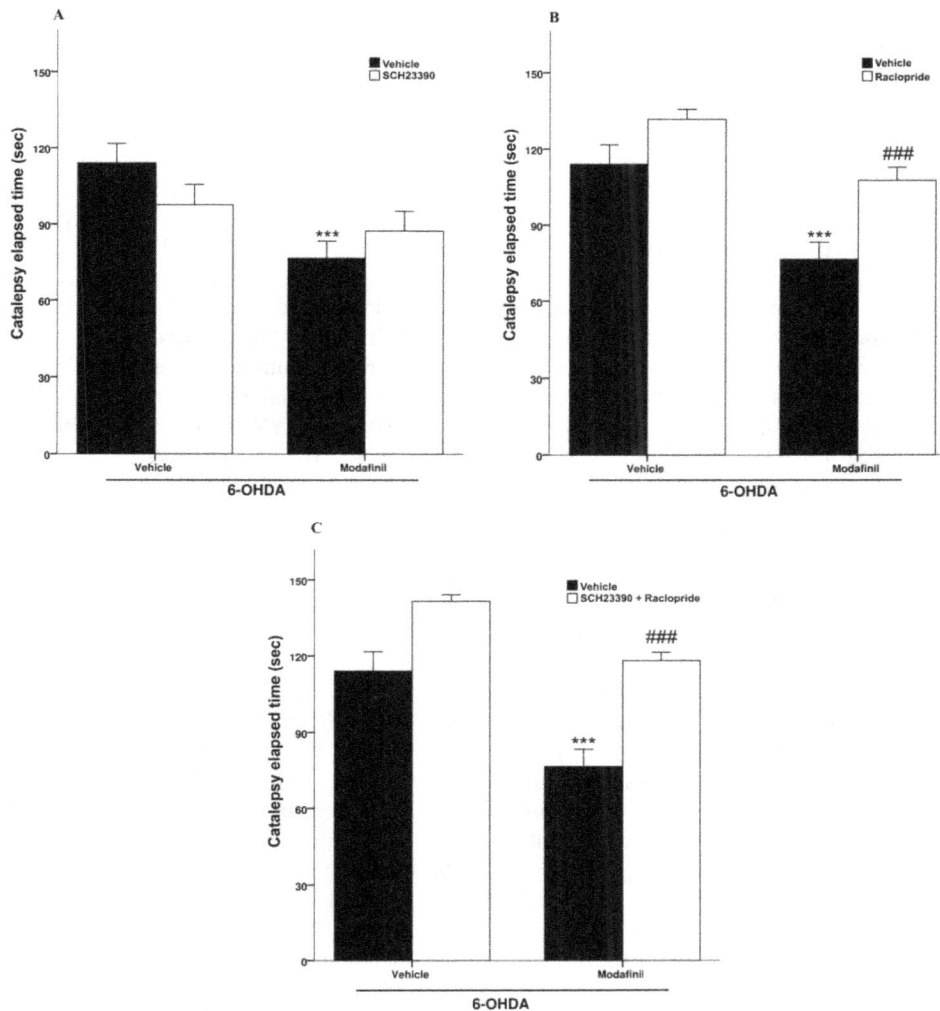

Figure 2. Effect of pretreatment with SCH23390 (0.75 mg/kg) (A), raclopride (1.25 mg/kg) (B) and/or SCH23390 + raclopride (0.75 + 1.25 mg/kg, respectively) (C) on the modafinil anti-cataleptic effect . Each bar represents the mean ± SEM. (n = 8) [***]$p<0.001$ and [###]$p<0.01$ as compared with the vehicle and the modafinil (100 mg/kg, ip) injected rats, respectively.

Nucleus accumbens which receives DAergic inputs from the ventral tegmental area and medial substantia nigra regulates normal motor function.[30,31] Modafinil increases DA efflux in this region[32] through inhibition of DA transports[16] as well as reduction of accumbal GABAergic tone. The inhibitory effect of modafinil on the GABAergic system also enhances the activity of the striatopallidal pathway.[33] This pathway governs normal motor function and is involved in the appearance of PD motor signs.[34]

In another portion of this study, parkinsonian rats pretreated with concomitant administration of D_1 and D_2 receptor antagonists (raclopride and SCH23390, respectively). This intervention increased immobility time in the BT and prevented the anti-parkinsonian effects of modafinil. Furthermore, blockade of D_2 receptors using raclopride reversed the anti-parkinsonian effect of modafinil in 6-OHDA lesioned rats.

Studies on the striatal D_2 receptor suggested that denervation of DAergic neurons by 6-OHDA might increase D_2 receptor densities from 2-8 weeks post-lesion in impacted animals.[35] Indeed, significant up-regulation of post synaptic D_2 receptor binding sites is accompanied by elevation of D_2 mRNA levels in 6-OHDA lesioned rats.[36,37] Moreover, postmortem studies in drug-naive PD patients have also confirmed such increase in striatal D_2 receptor binding sites.[38]

Contrary to D_2 receptors, there is contradictory evidence about D_1 receptor alterations in parkinsonian rats.[35-39] While there are no reports showing that alteration in D_1 density happens in PD,[38] Zhao et al. showed that a decline in mRNA levels for D_1 receptors in DA-lesioned striatum occurs in parkinsonian rats.[7] This reflects that denervation of DAergic structures is not able to increase D_1 receptors densities.[35]

Decline in striatal DA levels causes an imbalance in striatal functions and disrupts normal motor activity. Hence, pronounced up-regulation of D_2 receptors may potentiate responsiveness to decreased levels of striatal DA and normalize motor activity,[8] especially in *de novo* and young parkinsonian patients.[40] Moreover, when compared with D_2 receptors, D_1 receptors have less ability to increase locomotor activity.[41] Collectively, these data can explain why D_2 receptor activation may in part mediate anti-parkinsinian effects of modafinil.

Complications such as development of abnormal motor fluctuation and inadequate responses to standard anti-parkinsonian drugs remain major problems in parkinsonian patients.[20,42] In addition, non-motor comorbidities such as depression[43] and sleep disorders[44,45] are experienced by the majority of patients and impact their daily living activities.

Hence, application of regimens to overcome these problems is of great importance; the ability of modafinil to reduce PD symptoms in experimental models, as well as its potential for anti-depressant-like properties in preclinical research and treatment of sleep disorders in PD, suggests that modafinil may have potential to improve the effectiveness of current anti-PD medications.

Conclusion

In conclusion, this study showed that modafinil improves catalepsy behavior in a rat model of PD. Considering the role of DAergic neurotransmission in regulation of normal motor behavior and alterations of D_2 receptor densities in PD, it may be suggested that modafinil exert the anti-PD effect through modulation of DAergic system. Moreover, the complexity of modafinil's mechanism of action suggests that more experiments must be designed to reveal its neuropharmacological effects.

Acknowledgments

We would like to express our special gratitude to the Miyaneh branch of Islamic Azad University, Iran, for financial support.

Ethical Issues

The experiment was performed in accordance with the Guide and Use of Laboratory Animals (National Institutes of Health) and confirmed by the Ethical Committee for Animal Experimentation of the Miyaneh branch of Islamic Azad University.

Conflict of Interest

The authors declare no conflict of interests.

References

1. Haddadi R, Mohajjel Nayebi A, Brooshghalan SE. Pre-treatment with silymarin reduces brain myeloperoxidase activity and inflammatory cytokines in 6-ohda hemi-parkinsonian rats. *Neurosci Lett* 2013;555:106-11. doi: 10.1016/j.neulet.2013.09.022

2. Nagatsu T, Sawada M. Biochemistry of postmortem brains in Parkinson's disease: historical overview and future prospects. *J Neural Transm Suppl* 2007(72):113-20.

3. Shih MC, Hoexter MQ, Andrade LA, Bressan RA. Parkinson's disease and dopamine transporter neuroimaging: A critical review. *Sao Paulo Med J* 2006;124(3):168-75.

4. Beaulieu JM, Gainetdinov RR. The physiology, signaling, and pharmacology of dopamine receptors. *Pharmacol Rev* 2011;63(1):182-217. doi: 10.1124/pr.110.002642

5. Paul ML, Graybiel AM, David JC, Robertson HA. D1-like and D2-like dopamine receptors synergistically activate rotation and c-fos expression in the dopamine-depleted striatum in a rat model of parkinson's disease. *J Neurosci* 1992;12(10):3729-42.

6. Schwarting RK, Huston JP. The unilateral 6-hydroxydopamine lesion model in behavioral brain research. Analysis of functional deficits, recovery and treatments. *Prog Neurobiol* 1996;50(2-3):275-331. doi: 10.1016/s0301-0082(96)00040-8

7. Zhao R, Lu W, Fang X, Guo L, Yang Z, Ye N, et al. (6aR)-11-amino-N-propyl-noraporphine, a new dopamine D2 and serotonin 5-HT1A dual agonist, elicits potent antiparkinsonian action and attenuates levodopa-induced dyskinesia in a 6-OHDA-lesioned rat model of Parkinson's disease. *Pharmacol Biochem Behav* 2014;124:204-10. doi: 10.1016/j.pbb.2014.06.011

8. Ballion B, Frenois F, Zold CL, Chetrit J, Murer MG, Gonon F. D2 receptor stimulation, but not d1, restores striatal equilibrium in a rat model of parkinsonism. *Neurobiol Dis* 2009;35(3):376-84. doi: 10.1016/j.nbd.2009.05.019

9. Mahmoudi J, Farhoudi M, Reyhani-Rad S, Sadigh-Eteghad S. Dampening of serotonergic system through 5HT1A receptors is a promising target for treatment of levodopa induced motor problems. *Adv Pharm Bull* 2013;3(2):439-41. doi: 10.5681/apb.2013.071

10. Xiao YL, Fu JM, Dong Z, Yang JQ, Zeng FX, Zhu LX, et al. Neuroprotective mechanism of modafinil on Parkinson disease induced by 1-methyl-4-phenyl-1,2,3,6-tetrahydropyridine. *Acta Pharmacol Sin* 2004;25(3):301-5.

11. Dopheide MM, Morgan RE, Rodvelt KR, Schachtman TR, Miller DK. Modafinil evokes striatal [(3)H]dopamine release and alters the subjective properties of stimulants. *Eur J Pharmacol* 2007;568(1-3):112-23. doi: 10.1016/j.ejphar.2007.03.044

12. Qu WM, Huang ZL, Xu XH, Matsumoto N, Urade Y. Dopaminergic D1 and D2 receptors are essential for the arousal effect of modafinil. *J Neurosci* 2008;28(34):8462-9. doi: 10.1523/JNEUROSCI.1819-08.2008

13. Mahmoudi J, Farhoudi M, Talebi M, Sabermarouf B, Sadigh-Eteghad S. Antidepressant-like effect of modafinil in mice: Evidence for the involvement of the dopaminergic neurotransmission. *Pharmacol Rep* 2015;67(3):478-84. doi: 10.1016/j.pharep.2014.11.005

14. Van Vlieta SA, Blezer EL, Jongsma MJ, Vanwersch RA, Olivier B, Philippens IH. Exploring the

neuroprotective effects of modafinil in a marmoset parkinson model with immunohistochemistry, magnetic resonance imaging and spectroscopy. *Brain Res* 2008;1189:219-28. doi: 10.1016/j.brainres.2007.10.059

15. Madras BK, Xie Z, Lin Z, Jassen A, Panas H, Lynch L, et al. Modafinil occupies dopamine and norepinephrine transporters in vivo and modulates the transporters and trace amine activity in vitro. *J Pharmacol Exp Ther* 2006;319(2):561-9. doi: 10.1124/jpet.106.106583

16. Zolkowska D, Jain R, Rothman RB, Partilla JS, Roth BL, Setola V, et al. Evidence for the involvement of dopamine transporters in behavioral stimulant effects of modafinil. *J Pharmacol Exp Ther* 2009;329(2):738-46. doi: 10.1124/jpet.108.146142

17. Reyhani-Rad S, Mohajjel Nayebi A, Mahmoudi J, Samini M, Babapour V. Role of 5-Hydroxytryptamine 1A Receptors in 6-Hydroxydopmaine-induced Catalepsy-like Immobilization in Rats: a Therapeutic Approach for Treating Catalepsy of Parkinson's Disease. *Iran J Pharm Res* 2012;11(4):1175-81.

18. Hauber W, Neuscheler P, Nagel J, Muller CE. Catalepsy induced by a blockade of dopamine D1 or D2 receptors was reversed by a concomitant blockade of adenosine A(2A) receptors in the caudate-putamen of rats. *Eur J Neurosci* 2001;14(8):1287-93. doi: 10.1046/j.0953-816x.2001.01759.x

19. Paxinos GW, Charles W. The rat brain in stereotaxic coordinates. 5th ed. Burlington, MA: Elsevier Academic Press; 2005.

20. Mahmoudi J, Mohajjel Nayebi A, Samini M, Reyhani-Rad S, Babapour V. Buspirone improves the anti-cataleptic effect of levodopa in 6-hydroxydopamine-lesioned rats. *Pharmacol Rep* 2011;63(4):908-14. doi: 10.1016/s1734-1140(11)70606-5

21. Bazhenova EY, Kulikov AV, Tikhonova MA, Bazovkina DV, Fursenko DV, Popova NK. On the association between lipopolysaccharide induced catalepsy and serotonin metabolism in the brain of mice genetically different in the predisposition to catalepsy. *Pharmacol Biochem Behav* 2013;111:71-5. doi: 10.1016/j.pbb.2013.08.009

22. Fink-Jensen A, Schmidt LS, Dencker D, Schülein C, Wess J, Wörtwein G, et al. Antipsychotic-induced catalepsy is attenuated in mice lacking the M4 muscarinic acetylcholine receptor. *Eur J Pharmacol* 2011;656(1-3):39-44.

23. Tostes JG, Medeiros P, Melo-Thomas L. Modulation of haloperidol-induced catalepsy in rats by GABAergic neural substrate in the inferior colliculus. *Neuroscience* 2013;255:212-8. doi: 10.1016/j.neuroscience.2013.09.064

24. Di Matteo V, Pierucci M, Esposito E, Crescimanno G, Benigno A, Di Giovanni G. Serotonin modulation of the basal ganglia circuitry: Therapeutic implication for parkinson's disease and other motor disorders. *Prog Brain Res* 2008;172:423-63. doi: 10.1016/s0079-6123(08)00921-7

25. Mohajjel Nayebi A, Sheidaei H. Buspirone improves haloperidol-induced parkinson disease in mice through 5-HT(1A) recaptors. *Daru* 2010;18(1):41-5.

26. Schober A. Classic toxin-induced animal models of parkinson's disease: 6-OHDA and MPTP. *Cell Tissue Res* 2004;318(1):215-24. doi: 10.1007/s00441-004-0938-y

27. Nayebi AM, Rad SR, Saberian M, Azimzadeh S, Samini M. Buspirone improves 6-hydroxydopamine-induced catalepsy through stimulation of nigral 5-HT(1A) receptors in rats. *Pharmacol Rep* 2010;62(2):258-64.

28. de Saint Hilaire Z, Orosco M, Rouch C, Blanc G, Nicolaidis S. Variations in extracellular monoamines in the prefrontal cortex and medial hypothalamus after modafinil administration: A microdialysis study in rats. *Neuroreport* 2001;12(16):3533-7.

29. Ferraro L, Tanganelli S, O'Connor WT, Antonelli T, Rambert F, Fuxe K. The vigilance promoting drug modafinil increases dopamine release in the rat nucleus accumbens via the involvement of a local GABAergic mechanism. *Eur J Pharmacol* 1996;306(1-3):33-9. doi: 10.1016/0014-2999(96)00182-3

30. Swanson CJ, Kalivas PW. Regulation of locomotor activity by metabotropic glutamate receptors in the nucleus accumbens and ventral tegmental area. *J Pharmacol Exp Ther* 2000;292(1):406-14.

31. Kalivas PW, Alesdatter JE. Involvement of n-methyl-d-aspartate receptor stimulation in the ventral tegmental area and amygdala in behavioral sensitization to cocaine. *J Pharmacol Exp Ther* 1993;267(1):486-95.

32. Minzenberg MJ, Carter CS. Modafinil: A review of neurochemical actions and effects on cognition. *Neuropsychopharmacology* 2008;33(7):1477-502. doi: 10.1038/sj.npp.1301534

33. Ferraro L, Antonelli T, O'Connor WT, Tanganelli S, Rambert FA, Fuxe K. The effects of modafinil on striatal, pallidal and nigral GABA and glutamate release in the conscious rat: Evidence for a preferential inhibition of striato-pallidal GABA transmission. *Neurosci Lett* 1998;253(2):135-8. doi: 10.1016/s0304-3940(98)00629-6

34. Augustin SM, Beeler JA, McGehee DS, Zhuang X. Cyclic AMP and afferent activity govern bidirectional synaptic plasticity in striatopallidal neurons. *J Neurosci* 2014;34(19):6692-9. doi: 10.1523/JNEUROSCI.3906-13.2014

35. Araki T, Tanji H, Kato H, Itoyama Y. Sequential changes of dopaminergic receptors in the rat brain after 6-hydroxydopamine lesions of the medial forebrain bundle. *J Neurol Sci* 1998;160(2):121-7. doi: 10.1016/s0022-510x(98)00248-2

36. Narang N, Wamsley JK. Time dependent changes in da uptake sites, D1 and D2 receptor binding and mrna after 6-ohda lesions of the medial forebrain bundle in

the rat brain. *J Chem Neuroanat* 1995;9(1):41-53. doi: 10.1016/0891-0618(95)00064-e

37. Przedborski S, Levivier M, Jiang H, Ferreira M, Jackson-Lewis V, Donaldson D, et al. Dose-dependent lesions of the dopaminergic nigrostriatal pathway induced by instrastriatal injection of 6-hydroxydopamine. *Neuroscience* 1995;67(3):631-47. doi: 10.1016/0306-4522(95)00066-r

38. Bezard E, Brotchie JM, Gross CE. Pathophysiology of levodopa-induced dyskinesia: Potential for new therapies. *Nat Rev Neurosci* 2001;2(8):577-88. doi: 10.1038/35086062

39. Blunt SB, Jenner P, Marsden CD. Autoradiographic study of striatal D1 and D2 dopamine receptors in 6-OHDA-lesioned rats receiving foetal ventral mesencephalic grafts and chronic treatment with L-DOPA and carbidopa. *Brain Res* 1992;582(2):299-311. doi: 10.1016/0006-8993(92)90147-2

40. Hisahara S, Shimohama S. Dopamine receptors and Parkinson's disease. *Int J Med Chem* 2011;2011:403039. doi: 10.1155/2011/403039

41. Beninger RJ, Mazurski EJ, Hoffman DC. Receptor subtype-specific dopaminergic agents and unconditioned behavior. *Pol J Pharmacol Pharm* 1991;43(6):507-28.

42. Mahmoudi J, Mohajjel Nayebi A, Reyhani-Rad S, Samini M. Fluoxetine improves the effect of levodopa on 6-hydroxy dopamine-induced motor impairments in rats. *Adv Pharm Bull* 2012;2(2):149-55. doi: 10.5681/apb.2012.023

43. Lemke MR. Dopamine agonists in the treatment of non-motor symptoms of parkinson's disease: Depression. *Eur J Neurol* 2008;15 Suppl 2:9-14. doi: 10.1111/j.1468-1331.2008.02213.x

44. Kumar S, Bhatia M, Behari M. Sleep disorders in Parkinson's disease. *Mov Disord* 2002;17(4):775-81. doi: 10.1002/mds.10167

45. Happe S, Pirker W, Sauter C, Klosch G, Zeitlhofer J. Successful treatment of excessive daytime sleepiness in parkinson's disease with modafinil. *J Neurol* 2001;248(7):632-4. doi: 10.1007/s004150170148

14

Voltammetric Determination of Ivabradine Hydrochloride Using Multiwalled Carbon Nanotubes Modified Electrode in Presence of Sodium Dodecyl Sulfate

Ali Kamal Attia*, **Nisreen Farouk Abo-Talib**, **Marwa Hosny Tammam**

National Organization for Drug Control and Research, P.O. Box 29, Cairo, Egypt.

Keywords:
· Multiwalled carbon nanotubes
· Sodium dodecyl sulfate
· Ivabradine hydrochloride
· Voltammetry
· Plasma

Abstract

Purpose: A new sensitive sensor was fabricated for the determination of ivabradine hydrochloride (IH) based on modification with multiwalled carbon nanotubes using sodium dodecyl sulfate as micellar medium to increase the sensitivity.
Methods: The electrochemical behavior of IH was studied in Britton-Robinson buffer (pH: 2.0-11.0) using cyclic and differential pulse voltammetry.
Results: The voltammetric response was linear over the range of 3.984×10^{-6}-3.475×10^{-5} mol L^{-1}. The limits of detection and quantification were found to be 5.160×10^{-7} and 1.720×10^{-6} mol L^{-1}, respectively.
Conclusion: This method is suitable for determination of IH in tablets and plasma.

Introduction

Ivabradine HCl (IH) is used to reduce the heart rate through inhibition of the pacemaker current (I_f). IH is used in the treatment of heart failure, in sinus rhythm and angina pectoris when beta blockers are not responding.[1-3] Several methods have been reported to determine IH such as spectrophotometric method,[4] chromatographic methods,[4-11] spectrofluorimetric method,[12] and potentiometric method.[13]

The electroanalytical methods are simple, rapid, and in expensive techniques, they have great importance in environmental monitoring and pharmaceutical analysis.[14-20]

Carbon nanotubes (CNTs) have matchless geometrical, mechanical, electronic and chemical properties. Multi-walled carbon nanotubes (MWNTs) modified electrodes have plentiful characteristics compared with bare electrode according to their unrivaled properties. Nanoparticles increase the number of active sites and the rate of mass transport to the electrode surface.[21-24]

This study aims to determine IH at multiwalled carbon nanotubes modified carbon paste electrode (MWCNTCPE) utilizing voltammetric method based on the electrochemical oxidation of IH.

Materials and Methods

Apparatus

SP-150 (Biologic Science Instruments, France) was used for voltammetric experiments. The results were analyzed using EC-Lab software. Ag/AgCl (3.0 mol L^{-1} NaCl) reference electrode and a platinum wire counter electrode were purchased from BASi (USA), pH meter (JENWAY 3510, UK) was used to adjust buffer solutions. JSM-6700F scanning electron microscope (Japan Electro Company) was used to do scanning electron microscopy (SEM) experiments. FTIR-8400S spectrophotometer (Shimadzu, Japan) was used to obtain FTIR spectra of MWCNTCPE and MWCNTCPE/SDS. The charges of atoms of IH were calculated using Huckel's method (ChemBio 3D Ultra program).

Materials and reagents

IH (98.5%) and Procoralan® tablets (5.39 mg of IH per tablet) were provided by Servier Egypt Industries Limited.

MWCNTs (6-13 nm in diameter and 2.5-20 µm in length; purity >98%), sodium dodecyl sulfate (SDS), Graphite and paraffin oil were supplied from Sigma-Aldrich. IH stock solution (1.0×10^{-3} mol L^{-1}) and SDS solution (1.0×10^{-2} mol L^{-1}) was prepared using deionized water.

Britton-Robinson (BR) buffer solutions (pH: 2.0-11.0) were prepared as mentioned before.[16] Plasma was purchased from blood bank of VACSERA (Egypt).

Working electrodes

MWCNTCPE was made by mixing and stirring 1.0% (w/w) MWCNTs and 99% (w/w) graphite powder in ethyl ether to get good homogeneity, and then dry this mixture in air. The dried mixture was mixed with paraffin oil to obtain a uniformly wetted paste. The hole of the electrode was filled with paste and smoothed on a filter paper until a shiny appearance was obtained. A carbon paste electrode (CPE) was obtained using the same procedures without MWCNTs addition.

Effect of SDS
The cyclic voltammograms of IH (1.43×10^{-4} mol L^{-1}) in BR buffer (pH 3) were recorded at MWCNTCPE upon successive addition of different volumes of SDS (1.0×10^{-2} mol L^{-1}) to the voltammetric cell.

Calibration curve of IH
Different volumes of IH solution (1.0×10^{-3} mol L^{-1}) were added to 5 mL of BR buffer of pH 3.0. The solution was stirred for 5 s and the differential pulse voltammograms were done using scan rate of 10 mV s^{-1} at MWCNTCPE/SDS.

Analysis of IH in tablets
Fifteen Procoralan tablets were grounded. Suitable amount needed to get IH solution of 1.0×10^{-3} mol L^{-1} was added to flask containing 60 mL deionized water, then dissolved by sonication for 15 min and the volume was completed to 100 mL with deionized water. The solution was filtered to remove the insoluble excipients. Standard addition method was performed to determine IH in dosage form.

Analysis of IH in plasma
One mL of human plasma and 2 mL of acetonitrile were added to a series of 10 mL centrifuge tubes containing different volumes of IH (1.0×10^{-3} mol L^{-1}), the mixture was centrifuged at 5000 rpm for 10 min to get rid of protein residues. 0.5 mL from the supernatant was transferred into voltammetric cell containing 4.5 mL of BR buffer (pH 3.0) and SDS solution (3.58×10^{-4} mol L^{-1}). The procedures mentioned in calibration curve were done. The institutional board (NODCAR, Egypt) have agreed for testing with human subjects. Agreement was acquired from all contributors.

Results and Discussion
Voltammetric behavior of IH
Figure 1A displays the cyclic voltammograms of IH (1.43×10^{-4} mol L^{-1}) at CPE in BR buffer of different pH values. The forward scan shows anodic peak due to the oxidation process, while the reverse scan shows no peaks, indicating the irreversibility of the electrochemical process.

Influence of pH
The electrochemical action of IH (1.43×10^{-4} mol L^{-1}) was studied in different pH solutions (2.0-11.0) at CPE using cyclic voltammetry (CV) and scan rate of 100 mV

s^{-1} as shown in Figure 1. Figure 1A shows that well defined and sharp anodic peaks in acidic medium (pH: 2.0-6.0) and broad peaks in neutral and basic medium (pH: 7.0-11.0). Figure 1 (A, B) shows that the anodic peak current presents the highest value at pH 3.0. Therefore, pH 3.0 was chosen to determine IH. Figure 1 (A, C) shows that the anodic peak potentials increases as pH increases up to pH 6.0, and decreases as pH increases up to pH 11.0.

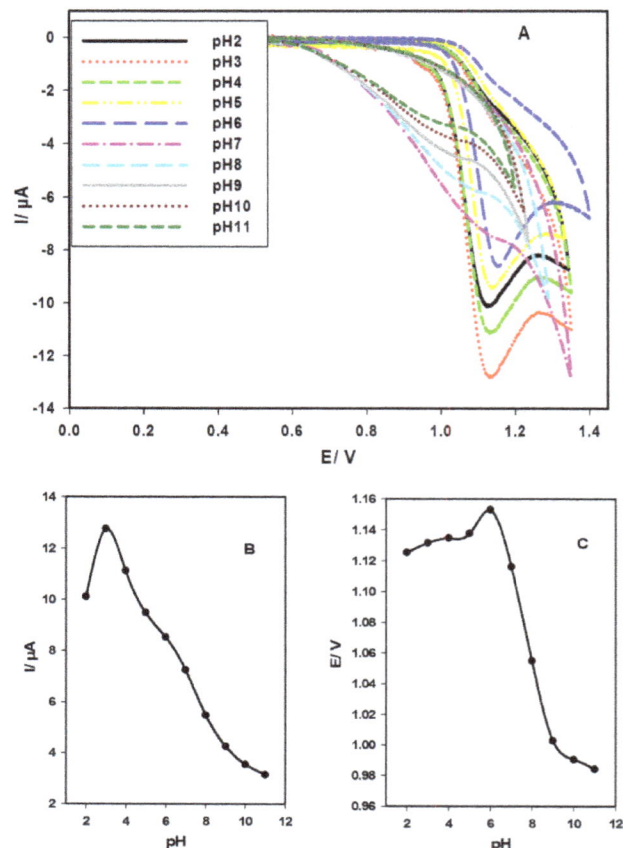

Figure 1. Cyclic voltammograms of the effect of solution pH on the oxidation of IH (1.43×10^{-4} mol L^{-1}) at CPE using BR buffers (pH 2.0-11.0) at scan rate of 100 mV s^{-1} (A). Linear plots of anodic peak currents (B) and potentials (C) as a function of pH.

Figure 2A shows that the anodic peak currents (I) are 12.755 μA (at 1.131V), 28.641 μA (at 1.117 V) and 63.543 μA (at 1.171 V) at CPE, MWCNTCPE and MWCNTCPE/SDS, respectively. Graphite and multiwalled carbon nanotubes have hydrophobic surface and SDS molecule has hydrophobic tail giving hydrophobic interactions between the electrode surface and SDS molecules.[25,26] SDS molecules were adsorbed on electrode surface to form negatively charged film which attract the positively charged drug and the drug concentration increases at the electrode surface leading to the increase of peak current.

Therefore, MWCNTCPE/SDS is the optimum electrode for the determination of IH according to its larger active surface area than CPE, and SDS works as micellar medium which increase the sensitivity and selectivity of

IH. Electronic Supplementary Information 1 (ESI 1) shows the difference in the surface shape between CPE and MWCNTCPE according to their SEM. ESI 2 shows the FTIR spectra of MWCNTCPE and MWCNTCPE/SDS. MWCNTCPE does not show clear absorption peaks in its FTIR spectrum.[27,28] MWCNTCPE/SDS shows S-O-C vibration peaks at 850

cm[-1] and 980 cm[-1], C-O stretching vibration peak at 1040 cm[-1], SO_2 symmetric vibration peak at 1100 cm[-1], CH_2 scissoring at 1460 cm[-1], CH_2 stretching at 2890 (asymmetric) and 2830 cm[-1] (symmetric), and a broad band between 3000 and 3650 cm[-1] due to O-H stretching vibration.[29]

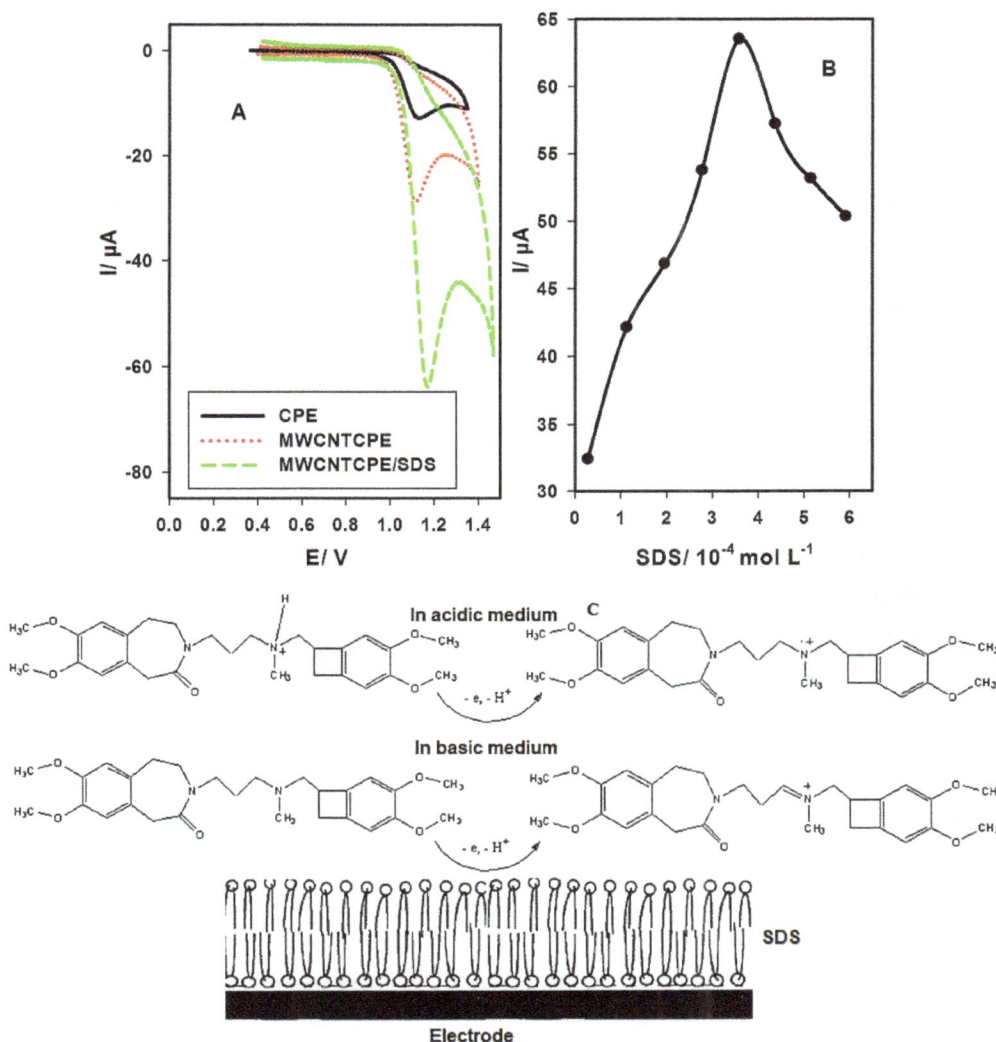

Figure 2. Cyclic voltammograms of IH (1.43×10^{-4} mol L[-1]) at CPE, MWCNTCPE and MWCNTCPE/SDS in BR buffer of pH 3.0 at scan rate of 100 mV s[-1] (A), effect of SDS concentration on the anodic peak current of IH (B), the oxidation mechanism of IH at MWCNTCPE/SDS (C).

Influence of SDS

Since IH is positively charged in acidic medium, SDS (as anionic surfactant) was used to enhance the peak current giving better sensitivity in the analysis of IH. Different volumes of SDS solution of concentrations varied from 2.85×10^{-5} to 5.91×10^{-4} mol L[-1] were added to the electrolytic cell containing IH (1.43×10^{-4} mol L[-1]) in BR buffer (pH 3.0). Figure 2B shows that the peak current increases as the concentration of SDS increases up to 3.58×10^{-4} mol L[-1] then after this concentration the peak current decreases as the concentration of SDS increases.

Hence, the optimum SDS concentration was 3.58×10^{-4} mol L[-1].

The mechanism of oxidation of IH is through the loss of one electron and one proton to form cation radical and cation in acidic and basic medium, respectively as shown in Figure 2C. The charges of atoms of IH were shown in ESI 3; N (amine) has the smallest negative value of -0.0586 (highest positive value) than those of the other atoms. Thus, it is the center of oxidation which loss one electron and its attached proton to form cation radical in acidic medium, while in basic medium this nitrogen atom loss one electron and the carbon atom C (18) which has the highest positive charge (0.0243) than those of the other carbon atoms loss one proton to form cation.

Influence of scan rate

Figure 3 represents the oxidation of IH (1.43×10^{-4} mol L^{-1}) in BR buffer (pH 3.0) as a function of scan rate (v) (10-400 mV s^{-1}) at MWCNTCPE/SDS. As v increases, the peak current increases, and the peak potentials increases (Figure 3A). Figure 3B, 3C show linear relationships were found between the peak currents and $v^{1/2}$ and between the logarithms of the peak current and v (log I = 0.80 + 0.48 log v, R (Correlation coefficient) = 0.9997), the slope 0.48 is near to 0.50 (theoretical value) suggesting diffusion controlled process of the oxidation of IH. [30]

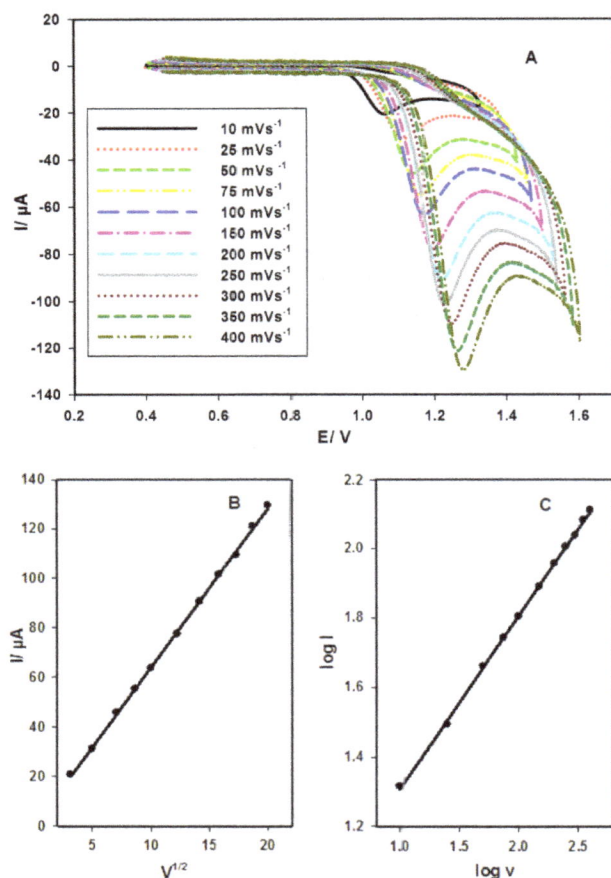

Figure 3. Effect of scan rate (10-400 mV s^{-1}) on the anodic peak current of IH at MWCNTCPE/SDS, cyclic voltammograms (A), I vs. $v^{1/2}$ (B) and log I vs. log v (C).

Chronoamperometry study

The diffusion coefficient of IH was determined in BR buffer (pH 3.0) at MWCNTCPE/SDS; the potential was set at 1.167 V. The diffusion coefficient of IH was determined using Cottrell equation: I = nFAC $(D/\pi t)^{1/2}$ where, I, n, F, C, D, and A are the current, the number of electrons (n = 1 for IH), Faraday constant (96480 C mol^{-1}), analyte concentration (mol cm^{-3}), the diffusion coefficient (cm^2 s^{-1}), and electroactive area of the working electrode, respectively. [31] A was obtained using

the diffusion coefficient of K_3Fe $(CN)_6$ which is equal to 7.6×10^{-6} cm^2 s^{-1}, [27] and thus A was calculated to be 0.115 cm^2.

Figure 4A represents the chronoamperograms of IH at MWCNTCPE/SDS in BR buffer of pH 3.0. It was shown that the chronoamperometric signal increases as the concentration of IH increases. It was found that 16 s is a sufficient electrolysis time to reach steady state. Figure 4B shows the linear relationships between I and $t^{-1/2}$. The plot of the slopes of straight lines obtained in Figure 4B against the concentration of IH gives a straight line as shown in Figure 4C; the slope of this relation is used to calculate D based on Cottrell equation. D of IH was found to be 3.175×10^{-5} cm^2 s^{-1}.

The reaction rate constant (K) was determined using the following equation: $I_C/I_L = (\pi K C t)^{1/2}$ where I_C and I_L are the catalytic and limited currents in the presence and in the absence of IH, respectively. [32] The value of K above equation was calculated from the slope of the plot of I_C/I_L vs. $t^{1/2}$ for 3.0×10^{-6} mol L^{-1} IH (Figure 4D), K was determined as 1.92×10^4 mol^{-1} L s^{-1}.

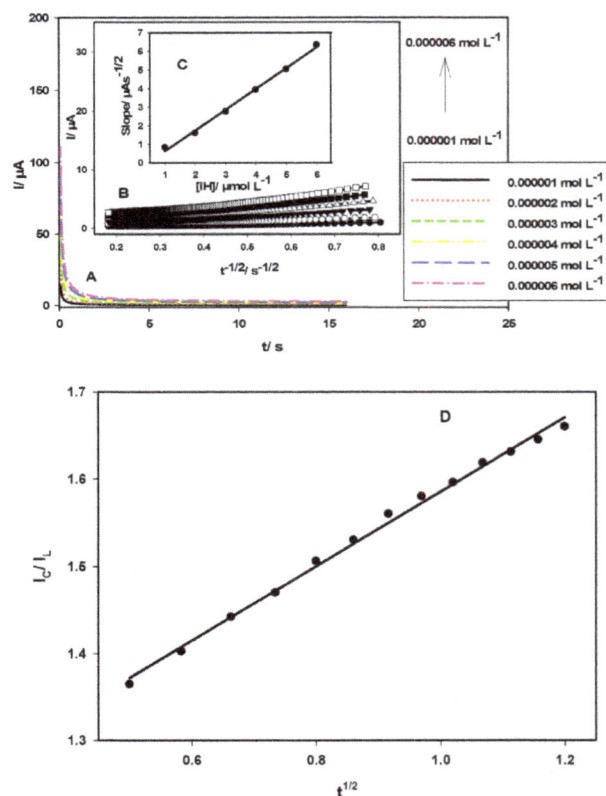

Figure 4. Chronoamperograms for IH at MWCNTCPE/SDS in BR buffer of pH 3.0 (A). Insets: I vs. $t^{1/2}$ from Cottrell's plot obtained from chronoamperograms (B) and the plot of the slopes of the straight lines against IH concentrations (C). Plot of I_C/I_L vs. $t^{1/2}$ in presence and absence of IH (3.0×10^{-6} mol L^{-1}) in BR buffer of pH 3.0 (D).

Determination of IH

Linear range, limits of detection (LOD) and quantification (LOQ) of IH were obtained using differential pulse voltammetry (DPV) at the

MWCNTCPE/SDS. Figure 5 depicts the calibration curve of IH (3.984×10^{-6} - 3.475×10^{-5} mol L^{-1}), I (μA) = $3.51 + 0.52$ C (μmol L^{-1}), R = 0.9994. LOD and LOQ were found to be 5.160×10^{-7} and 1.720×10^{-6} mol L^{-1}, respectively.

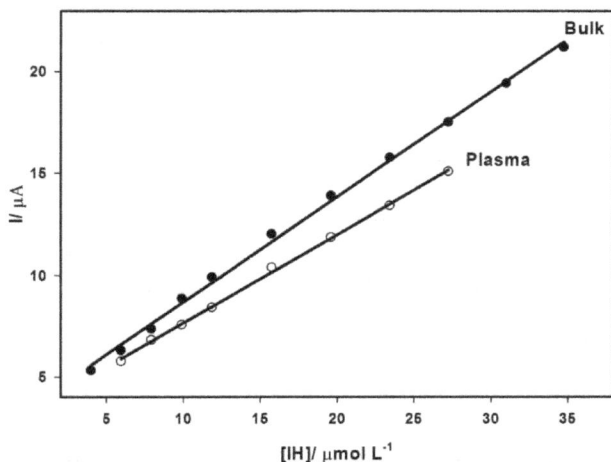

Figure 5. Calibration curves of IH in bulk and plasma using DPV at MWCNTCPE/SDS in BR buffer solution of pH 3.0, $\upsilon = 10$ mV s^{-1}.

Table 1 shows comparison between the proposed method and some reported methods used for analysis of IH. The proposed DPV method is more sensitive than these methods.

Statistical comparison between the results obtained by proposed voltammetric method and reported method,[11] was performed using t- test and F-ratio.[33] There is no significance difference between them as shown in Table 1. Table 2 shows the repeatability of the proposed method using different concentrations of IH which each of them was measured three times a day for three successive days.

The proposed method shows good repeatability as shown in Table 2.

The reproducibility of the proposed method was done by two different analysts using the same procedures for analysis of IH (9.9×10^{-6} mol L^{-1}). The recovery values were 99.65% and 100.48% for the first and the second analyst, respectively. The relative standard deviations of three replicate measurements were 0.61% and 0.74% for the first and the second analyst, respectively, suggesting good agreement of results.

Table 1. Comparison between the proposed DPV method and some other reported methods used to determine IH. Statistical analysis of the proposed method and the reported HPLC method for determination of IH.[11]

Method	Linear range	Reference
DPV (mol L^{-1}) (μg mL^{-1})	3.984×10^{-6} - 3.475×10^{-5} (2.012 - 17.550)	This work
Spectrophotometry (μg mL^{-1})	4.2 - 31.6	[4]
Chromatography (μg mL^{-1})	4.2 - 31.6	[4]
	70.69 - 131.29	[11]
Potentiometry (mol L^{-1})	1.0×10^{-5} - 1.0×10^{-2}	[13]

Statistical term	Proposed method	Reported method[11]
%Mean recovery	100.316	100.852
SD	1.593	1.450
Variance	2.537	2.163
n	5	5
t-test (2.306)*	0.553	
F-ratio (6.39)*	1.173	

*Figures in parenthesis are the theoretical values of t and F at confidence limit 95%.

Interference study

Lactose, microcrystalline cellulose, titanium dioxide and magnesium stearate are used as excipients in pharmaceutical industry. Interference studies were performed prior to analysis of IH in dosage forms using 1.0×10^{-5} mol L^{-1} and 1.0×10^{-4} mol L^{-1} of IH and all excipients, respectively. The presence of excipient not affect drug estimate.

Analysis of IH in tablets

Standard addition method was applied for analysis of IH in Procoralan tablets without any extraction steps prior to the analysis. The results showed that interference from the matrix was negligible (Table 2). IH can be determined in pharmaceutical formulation within the linear range (3.984×10^{-6} - 3.475×10^{-5} mol L^{-1}).

Analysis of IH in plasma

DPV method was successfully used to determine IH in spiked human plasma over the range of 5.964×10^{-6} - 2.723×10^{-5} mol L^{-1} (Figure 5) obeying analytical equation: I (μA) = $3.29 + 0.43$ C (μmol L^{-1}), R = 0.9991. LOD and LOQ were 1.15×10^{-6} and 3.82×10^{-6} mol L^{-1}, respectively. The recovery values were in the range of 99.16-102.32%. The relative standard deviation was 0.996%.

Table 2. Precision data for the proposed method. Determination of IH in Procoralan tablets by applying standard addition method.

Concentration (mol L^{-1})	Intra-day precision		%Mean Recovery±SD	%RSD
	Amount found[a]	%Recovery[a]		
7.936×10^{-6}	7.938×10^{-6}	100.025		
1.574×10^{-5}	1.565×10^{-5}	99.428	99.854±0.372	0.372
2.723×10^{-5}	2.726×10^{-5}	100.110		

Concentration (mol L^{-1})	Inter-day precision		%Mean Recovery±SD	%RSD
	Amount Found[a]	%Recovery[a]		
7.936×10^{-6}	7.931×10^{-6}	99.937		
1.574×10^{-5}	1.561×10^{-5}	99.174	99.630±0.403	0.404
2.723×10^{-5}	2.717×10^{-5}	99.780		

Dosage form	IH (mol L^{-1}) Taken	IH (mol L^{-1})		Recovery (%)
		Added	Found	
		1.984×10^{-6}	7.880×10^{-6}	99.144
Procoralan	5.964×10^{-6}	3.964×10^{-6}	9.898×10^{-6}	99.698
		5.940×10^{-6}	11.95×10^{-6}	100.386
		7.912×10^{-6}	13.78×10^{-6}	99.308
Mean recovery ± RSD*%				99.634±0.553

[a] Mean of three different samples for each concentration.
SD: Standard deviation of three different determinations
RSD: Relative standard deviation

Conclusion
The proposed method used MWCNTs and SDS based on their properties for the quantitative determination of IH in bulk, tablets and plasma. The sensor sensitivity and selectivity were enhanced using MWCNTs and SDS in comparison with CPE. The proposed DPV method is not time consuming method, there is no extraction stage. It can be used for quality control of IH.

Acknowledgments
The authors would like to express their gratitude to the National Organization for Drug Control and Research (NODCAR, Egypt) for providing instruments and the means necessary to accomplish this work.

Ethical Issues
Not applicable.

Conflict of Interest
Authors declare no conflict of interest in this study.

References
1. Sweetman SC. Martindale: The Complete Drug Reference. 36th ed. London, UK: Pharmaceutical Press; 2009.
2. Vilaine JP. The discovery of the selective I$_f$ current inhibitor ivabradine. A new therapeutic approach to ischemic heart disease. *Pharmacol Res* 2006;53(5):424-34. doi: 10.1016/j.phrs.2006.03.016
3. Tubati VP, Murthy TEGK, Rao ASS. Comparision of different techniques involved in the development of ivabradine HCl floating pulsatile multiparticulate systems for chronotherapeutic delivery. *Br J Pharm Res* 2016;9(4):1-12. doi: 10.9734/BJPR/2016/22566
4. Maheshwari S, Khandhar AP, Jain A. Quantitative determination and validation of ivabradine HCl by stability indicating RP-HPLC method and spectrophotometric method in solid dosage form. *Eurasian J Anal Chem* 2010;5(1):53-62.
5. Klippert P, Jeanniot JP, Polve S, Lefevre C, Merdjan H. Determination of ivabradine and its N-demethylated metabolite in human plasma and urine, and in rat and dog plasma by a validated high-performance liquid chromatographic method with fluorescence detection. *J Chromatogr B Biomed Sci Appl* 1998;719(1-2):125-33. doi: 10.1016/S0378-4347(98)00406-X
6. Francois-Bouchard M, Simonin G, Bossant, Boursier-Neyret C. Simultaneous determination of ivabradine and its metabolites in human plasma by liquid chromatography--tandem mass spectrometry. *J Chromatogr B Biomed Sci Appl* 2000;745(2):261-9. doi: 10.1016/S0378-4347(00)00275-9
7. Lu C, Jia Y, Yang J, Jin X, Song Y, Liu W, et al. Simultaneous determination of ivabradine and N-desmethylivabradine in human plasma and urine using a LC-MS/MS method: application to a pharmacokinetic study. *Acta Pharm Sin B* 2012;2(2):205-12. doi: 10.1016/j.apsb.2012.01.004
8. Pikul P, Nowakowska J, Ciura K. Chromatographic analysis of ivabradine on polar, nonpolar and chemically modified adsorbents by HPTLC. *J Food Drug Anal* 2013;21(2):165-8. doi: 10.1016/j.jfda.2013.05.006
9. Damle MC, Bagwe RA. Development and validation of stability-indicating HPTLC method for ivabradine HCl. *Pharm Sci Monitor* 2015;6(1):141-52.

10. Motisariya MH, Patel KG, Shah PA. Validated stability-indicating high performance thin layer chromatographic method for determination of Ivabradine hydrochloride in bulk and marketed formulation: an application to kinetic study. *Bull Fac Pharm Cairo Univ* 2013;51(2):233-41. doi: 10.1016/j.bfopcu.2013.07.001

11. Kumar PS, Pandiyan K, Rajagopal K. Development and validation of stability indicating rapid HPLC method for estimation of ivabradine hydrochloride in solid oral dosage form. *Int J Pharm Pharm Sci* 2014;6(4):378-82.

12. Patel KG, Motisariya MH, Patel KR, Shah PA, Gandhi TR. Development and validation of spectrofluorimetric method for estimation of ivabradine hydrochloride in marketed formulation and its applicability in plasma. *Pharm Lett* 2014;6(5):8-13.

13. Abo-Talib NF, Tammam MH, Attia AK. Electrochemical study of ivabradine hydrochloride ion selective electrodes using different ionophores. *RSC Adv* 2015;5(116):95592-7. doi: 10.1039/c5ra21033j

14. Majidi MR, Pournaghi-Azar MH, Azar P, Fadakar Bajeh Baj R, Naseri A. Fabrication of ferrocene functionalised ionic liquid/carbon nanotube nanocomposite modified carbon-ceramic electrode: application to the determination of hydrazine. *Int J Environ Anal Chem* 2016;96(1):50-67. doi: 10.1080/03067319.2015.1114106

15. Shishehbore MR, Zare HR, Nematollahi D. Electrocatalytic determination of morphine at the surface of a carbon paste electrode spiked with a hydroquinone derivative and carbon nanotubes. *J Electroanal Chem* 2012;665:45-51. doi: 10.1016/j.jelechem.2011.11.018

16. Rizk M, Attia AK, Elshahed MS, Farag AS. Validated voltammetric method for the determination of antiparkinsonism drug entacapone in bulk, pharmaceutical formulation and human plasma. *J Electroanal Chem* 2015;743:112-9. doi: 10.1016/j.jelechem.2015.02.022

17. Babaei A, Afrasiabi M, Azim G. Nanomolar simultaneous determination of epinephrine and acetaminophen on a glassy carbon electrode coated with a novel Mg-Al layered double hydroxide-nickel hydroxide nanoparticles-multi-walled carbon nanotubes composite. *Anal Methods* 2015;7(6):2469-78. doi: 10.1039/C4AY02406K

18. Attia AK. Determination of antihypertensive drug moexipril hydrochloride based on the enhancement effect of sodium dodecyl sulfate at carbon paste electrode. *Talanta* 2010;81(1-2):25-9. doi: 10.1016/j.talanta.2009.11.031

19. Attia AK, Badawy AM, Abd-Elhamid SG. Determination of sparfloxacin and besifloxacin hydrochlorides using gold nanoparticles modified carbon paste electrode in micellar medium. *RSC Adv* 2016;6(46):39605-17. doi: 10.1039/C6RA04851J

20. Attia AK, Salem WM, Mona AM. Voltammetric assay of metformin hydrochloride using pyrogallol modified carbon paste electrode. *Acta Chim Solv* 2015;62(3):588-94. doi: 10.17344/acsi.2014.950

21. Rao CN, Satishkumar BC, Govindaraj A, Nath M. Nanotubes. *ChemPhysChem* 2001;2(2):78-105. doi: 10.1002/1439-7641(20010216)

22. Baughman RH, Zakhidov AA, de Heer WA. Carbon nanotubes--the route toward applications. *Science* 2002;297(5582):787-92. doi: 10.1126/science.1060928

23. Xiong H, Zhao Y, Liu P, Zhang X, Wang S. Electrochemical properties and the determination of nicotine at a multi-walled carbon nanotubes modified glassy carbon electrode. *Mikrochim Acta* 2010;168(1):31-6. doi: 10.1007/s00604-009-0258-8

24. Kasumov AY, Bouchiat H, Reulet B, Stephan O, Khodos II, Gorbatov YB, et al. Conductivity and atomic structure of isolated multiwalled carbon nanotubes. *Europhys Lett* 1998;43(1):89-94. doi: 10.1209/epl/i1998-00324-1

25. Shi G, Shen Y, Liu J, Wang C, Wang Y, Song B, et al. Molecular-scale hydrophilicity induced by solute: molecular-thick charged pancakes of aqueous salt solution on hydrophobic carbon-based surfaces. *Sci Rep* 2014;4:6793. doi: 10.1038/srep06793

26. Rusling JF. Molecular aspects of electron transfer at electrodes in micellar solutions. *Colloids Surf Physicochem Eng Aspects* 1997;123-124:81-8. doi: 10.1016/S0927-7757(96)03789-2

27. Muraliganth T, Murugan AV, Manthiram A. Nanoscale networking of $LiFePO_4$ nanorods synthesized by a microwave-solvothermal route with carbon nanotubes for lithium ion batteries. *J Mater Chem* 2008;18(46):5661-8. doi: 10.1039/B812165F

28. Morávková Z, Trchová M, Tomšík E, Čechvala J, Stejskal J. Enhanced thermal stability of multi-walled carbon nanotubes after coating with polyaniline salt. *Polym Degrad Stab* 2012;97(8):1405-14. doi: 10.1016/j.polymdegradstab.2012.05.019

29. Coates J. Interpretation of infrared spectra, a practical approach. Encyclopedia of analytical chemistry. USA: John Wiley & Sons; 2000.

30. Gosser DK. Cyclic voltammetry: Simulation and analysis of reaction Mechanism. New York: VCH; 1993.

31. Bard AJ, Faulkner LR. Electrochemical methods: Fundamentals and applications. 2nd ed. New York: Wiley; 2001.

32. Galus Z. Fundamentals of electrochemical analysis. New York: Ellis Horwood; 1994.

33. Miller JN, Miller JC. Statistics and chemometrics for analytical chemistry. 4th ed. Harlow, England: Prentice Hall; 2000.

15

The Impact of Amorphisation and Spheronization Techniques on the Improved *in Vitro* & *in Vivo* Performance of Glimepiride Tablets

Rana Refaat Makar[1], Randa Latif[2]*, Ehab Ahmed Hosni[3], Omaima Naim El Gazayerly[2]

[1] Faculty of Pharmacy, Ahram Canadian University, Egypt.
[2] Faculty of Pharmacy, Department of Pharmaceutics, Cairo University, Cairo, Egypt.
[3] Faculty of Pharmacy, Russian University, Egypt.

Keywords:
· Dissolution
· Pharmacodynamic study
· Blood glucose level
· Matrix tablets
· Spherical agglomeration
· Triple solid dispersion adsorbate

Abstract

Purpose: Triple solid dispersion adsorbates (TSDads) and spherical agglomerates (SA) present new techniques that extensively enhance dissolution of poorly soluble drugs.
The aim of the present study is to hasten the onset of hypoglycemic effect of glimepiride through enhancing its rate of release from tablet formulation prepared from either technique.

Methods: Drug release from TSDads or SA tablets with different added excipients was explored. Scanning electron microscopy (SEM) and effect of compression on dissolution were illustrated. Pharmacodynamic evaluation was performed on optimized tablets.

Results: TSDads & SA tablets with Cross Povidone showed least disintegration times of 1.48 and 0.5 min. respectively. Kinetics of drug release recorded least half-lives (54.13 and 59.83min for both techniques respectively). Cross section in tablets displayed an organized interconnected matrix under SEM, accounting for the rapid access of dissolution media to the tablet core. Components of tablets filled into capsules showed a similar release profile to that of tablets after compression as indicated by similarity factor. The onset time of maximum reduction in blood glucose in male albino rabbits was hastened to 2h instead of 3h for commercial tablets.

Conclusion: After optimization of tablet excipients that interacted differently with respect to their effect on drug release, we could conclude that both amorphisation and spheronization were equally successful in promoting in vitro dissolution enhancement as well as providing a more rapid onset time for drug action *in vivo*.

Introduction

A variety of technical problems are usually encountered in the pharmaceutical industry when dealing with the formulation of insoluble drugs,[1] often leading to a suboptimal drug product. Poor aqueous solubility of drugs affects both their *in vitro* dissolution rate,[2] as well as their pharmacological activity.[3] Therefore, continuous efforts have been dedicated for the treatment of such problem through a different design of particle technology[4] and particle engineering processes, such as spray freezing into liquids,[5] sonocrystallization,[6,7] and others.[8] In general, most preliminary pretreatment of particles relies upon making a change in the drug crystallinity, the so-called amorphisation techniques.[9] Amorphous forms of drugs are characterized by a disordered arrangement of molecules in the solid state. This is accompanied by a higher state of free energy, enabling faster extent and rate of drug dissolution.[10,11] Another well-known strategy for decreasing drug crystallinity is particle spheronization which was achieved in literature via different techniques and mechanisms;[12] thus, enabling dissolution enhancement of poorly soluble drugs.[13]

Direct tabletting of pharmaceutical materials involves dry blending and compaction of the active pharmaceutical ingredient with the necessary excipients and lubricants. The whole process is simple and saves time, costs and energy.[14,15]

Many excipients were found helpful in the design of a proper formulation when they were incorporated during tablet manufacture.

In some cases, the addition of diluents might contribute to enhancing the dissolution of poorly soluble drugs.[16] Lactose is one of the most famous diluents used in pharmaceutical formulation. It gained much popularity due to its good physical properties, being pleasant in taste, non hygroscopic, readily soluble in water and non-reactive with most excipients.[17] Khan and Zhu[18] revealed that tabletting with lactose resulted in a limited enhancement in the release rate of ibuprofen. Lin[19] also found an increase in the release rate of theophylline from tabletted microcapsules containing lactose. Mannitol (Pearlitol SD) was selected in some formulae as diluent owing to its low hygroscopicity and good flowability. Gonnissen et al.[20] believed that mannitol imparted an acceptable tensile strength to the tablets.

It was also shown that many binders had a very good influence on the dissolution profile of drugs. Chitosan, when used as a binder, affected the mechanical properties of granules, the disintegration time of tablets, and the whole dissolution profile of chlorpheniramine maleate was enhanced.[21] Avicel PH 102 as a direct compression excipient[22] produced tablets with lower crushing strength, shorter disintegration time and smaller weight variation as compared to Avicel PH101.[23] Low substituted hydroxypropyl cellulose (L-HPC) had also good binding and disintegrating properties when used in fast disintegrating tablets along with Avicel PH102.[24] Moreover, increased amount of L-HPC in the prepared granules of sparfloxacin resulted in increasing its dissolution rate. The polymer induced a considerable expansion in the matrix of the film-coated granules due to their uptake of water from the dissolution medium. The process resulted in film bursting after a short lag time.[25]

Many superdisintegrants were found to be successful in tablet formulations.[26,27] Generally, starch disintegrants tended to swell and disrupt the tablet or helped disintegration by particle-to-particle repulsion.[17] The pregelatinization process involved physical modification of the starch resulting in the combined benefits of the soluble and insoluble functions of starch. Its high swelling power could be achieved when hydrated with cold water. This produced viscous slurries that might have resulted in better wetting of drug matrices inside tablets.[28] Ac-Di-Sol, a well known superdisintegrant, swelled 4-9 times its original volume when it came in direct contact with water. This helped water uptake by the tablet, causing its rapid breakage. The individual fibers of Ac-Di-Sol acted as hydrophilic channels to absorb and transfer water into the tablet system, giving rapid solubilization of tablet constituents and a higher disintegration and dissolution rate.[29]

Cross Povidone (CP) is a water insoluble polymer. Its particles possessed a porous morphology that initiated rapid water absorption and volume expansion. A probable hydrostatic pressure was then exerted on tablets, causing their disintegration.[30, 20]

Generally, drugs may be incorporated inside tablets as simple powder[31,32] or preformulated in other forms. Solid dispersion of poorly soluble drugs prepared by several techniques were compressed into tablets in order to attain an enhancement in dissolution profiles of such drugs.[33-35] Spherical crystals of several drugs were also compressed in the form of tablets. A considerable increase in the rate and extent of drug release from such formulae was illustrated.[36-38]

Trial for dissolution enhancement of glimepiride was achieved through the preparation of solid dispersion with either sodium starch glycolate[39] or with PVPK30.[40] However, to our knowledge; literature available on glimepiride lacks research study on spheronization or surfactant-aided solid dispersion.

The present study aims to test and compare the applicability of new amorphisation and spheronization techniques viz: Triple solid dispersion adsorbate (TSDads) or spherical agglomerates (SA) in attaining best results in dissolution enhancement of glimepiride, as well as

studying the effect of compression on dissolution parameters. The work will involve an *in vitro* optimization of the tabletting process in the presence of different partially water-soluble to water-insoluble excipients. A pharmacodynamic evaluation is carried out on optimized formulae to test for the hastening in the onset of hypoglycemic action after oral administration compared to a marketed product.

Materials and Methods
Materials
Glimepiride was kindly supplied by Sedico Pharmaceuticals, Giza, Egypt. Sodium Lauryl Sulphate (SLS) was purchased from El-Nasr Pharmaceutical Chemicals Co., Cairo, Egypt. Pregelatinized starch (PreGelSt) was a gift from Colorcon Limited, UK. Ac-Di-Sol (Crosscarmellose sodium) was purchased from E. Merck, Germany. Crosspovidone XL (CP) and Avicel pH 102 were purchased from FMC Corporation, Philadelphia, USA. Starlac (lactose and maize starch), Pearlitol SD (Mannitol) and Pearlitol flash (mannitol and maize starch) were a gift from Roquette, France. Gelucire 50/13 was obtained from Gattefosé, France. Colloidal Silicon dioxide (Aerosil 200) hydrophilic was obtained from Degussa, USA. Polyvinylpyrrolidone (PVP K30) was obtained from Fluka, Switzerland. Low substituted Hydroxypropylcellulose (L-HPC) was purchased from Shin-Etsu Chemical Co., Ltd Tokyo, Japan. Spray-dried lactose was a gift from Ph. Francaise Co., France. Carbon tetrachloride and magnesium stearate were obtained from El-Nasr Pharmaceutical Chemicals Company, Cairo, Egypt. Aspartame was purchased from Sigma, St.Louis, USA. Amaryl® tablets (3 mg): Batch No. 2EG008 was obtained from Sanofi-Aventis, Cairo, Egypt.

Methods
Preparation of ternary solid dispersion (TSD)
Glimepiride TSD was prepared with PreGelSt as a carrier by the melting method using Gelucire 50/13 as surfactant at a drug-to-carrier-to-surfactant ratio of 1:5:15, respectively. The drug and carrier were added consecutively with continuous stirring in the molten Gelucire until a homogenous dispersion was obtained. The mixture was then allowed to cool on an ice bath until solidification.

Preparation of ternary solid dispersion adsorbates (TSDads)
The melt adsorption technique described by Parmar et al.[41] was used to prepare TSDads. In brief TSD was dropped (while in the molten state) onto lactose powder (preheated to 70 °C) with continuous stirring to obtain the respective TSDads at a drug-to-carrier-to-surfactant-to-adsorbent ratio of 1:5:15:30, respectively. The mixture was allowed to cool to room temperature where it continued to have the appearance of free flowing powder.

Evaluation and characterization of TSD &TSDads
Drug content uniformity: To test for homogeneity of drug content within batches of TSD & their adsorbates, ten

random samples were taken from each batch. A fixed weight was stirred in methanol for 15 min, filtered and assayed spectrophotometrically for glimepiride content. Each experiment was done in triplicates.

Scanning electron microscopy: The surface morphology of glimepiride and formulae based on solid dispersion with the drug were visualized by scanning electron microscopy (SEM JSM-6390 LV, JEOL, Tokyo, Japan) at a working distance of 20 mm and an accelerated voltage of 15 kV. Samples were gold-coated with a sputtercoater (Desk V, Denton Vacuum, NJ, USA) before SEM observation under high vacuum of 45 mTorr and high voltage of 30 mV.

Preparation of spherical agglomerates (SA)
SA were prepared by a slight modification to the quasi-emulsion[42] and crystallo-co-agglomeration.[43,44] Glimepiride (150mg) was dissolved in 2ml dimethyl formamide at 25°C. To this solution were added Aerosil 200 (150mg) as dispersing agent[45] and Starlac (0.5% w/v) as carrier[46] with continuous agitation using a three-blade mechanical stirrer at 500 rpm to keep the suspension uniformly dispersed. PVP K30 was dissolved in water (4 ml) until a saturated solution (data not shown) was formed at room temperature, then the prepared aqueous solution, acting as poor solvent for the drug, was added to the drug solution with continuous agitation in order to precipitate the drug. Carbon tetrachloride (0.85ml), acting as a bridging liquid, was added drop-wise to the agitated dispersion. Formed agglomerates were collected after a further 10-minute agitation, washed with distilled water, filtered, dried in a hot air oven at 45°C for 24h and stored in tightly closed containers in a desiccator for further investigations.

Evaluation and characterization of SA
Drug content uniformity: Glimepiride content was tested within batches of SA. Ten random samples were taken from each batch. Spherical agglomerates were crushed in a glass mortar. A fixed weight was then stirred in methanol for 15 min, filtered and assayed spectrophotometrically for glimepiride. Each experiment was done in triplicates.

Scanning electron microscopy: Surface topography of glimepiride particles, pure excipients and prepared SAs were observed and compared through a scanning electron microscope (Joel Corp., Mikaka, Japan) operated at 15 Kv after coating with gold. Different magnification powers were illustrated.

Formulation of tablets
Previously prepared TSDads and SA were compressed into tablets. Some superdisintegrants viz: PreGelSt, Starlac, Ac-Di-Sol, CP and Pearlitol flash were tried during compression. All added excipients were mixed with previously prepared TSDads or SA by the geometric dilution method; lactose was added as a diluent to adjust the final weight of the tablet to 250 mg. Powder mixtures was compressed using a single punch tablet press (Korsch EKO, Germany) using 6mm flat level edged punch. A compression force of (3-5 KN) was applied so as to

provide a constant value for hardness for all tested formulae, and measured with tablet hardness tester (Coplay scientific type TH3/500 Nottingham, United Kingdom NG42J).

Evaluation of prepared tablets containing TSDads or SA
Prepared tablets were subjected to quality control tests following USP Pharmacopeial regulations, namely: weight variation,[47] friability,[48] and content uniformity.

Disintegration time (D.T.): The D.T. for six tablets from each formula was determined in distilled water at 37°C using USP disintegration tester (Coplay Scientific, NE4-COP, UK). The initial disintegration time (I.D.T.) was recorded at the beginning of disintegration. The time at which complete tablet disintegration occurred was recorded as total disintegration time (T.D.T.).

In vitro drug release: The release profile of the drug from prepared formulae was determined using USP dissolution tester (Hanson Research, 64-705-045, USA) type I at 100 rpm. Release was carried out at 37°C in 900ml 0.5% aqueous solution of SLS. Two ml samples were withdrawn at different time intervals and replaced with fresh media. Absorbance of the samples was measured spectrophotometrically at λ_{max} 228nm. Results were mean of three determinations.

Kinetic analysis of release data: Data obtained from release experiments were treated statistically according to linear regression analysis. Data were fitted to zero order, first order and Higushi diffusion model.
Equation for zero order: $C = C_\circ - K_\circ t$
Equation for first order: $\log C = \log C_\circ - Kt/2.303$
Simplified equation for Higuchi diffusion model:
$$Q = K \times t^{1/2}$$
Physicochemical characterization of optimized tablet formulae containing TSDads or SA
Tablet formulae with TSDads or SA showing best results with respect to DT and dissolution profile were selected for further characterization.

Scanning Electron Microscopy (SEM): The surface topography and cross section of optimum tablet formulae T5 and TS2 were observed through a scanning electron microscope (Joel Corp., Mikaka, Japan) operated at 15 kv after coating with gold.

Effect of compression on glimepiride release: The components of tablet formulae T5 and TS2 were filled in hard gelatin capsules size 1 and subjected to release study under the same conditions as their respective tablets. Kinetic treatment of drug release data was then matched with results obtained from their respective tablets.

Pharmacodynamic evaluation of optimized tablet formulae
Optimized tablet formulae with the least recorded release $t_{1/2}$ were further evaluated with respect to their pharmacodynamic effect on male albino rabbits.
The study protocol was approved by the institutional review board of the Faculty of Pharmacy, Cairo University (PI 1144).

The study was based on single dose and parallel group design. Male albino rabbits weighing 3.5-4kg were kept on standard diet and then made to fast overnight before carrying the experiment. They were divided into three groups, each of eight animals. Groups I, II and III for administration of marketed product Amaryl®, TS2 and T5 tablets respectively. All tested tablets contained an amount equivalent to 3 mg glimepiride. Blood samples after oral intake of glimepiride were withdrawn from the marginal ear vein of rabbits at specific time intervals; every 15 min. during the first hour, every 30 min. up to 3h, and then every hour up to 12h. Samples were measured for blood glucose level (BGL) using *ACCU CHEK® Go* system.[49,50] Initial BGL was measured at zero time (just before the administration of the respective tablets). Each animal was considered as its own control and the hypoglycemic response was calculated as the percent reduction in blood glucose level according to the following equation

$$\text{Decrease BGL (\%)} = \frac{BGL\ at\ t = 0 - BGL\ at\ t = t \times 100}{BGL\ at\ t = 0}$$

Mean percent reduction in BGL versus time was drawn and the area under the Curve (AUC $_{0-12}$) was calculated adopting the trapezoidal rule.[51] Maximum reduction (Red max) was attained in BGL and the time to reach Red max was denoted as Tmax was compared for both formulae and the marketed product. Statistical analysis of the results was performed using one-way analysis of variance (ANOVA) to determine the least significant difference between tested formulae.

Results and Discussion
Drug content evaluation in TSD, TSDads & SA
All assayed samples of TSD & TSDads resulted in 98-100% glimepiride content, indicating uniformity of drug distribution within different matrices. Samples of SA gave around 97-99% glimepiride content, indicating the absence of drug loss during the dispensing procedures.

Scanning electron microscopy for TSD, TSDads & SA
Figure1 shows the strong crystal habit of glimepiride platelets with distinct sharp edges and the gradual transformation that occurred into an amorphous structure with smooth to round edges through the formulation of TSD & TSDads. The surface of TSD acquired an amorphous shape with smooth texture similar to the surface topography of intact gelucire pellets. This obviously demonstrated the contribution of gelucire in the final amorphisation of the triple dispersion. TSDads showed a perfect spherical morphology with complete rounded edges coinciding to the surface structure of lactose. It could be, thus, clearly identified that the role of the adsorbent was not only restricted to disaggregation and micronization of particles, but also to promoting their spheronization.

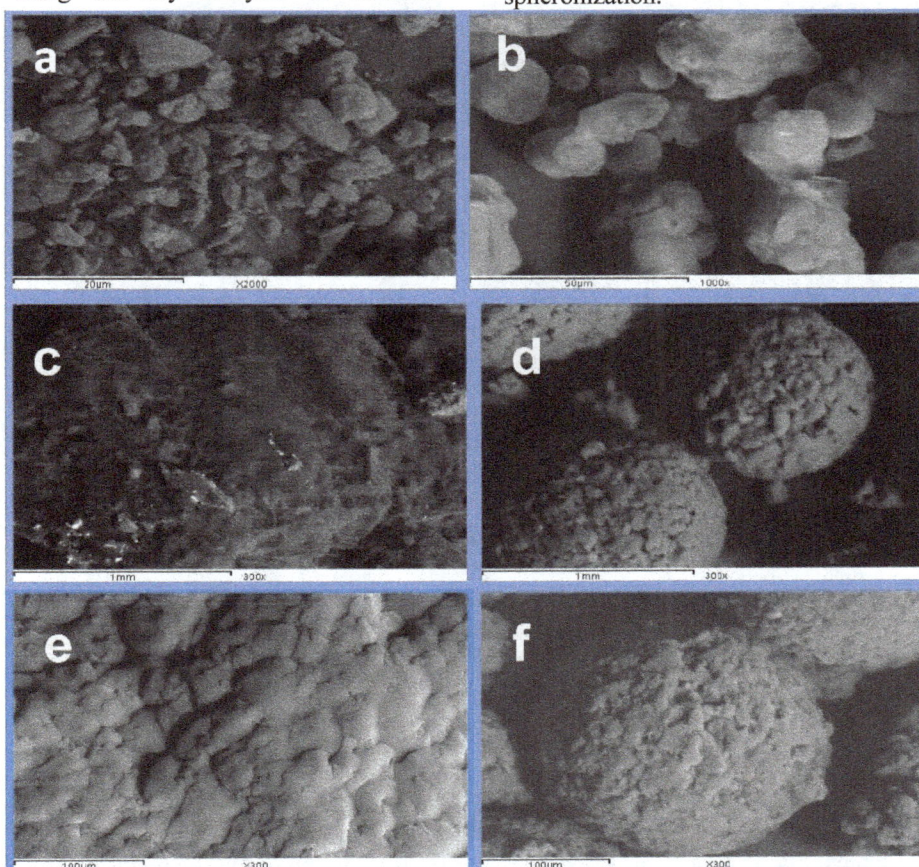

Figure 1. SEM of (a) glimepiride particles; (b) pregelatinized starch [PreGelSt]; (c) gelucire 50/13 ; (d) lactose; (e) triple solid dispersion[TSD] ; (f) triple solid dispersion adsorbate [TSD ads]

Figure 2 illustrates the elements used in the preparation of SA. Starlac particles were globular in shape with an irregular surface similar to lactose globules (which constitutes the larger percentage of such carrier). PVP K30 appeared as large smooth spheres while Aerosil 200 appeared as fine particles. The prepared SAPVPst agglomerates were much larger in size compared with the single components, perfectly spherical with a distinct rough surface. Higher magnification of agglomerate surfaces showed the aggregation of drug platelets together with occasional small spherical patches that might be due to the surface adsorption of Starlac particles.

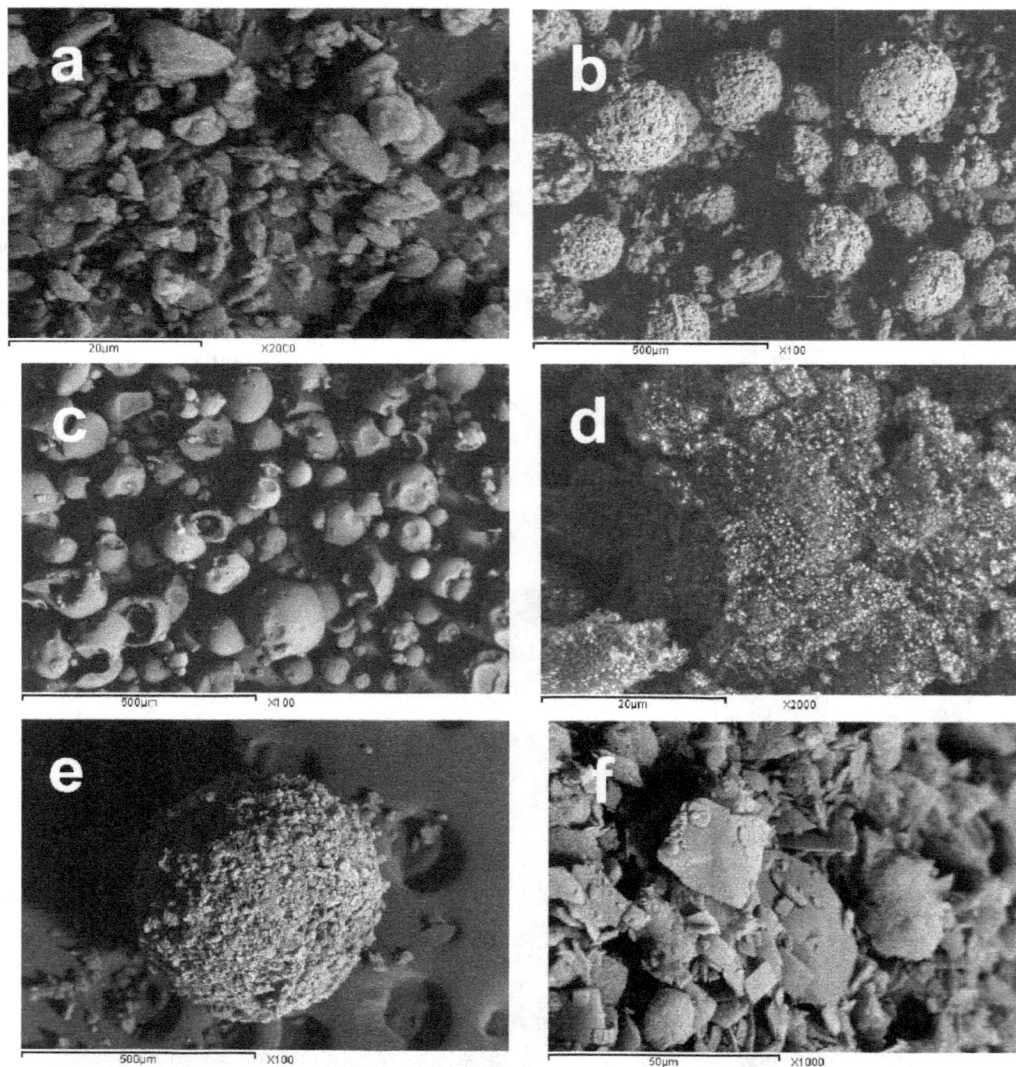

Figure 2. SEM micrographs of (a) pure glimepiride; (b) Starlac at 100 x; (c) PVP K30 at 100x; (d) Aerosil 200 at 2000x (e) spherical agglomerates with PVP & starlac [SAPVPst] whole spheres at 100x; (f) SAPVPst surface at 10000x

Optimization of tablet formulations prepared with TSDads & SA

Quality control tests for the prepared tablets showed acceptable results within the US Pharmacopeial limits (data not shown).

Disintegration time

Initial disintegration time (I.D.T) was thought to be the rate-limiting step in drug dissolution; therefore, it was mainly considered in tablet optimization.

Formulae T1-T4 (Table 1) containing PreGelSt as an externally added superdisintegrant showed variation in I.D.T. The best value was recorded in T4 (1.51 min.)

(Table 2). The high concentration of PreGelSt present in T4 might have added value to the swelling properties of the starch, helping the rapid uptake of water into the tablet core and causing its rapid disintegration. Tablets containing CP in T5 had the least value for I.D.T. (1.48 min). These results confirmed the superiority of CP over all tested superdisintegrants.[52-54] Its unique porous structure along with its high hydration capacity[55] resulted in a high swelling volume and an increase in the internally applied pressure inside tablet matrices. Thus, the rapid disintegration of tablets occurred at a much higher rate.

Tablets containing CP in TS2 (Table 2) also had the least value for D.T. (0.5 min), confirming its superiority. Other superdisintegrants, either in TSDads or SA tablets, were ranked with respect to their efficiency in the following order Ac-Di-Sol> Starlac> Pearlitol flash. Although the marketed tablets Amaryl® showed spontaneous disintegration, yet the low release rate of its tablet overshadowed the good result for its D.T.

Table 1. Composition of triple solid dispersion adsorbate [TSDads] & spherical agglomerates [SA] tablets

Formula Code	Superdisintegrant		Lubricant	Sweetener	Compression aid	Binder	
	Type	Weight (mg)	Mg Stearate(mg)	Aspartame (mg)	Pearlitol SD (mg)	Avicel (mg)	L-HPC (mg)
T1*	PreGelSt#	25	2.5	5	25	32.9	6.6
T2*	PreGelSt#	25	0.625	5	25	34.47	6.89
T3*	PreGelSt#	50	0.625	5	25	13.64	2.72
T4*	PreGelSt#	50	0.625	5	20	15	5
T5*	CP##	50	0.625	5	20	15	5
T6*	Ac-Di-Sol	50	0.625	5	20	15	5
T7*	Pearlitol flash	50	0.625	5	20	15	5
T8*	Starlac	50	0.625	5	20	15	5
TS1**	PreGelSt#	50	0.625	5	20	15	5
TS2**	CP##	50	0.625	5	20	15	5
TS3**	Starlac	50	0.625	5	20	15	5
TS4**	Ac-Di-Sol	50	0.625	5	20	15	5
TS5**	Pearlitol flash	50	0.625	5	20	15	5

*All formulae contain 153 mg of the optimized TSDads equivalent to 3 mg glimepiride
**All formulae contain 6.6 mg of the optimized SA equivalent to 3 mg glimepiride and 143.7 mg lactose as diluents
Pregelatinized starch
Crosspovidone

Table 2. In-vitro disintegration time for tablet formulae containing triple solid dispersion adsorbate [TSDads] & spherical agglomerates [SA]

Formula Code	Initial disintegration time I.D.T. (min.)	Total disintegration time T.D.T (min.)
Amaryl®	0.25	2.00
T1*	3.01	16.20
T2*	2.56	14.12
T3*	2.30	10.50
T4*	1.51	8.42
T5*	1.48	6.29
T6*	2.07	9.16
T7*	3.53	9.39
T8*	3.11	8.12
TS1**	1.34	4.75
TS2**	0.50	1.09
TS3**	1.02	3.24
TS4**	0.86	3.19
TS5**	1.02	2.41

* Triple solid dispersion adsorbate TSDads tablets
** Spherical agglomerates SA tablets

Kinetic analysis of release data

Kinetic treatment of glimepiride release data (Table 3) showed that a diffusion model prevailed in most of the TSDads tablets except for T6 (with Ac-Di-Sol), where a first order release and a small percentage of flush release occurred. The other formulae demonstrated different lag time values. This variation might be a result of a difference in the wetting capability within the tablet core. T1 possessed the longest lag time (7.9 min) While proceeding in optimization, lag time values decreased sequentially with the successive decrease in binder weights along with the increase in the amount of added

PreGelSt.[56,57] It seemed that the concomitant variation in these two excipients was a promising factor that predisposes the particles earlier to the wetting effect of the dissolution medium. The least value was attained in

T5 (1.01 min) containing CP. This proved its superiority in achieving the highest rate of wetting to tablet matrix before the release began to proceed.

Table 3. Kinetic treatment of release data of glimepiride from triple solid dispersion adsorbate [TSDads] & spherical agglomerates [SA] tablets

Formula Code	Order of release	K***	Half- life (min.)	Y-intercept	Significance of Y-intercept	
					Flush release (mg%)	Lag time (min.)
T1*	diffusion	8.75	72.62	-24.63	-	7.92
T2*	diffusion	9.12	66.90	-24.67	-	7.31
T3*	diffusion	9.78	59.70	-25.71	-	6.90
T4*	diffusion	8.03	60.82	-12.62	-	2.47
T5*	diffusion	7.86	54.13	-7.93	-	1.02
T6*	first	0.01	61.43	1.99	1.67	-
T7*	diffusion	7.45	66.27	-10.84	-	2.12
T8*	diffusion	8.33	57.50	-13.25	-	2.53
TS1**	diffusion	6.74	75.17	-8.44	-	1.57
TS2**	diffusion	7.90	59.83	-11.11	-	1.98
TS3**	diffusion	7.29	72.35	-12.01	-	2.72
TS4**	first	0.01	64.02	1.98	4.50	-
TS5**	first	9.902×10^{-3}	69.98	1.97	5.16	-
Amaryl®	zero	0.37	122.98	4.02	4.03	-

* triple solid dispersion adsorbate TSDads Tablets, ** spherical agglomerates SA tablets
***Units of K (rate constant) is mg/min for zero order, min^{-1} for first order & mg/ min$^{1/2}$ for Higushi diffusion model

Tested superdisintegrants in SA tablets acted differently within their respective matrices. Tablets with Ac-di-sol (TS4) and Pearlitol flash (TS5) showed a similar behavior, where a first order kinetics prevailed with a similar magnitude of flush release. On the contrary, release from tablets containing PreGelSt (TS1), CP (TS2) and Starlac (TS3) matched with a perfect diffusion model with different lag time values. All SA tablets showed variable release rates. This variation might be a result of a difference in the wetting capability within their tablet cores. Different types of added superdisintegrants contributed to that difference. The tablet formula (TS2) containing CP was considered optimum, as it showed the least release $t_{1/2}$ (59.8 min), as well as an acceptable short lag time value (1.98 min).

Physicochemical characterization of optimized tablet formulae containing TSDads and SA
Scanning Electron Microscopy (SEM)
A surface view of tablets containing TSDads showed a rough non-planar surface with occasional protrusions (Figure 3a). Occasional pores were clearly identified at a higher magnification power (1500x). The pores were extending to the interior of the core structure, as illustrated in the cross-sectional view (Figure 3b). Tablets containing SA showed a more extensive rough reticulated surface with more frequent pores extending to the tablet core (Figure 3c,3d). Spherical crystals of the drug might account for the obvious reticulation on the surface of their respective tablets. As clearly demonstrated, tablets with either TSDads or SA with CP

as an external superdisintegrant gave upon compression a perfect design for a well-organized interconnected porous matrix. This was confirmed by the kinetic treatment of the release data in which glimepiride release from such matrices obeyed Higuchi diffusion model (Table 3).

Effect of compression on glimepiride release
An important reason which prevents the scaling up of both solid dispersion and spherical crystal techniques industrially was the fragility of their matrices and the high probability of destruction upon compression. That is why tablets were compressed at a low compression force, and the effect of compression on release was depicted. Results shown in Figure 4 illustrate similar release rates for capsules of T5, TS2 and their respective tablets as indicated by the nearly parallel curves in either case. A high value for similarity factor (Table 4) confirmed the results in both cases. Also, a similar extent of release after 120 min. was demonstrated, where T5 gave 88% and 80% release for capsules and tablets, respectively, & TS2 gave 84% and 79% release, respectively, before and after tabletting. This result confirmed the success of glimepiride tablet formulation to provide high extent of drug release by either technique adopted, and it can be postulated that the low compression force applied protected the integrity of the solid dispersion and spherical crystals upon tabletting, offering a great opportunity for the success of both techniques on industrial scale production.

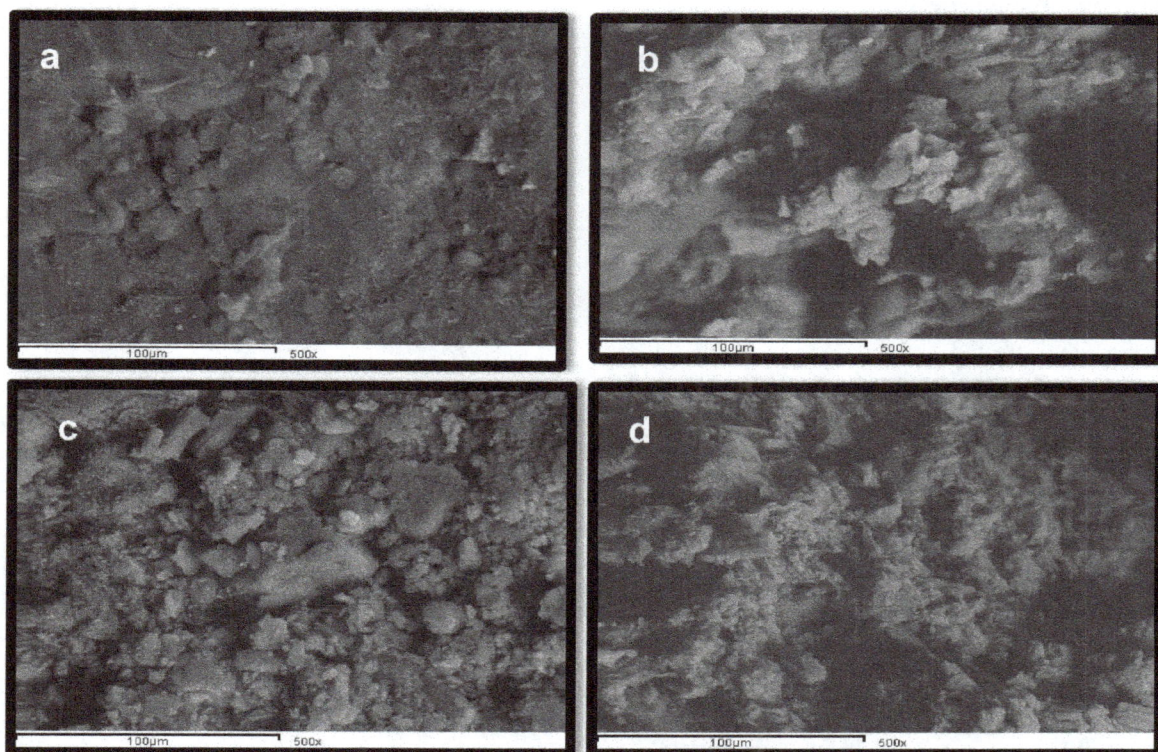

Figure 3. SEM for optimized triple solid dispersion adsorbate [TSDads] tablet formula (T5) (a) Surface view, (b) Cross section view; optimized spherical agglomerates [SA] tablet formula (TS2) (c) Surface view, (d) Cross section view

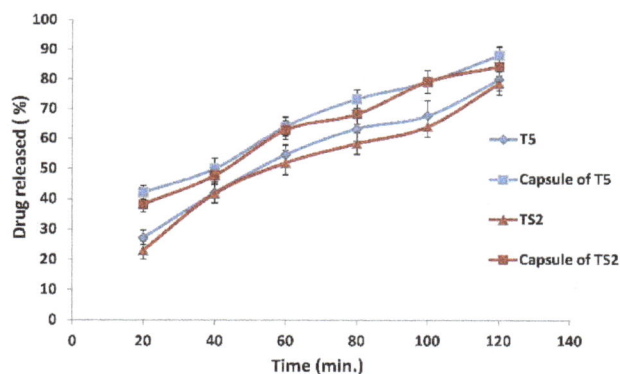

Figure 4. Comparison of release profile of glimepiride from capsules containing the constituents of T5 or TS2 to their respective tablets T5 or TS2

Kinetic data of release for both formulae before and after compression (Table 4) revealed a common release mechanism in capsule form for T5 and TS2 (zero order), which was shifted to a diffusion model in the tablet form. Furthermore, capsules of T5 and TS2 showed a similar flush release which, upon tabletting, turned to similar lag times values. As stated before, an organized matrix structure was illustrated in tablet form (Figure 3b, d) from which the diffusion-controlled release predominated. The time necessary for the dissolution medium to access drug particles inside respective matrices accounted for the encountered lag time.

Table 4. Kinetic treatment of release data of glimepiride from optimized triple solid dispersion adsorbate [TSDads] & spherical agglomerates [SA] before and after compression

Formula Code		Order of release	K****	Similarity Factor f_2***	Half-life (min.)	Y-intercept	Significance of Y-intercept	
							Flush release (%)	Lag time (min.)
T5*	Tablet	diffusion	7.86	99.668	54.13	-7.93	-	1.02
	Capsule	zero	0.47		36.79	32.65	32.65	-
TS2**	Tablet	diffusion	7.90	98.837	59.83	-11.11	-	1.98
	Capsule	zero	0.47		43.69	29.07	29.07	-

*TSDads, **SA　　***$f_2 = 50.\,log \left[\dfrac{100}{\sqrt{1+\sum \frac{(capsule-tablet)^2}{n}}} \right]$

****Units of K (rate constant) is mg/min for zero order, min-1 for first order & mg/ min1/2 for Higushi diffusion model

The similarity in results between the two optimized formulae based on either TSDads or SA might rely upon the same type and percentage of the added superdisintegrant. CP acted upon the formulae in capsule form through a strong wetting and swelling action. It acted also on both tablet formulae by creating similar interconnecting channels from which a similar release rate was shown (Table 4).

Pharmacodynamic evaluation of optimized tablet formulae

The mean percent reduction in blood glucose level (BGL) for the treated rabbits versus time after administration of the marketed product Amaryl®, formula TS2 and formula T5 is represented in Figure 5. Maximum percent reduction in BGL (Red max), the corresponding time (Tmax) and the Area under the Curve (AUC $_{0-12}$) were calculated using *Kinetica®* software.

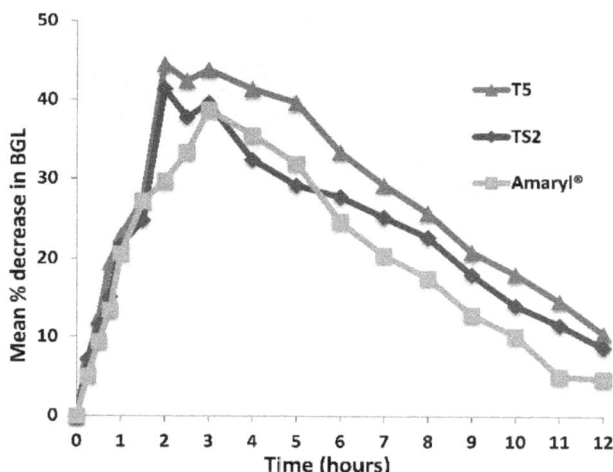

Figure 5. Mean percent decrease in blood glucose level [BGL] of normal rabbits receiving Amaryl®, formula TS2 and formula T5

Both tablet formulae gave higher values for Red max and Tmax was attained earlier than that of the marketed product. Therefore, the two new tablet formulations were thought to be more efficient in their hypoglycemic effect, as illustrated in Table 5 & Figure 5. Results were then analyzed statistically using the one-way analysis of variance (*ANOVA*) to determine the least significant difference, if any, between the tested formulae and the marketed product. The difference between formula T5 and TS2 in Red max, AUC$_{0-12}$ and Tmax was found to be non-significant ($p > 0.05$), suggesting an equivalent therapeutic efficacy for either tested formula. However, there was a significant difference between the value of Tmax of the tablet formula and that of the marketed product ($p < 0.05$). This could support the goal of our work in which the enhancement in glimepiride dissolution through tablet formulation had contributed to a more rapid onset of action, which could be of value in acute cases of hyperglycemia.

Table 5. Comparison between pharmacokinetic parameters of optimized tablets with marketed product

Pharmacokinetic parameters	Amaryl®	TS2	T5
Red max (maximum % decrease in BGL*) ± S.D.	40.07±10.14	42.89±4.49	48.58±3.84
Tmax (time to attain maximum % decrease in BGL) ± S.D.	2.87±0.25	2.12±0.25	2.50±0.57
AUC $_{0-12}$ ± S.D.	244.07±56.02	277.34±72.55	328.43±118.73

S.D.: Standard Deviation.
* BGL: Blood glucose level

Conclusion

The inclusion of glimepiride in a matrix of either triple solid dispersion adsorbates or spherical agglomerates appeared to be equally successful in achieving the target of experimental work. An extensive enhancement in glimepiride release from such formulae occurred, accounting for an average t$_{1/2}$ less than 60 min, while that of the marketed product extended to about 123 min. Furthermore, an *in vivo* hastening in the onset time occurred, where the hypoglycemic effect appeared about 2h after the oral administration of either formula to male albino rabbits relative to 3h in case of the marketed product. Hence, the results of this study demonstrate the potential of either studied techniques in enhancing both the *in vitro* and *in vivo* performance of glimepiride through oral tablet formulation.

Ethical Issues
Not applicable

Conflict of Interest
The authors declare no conflict of interests.

References

1. Kalepu S, Nekkanti V. Insoluble drug delivery strategies: Review of recent advances and business prospects. *Acta Pharm Sin B* 2015;5(5):442-53. doi: 10.1016/j.apsb.2015.07.003
2. Gowthamarajan K, Singh SK. Dissolution Testing for Poorly Soluble Drugs: A Continuing Perspective. *Dissol Tech* 2010; 8:24-32. doi:10.14227/DT170310P24
3. Savolainen J, Forsberg M, Taipale H, Männistö PT, Järvinen K, Gynther J, et al. Effects of Aqueous Solubility and Dissolution Characteristics on Oral Bioavailability of Entacapone. *Drug Dev Res* 2000; 49(4):238–44. doi: 10.1002/1098-2299(200004)49:4<238::AID-DDR2>3.0.CO;2-V
4. Khadka P, Ro J, Kim H, Kim I, Kim JT, Kim H, et al. Pharmaceutical particle technologies: An approach to improve drug solubility, dissolution and bioavailability. *Asian J Pharm Sci* 2014; 9(6): 304-16. doi. 10.1016/j.ajps.2014.05.005
5. Rogers TL, Nelsen AC, Hu J, Brown JN, Sarkari M, Young TJ, et al. A novel particle engineering technology to enhance dissolution of poorly water soluble drugs: Spray-freezing into liquid. *Eur J Pharm Biopharm* 2002;54(3):271-80.

6. Sander JR, Zeiger BW, Suslick KS. Sonocrystallization and sonofragmentation. *Ultrason Sonochem* 2014;21(6):1908-15. doi: 10.1016/j.ultsonch.2014.02.005

7. Cintas P, Tagliapietra S, Caporaso M, Tabasso S, Cravotto G. Enabling technologies built on a sonochemical platform: Challenges and opportunities. *Ultrason Sonochem* 2015;25:8-16. doi: 10.1016/j.ultsonch.2014.12.004

8. Shoyele SA, Cawthorne S. Particle engineering techniques for inhaled biopharmaceuticals. *Adv Drug Deliv Rev* 2006;58(9-10):1009-29. doi: 10.1016/j.addr.2006.07.010

9. Wlodarski K, Sawicki W, Paluch KJ, Tajber L, Grembecka M, Hawelek L, et al. The influence of amorphization methods on the apparent solubility and dissolution rate of tadalafil. *Eur J Pharm Sci* 2014;62:132-40. doi: 10.1016/j.ejps.2014.05.026

10. Graeser KA, Patterson JE, Zeitler JA, Rades T. The role of configurational entropy in amorphous systems. *Pharmaceutics* 2010;2(2):224-44. doi: 10.3390/pharmaceutics2020224

11. Jadhav KR, Pacharane SS, Pednekar PP, Praveen V, Koshy PV, Kadam VJ. Approaches to stabilize amorphous form - a review. *Curr Drug Therapy* 2012; 7(4): 255-62. doi: 10.2174/1574885511207040004

12. Kondo K, Kido K, Niwa T. Spheronization mechanism of pharmaceutical material crystals processed by extremely high shearing force using a mechanical powder processor. *Eur J Pharm Biopharm* 2016;107:7-15. doi: 10.1016/j.ejpb.2016.06.021

13. Ibrahim MA, Al-Anazi FK. Enhancement of the dissolution of albendazole from pellets using mtr technique. *Saudi Pharm J* 2013;21(2):215-23. doi: 10.1016/j.jsps.2012.03.001

14. Maghsoodi M, Hassan-Zadeh D, Barzegar-Jalali M, Nokhodchi A, Martin G. Improved compaction and packing properties of naproxen agglomerated crystals obtained by spherical crystallization technique. *Drug Dev Ind Pharm* 2007;33(11):1216-24. doi: 10.1080/03639040701377730

15. Meeus L. Direct compression versus granulation. *Pharm Tech Europe* 2011;23(3).

16. Phaechamud T, Ritthidej GC. Formulation variables influencing drug release from layered matrix system comprising chitosan and xanthan gum. *AAPS PharmSciTech* 2008;9(3):870-7. doi: 10.1208/s12249-008-9127-8

17. Aulton ME, Taylor K. Aulton's pharmaceutics: The design and Manufacture of Medicines. Philadelphia: Churchill Livingstone Elsevier; 2007.

18. Khan GM, Zhu JB. Studies on drug release kinetics from ibuprofen-carbomer hydrophilic matrix tablets: Influence of co-excipients on release rate of the drug. *J Control Release* 1999;57(2):197-203.

19. Lin SY. Effect of excipients on tablet properties and dissolution behavior of theophylline-tableted

microcapsules under different compression forces. *J Pharm Sci* 1988;77(3):229-32.

20. Gonnissen Y, Remon JP, Vervaet C. Effect of maltodextrin and superdisintegrant in directly compressible powder mixtures prepared via co-spray drying. *Eur J Pharm Biopharm* 2008;68(2):277-82. doi: 10.1016/j.ejpb.2007.05.004

21. Upadrashta SM, Katikaneni PR, Nuessle NO. Chitosan as a tablet binder. *Drug Dev Ind Pharm* 1992; 18(15): 1701-8. doi:10.3109/03639049209040896

22. Ishikawa T, Watanabe Y, Utoguchi N, Matsumoto M. Preparation and evaluation of tablets rapidly disintegrating in saliva containing bitter-taste-masked granules by the compression method. *Chem Pharm Bull (Tokyo)* 1999;47(10):1451-4.

23. Lahdenpää E, Niskanen M, Yliruusi J. Crushing strength, disintegration time and weight variation of tablets compressed from three Avicel® PH grades and their mixtures. *Eur J Pharm Biopharm* 1997;43(3): 315-22. doi:10.1016/S0939-6411(97)00053-2

24. Bi Y, Sunada H, Yonezawa Y, Danjo K, Otsuka A, Iida K. Preparation and evaluation of a compressed tablet rapidly disintegrating in the oral cavity. *Chem Pharm Bull (Tokyo)* 1996;44(11):2121-7.

25. Shirai Y, Sogo K, Yamamoto K, Kojima K, Fujioka H, Makita H, et al. A novel fine granule system for masking bitter taste. *Biol Pharm Bull* 1993;16(2):172-7.

26. Balasubramaniam J, Bee T. Influence of superdisintegrants on the rate of drug dissolution from oral solid dosage forms. *Pharmaceut Tech* 2009; Suppl(1).

27. Shoukri RA, Ahmed IS, Shamma RN. In vitro and in vivo evaluation of nimesulide lyophilized orally disintegrating tablets. *Eur J Pharm Biopharm* 2009;73(1):162-71. doi: 10.1016/j.ejpb.2009.04.005

28. Visavarungroj N, Remon JP. Crosslinked starch as a disintegrating agent. *Int J Pharmaceut* 1990;62(2-3):125-31. doi:10.1016/0378-5173(90)90226-T

29. Zhao N, Augsburger LL. The influence of swelling capacity of superdisintegrants in different ph media on the dissolution of hydrochlorothiazide from directly compressed tablets. *AAPS PharmSciTech* 2005;6(1):E120-6. doi: 10.1208/pt060119

30. Zhao N, Augsburger LL. Functionality comparison of 3 classes of superdisintegrants in promoting aspirin tablet disintegration and dissolution. *AAPS PharmSciTech* 2005;6(4):E634-40. doi: 10.1208/pt060479

31. D McCormick. Evolutions in direct compression. *Pharmaceut Tech* 2005;4:52-62.

32. Yuan J, Shi L, Sun WJ, Chen J, Zhou Q, Sun ChC. Enabling direct compression of formulated Danshen powder by surface engineering. *Powder Tech* 2013;241(6):211-8. doi:10.1016/j.powtec.2013.03.010

33. Fujii M, Okada H, Shibata Y, Teramachi H, Kondoh M, Watanabe Y. Preparation, characterization, and

tableting of a solid dispersion of indomethacin with crospovidone. *Int J Pharm* 2005;293(1-2):145-53. doi: 10.1016/j.ijpharm.2004.12.018

34. Chaulang G, Patil K, Ghodke D, Khan S, Yeole P. Preparation and characterization of solid dispersion tablet of furosemide with crospovidone. *Res J Pharm Tech* 2008;1(4):386-9.

35. Rahman Z, Zidan AS, Khan MA. Risperidone solid dispersion for orally disintegrating tablet: Its formulation design and non-destructive methods of evaluation. *Int J Pharm* 2010;400(1-2):49-58. doi: 10.1016/j.ijpharm.2010.08.025

36. Nokhodchi A, Maghsoodi M, Hassanzadeh D. An improvement of physicomechanical properties of carbamazepine crystals. *Iran J Pharm Res* 2007;6(2):83-93

37. Usha AN, Mutalik S, Reddy MS, Ranjith AK, Kushtagi P, Udupa N. Preparation and, in vitro, preclinical and clinical studies of aceclofenac spherical agglomerates. *Eur J Pharm Biopharm* 2008;70(2):674-83. doi: 10.1016/j.ejpb.2008.06.010

38. Dixit M, Kulkarni PK, Anis Sh, Kini AG. Preparation and characterization of spherical agglomerates of ketoprofen by neutralization method. *Int J Pharm Bio Sci* 2010; 1(4): 395-406.

39. Vidyadhara S, Babu JR, Sasidhar RLC, Ramu A, Prasad SS, Tejasree M. Formulation and evaluation of glimepiride solid dispersions and their tablet formulations for enhanced bioavailability. *Pharmanest* 2011; 2(1): 15-20

40. Ning X, Sun J, Han X, Wu Y, Yan Z, Han J, et al. Strategies to improve dissolution and oral absorption of glimepiride tablets: Solid dispersion versus micronization techniques. *Drug Dev Ind Pharm* 2011;37(6):727-36.   doi: 10.3109/03639045.2010.538061

41. Parmar KR, Shah SR, Sheth NR. Studies in dissolution enhancement of ezetimibe by solid dispersions in combination with a surface adsorbent. *Dissolut Technol*   2011;   18(3):   55-61. doi:10.14227/DT180311P55

42. Fodor-Kardos A, Toth J, Gyenis J. Preparation of protein loaded chitosan microparticles by combined precipitation and spherical agglomeration. *Powder Technol*   2013;   244(8):   16-25. doi:10.1016/j.powtec.2013.03.052

43. Garala KC, Patel JM, Dhingani AP, Dharamsi AT. Preparation and evaluation of agglomerated crystals by crystallo-co-agglomeration: An integrated approach of principal component analysis and box-behnken experimental design. *Int J Pharm* 2013;452(1-2):135-56.   doi: 10.1016/j.ijpharm.2013.04.073

44. Garala KC, Patel JM, Dhingani AP, Dharamsi AT. Quality by design (QbD) approach for developing agglomerates containing racecadotril and loperamide hydrochloride by crystallo-co-agglomeration. *Powder Technol*   2013;   247(10):128-46. doi:10.1016/j.powtec.2013.07.011

45. Maghsoodi M, Sadeghpoor F. Preparation and evaluation of solid dispersions of piroxicam and eudragit s100 by spherical crystallization technique. *Drug Dev Ind Pharm* 2010;36(8):917-25. doi: 10.3109/03639040903585127

46. Nokhodchi A, Maghsoodi M. Preparation of spherical crystal agglomerates of naproxen containing disintegrant for direct tablet making by spherical crystallization technique. *AAPS PharmSciTech* 2008;9(1):54-9. doi: 10.1208/s12249-007-9019-3

47. United States Pharmacopeia / The National Formulary. Physical Tests: Uniformity of dosage units (905).26/21ed. Rockville, MD: USP Convention Inc; 2003.

48. United States Pharmacopeia/ The National Formulary. Physical Tests: Tablet friability (1216), 26/21ed, Rockville, MD: USP Convention Inc; 2003.

49. Gabra BH, Sirois P. Hyperalgesia in non-obese diabetic (nod) mice: A role for the inducible bradykinin b1 receptor. *Eur J Pharmacol* 2005;514(1):61-7. doi: 10.1016/j.ejphar.2005.03.018

50. Ammar HO, Salama HA, Ghorab M, Mahmoud AA. Implication of inclusion complexation of glimepiride in cyclodextrin-polymer systems on its dissolution, stability and therapeutic efficacy. *Int J Pharm* 2006;320(1-2):53-7.   doi: 10.1016/j.ijpharm.2006.04.002

51. Wagner SG. Fundamentals of Clinical Pharmacokinetics. 1st ed. Hamilton, Illinois: Drug Intelligence Publications Inc; 1975.

52. Battu SK, Repka MA, Majumdar S, Madhusudan RY. Formulation and evaluation of rapidly disintegrating fenoverine tablets: Effect of superdisintegrants. *Drug Dev Ind Pharm* 2007;33(11):1225-32. doi: 10.1080/03639040701377888

53. Sammour OA, Hammad MA, Megrab NA, Zidan AS. Formulation and optimization of mouth dissolve tablets containing rofecoxib solid dispersion. *AAPS PharmSciTech* 2006;7(2):E55. doi: 10.1208/pt070255

54. Setty CM, Prasad DV, Gupta VR, Sa B. Development of fast dispersible aceclofenac tablets: Effect of functionality of superdisintegrants. *Indian J Pharm Sci* 2008;70(2):180-5. doi: 10.4103/0250-474x.41452

55. He X, Kibbe AH. Crospovidone. In: Rowe RC., Sheskey PJ, Weller PJ, editors. Handbook of Pharmaceutical Excipients, 4th ed. Washington, DC: American Pharmaceutical Association, London: Pharmaceutical Press; 2003.

56. Michailova V, Titeva S, Kotsilkova R, Krusteva E, Minkov E. Influence of hydrogel structure on the processes of water penetration and drug release from mixed hydroxypropylmethyl cellulose/thermally pregelatinized waxy maize starch hydrophilic matrices. *Int J Pharm* 2001;222(1):7-17.

57. Maghsoodi M. How spherical crystallization improves direct tableting properties: A review. *Adv Pharm Bull* 2012;2(2):253-7. doi: 10.5681/apb.2012.039

16

Immuno-biosensor for Detection of CD20-Positive Cells Using Surface Plasmon Resonance

Dariush Shanehbandi[1,2], **Jafar Majidi**[1]*, **Tohid Kazemi**[1,2]*, **Behzad Baradaran**[1], **Leili Aghebati-Maleki**[1,2], **Farzaneh Fathi**[2,3], **Jafar Ezzati Nazhad Dolatabadi**[3]

[1] *Immunology Research Center, Tabriz University of Medical Sciences, Tabriz, Iran.*
[2] *Student Research Committee, Tabriz University of Medical Sciences, Tabriz, Iran.*
[3] *Research Center for Pharmaceutical Nanotechnology, Tabriz University of Medical Sciences, Tabriz, Iran.*

Keywords:
· CD20
· Surface Plasmon Resonance
· Immobilization
· *Staphylococcus aureus* protein A
· 11-mercaptoundecanoic acid

Abstract

Purpose: Surface plasmon resonance (SPR) sensing confers a real-time assessment of molecular interactions between biomolecules and their ligands. This approach is highly sensitive and reproducible and could be employed to confirm the successful binding of drugs to cell surface targets. The specific affinity of monoclonal antibodies (MAb) for their target antigens is being utilized for development of immuno-sensors and therapeutic agents. CD20 is a surface protein of B lymphocytes which has been widely employed for immuno-targeting of B-cell related disorders. In the present study, binding ability of an anti-CD20 MAb to surface antigens of intact target cells was investigated by SPR technique.

Methods: Two distinct strategies were used for immobilization of the anti-CD20 MAb onto gold (Au) chips. MUA (11-mercaptoundecanoic acid) and *Staphylococcus aureus* protein A (SpA) were the two systems used for this purpose. A suspension of CD20-positive Raji cells was injected in the analyte phase and the resulting interactions were analyzed and compared to those of MOLT-4 cell line as CD20-negative control.

Results: Efficient binding of anti-CD20 MAb to the surface antigens of Raji cell line was confirmed by both immobilizing methods, whereas this MAb had not a noticeable affinity to the MOLT-4 cells.

Conclusion: According to the outcomes, the investigated MAb had acceptable affinity and specificity to the target antigens on the cell surface and could be utilized for immuno-detection of CD20-positive intact cells by SPR method.

Introduction

Surface plasmon resonance (SPR) technology is widely used for the study of the interactions between a variety of chemical compounds and various biomolecules such as proteins, peptides and nucleic acids.[1] Assessment of the interactions between analytes and immobilized ligands such as antibody/antigen and complementary nucleic acids is possible using this technology.[2,3] Membrane proteins as important targets for drug discovery have recently attracted a great deal of interest for binding studies by this system.[4] SPR based assessments are highly reproducible and permit the real-time investigation of probable interactions in label free form.[4] CD20 is a surface protein which has been extensively utilized for targeted therapy of hematologic malignancies and autoimmune disorders.[5] Rituximab was the first FDA approved anti-CD20 monoclonal antibody (MAb) for the targeted therapy of non-Hodgkin's lymphoma and chronic lymphocytic leukemia.[6] However, Rituximab and current therapeutics have not associated with complete remission in a considerable portion of the patients.[7]

Hence there is an urgent need for development and assessment of more efficient therapeutics. Targeted therapy, due to the reduced drug dosage and minimized harmful effects on unintended tissues has been considered as a more tolerable treatment approach.[8] In addition to MAbs with native format, antibody derivatives have been also introduced for targeting studies.[5] Bispecific antibodies (which simultaneously target two different antigens) and CAR T cells (engineered T cells with surface expression of chimeric antigen receptors) are examples of novel targeting agents.[9] These agents acquire their antigen binding parts from the single-chain variable fragments (scFvs) of the input MAbs. Consequently, efficient binding of the utilized MAb is a prerequisite for engineering of this type therapeutics.

In the present study, the antigen-binding capacity of an anti-CD20 MAb was assessed by SPR system. Since proper functionalizing and assembly of the SPR chips is an important step to enable reliable detection of biomolecule binding,[1] we optimized two distinct

*Corresponding authors: Jafar Majidi and Tohid Kazemi, Emails: majidij@tbzmed.ac.ir, kazemit@tbzmed.ac.ir

strategies for detection of a CD20-positive Burkitt's lymphoma cell line.

Materials and Methods

N-hydroxysuccinimide (NHS), 11-mercaptoundecanoic acid (MUA), Bovine serum albumin (BSA) and PBS 10X were purchased from Sigma–Aldrich (Steinheim, Germany). Fetal bovine serum, penicillin and streptomycin were obtained from Gibco (Thermo Fisher Scientific, USA). Pure gold (Au) chips were acquired from bionavis company (Tampere, Finland). The recombinant *Staphylococcus aureus* protein A (SpA) was kindly provided by Dr. Gholamreza Ahmadian and Dr. Garshasb Rigi (Department of Molecular Genetics, National Institute of Genetic Engineering and Biotechnology, NIGEB). The murine IgG2a anti-CD20 MAb was acquired from our previous works.[9,10] Raji (a Burkitt's lymphoma cell line) and MOLT-4 (human T lymphoblast related to acute lymphoblastic leukemia) were purchased from the National Cell Bank of Iran (Pasteur Institute, Tehran, Iran).

Cell culture

CD20-positive Raji cells and MOLT-4 cells as representative of CD20-negative T lymphoblasts were cultured in RPMI-1640 medium supplemented with 100U/ml penicillin, 100 µg/ml streptomycin and 10% fetal bovine serum and incubated at 37 °C in a humidified incubator with 5% CO_2.

Sensor surface cleaning

SPR-Navi Au-slides are made of BK7- glass and coated with 50 nm of gold layer. For cleaning the Au surface, a solution composed of ammonia and hydrogen peroxide was used. In Brief, a solution containing 4 ml of ammonia (NH_4OH), 4 ml of hydrogen peroxide (H_2O_2) and 12 ml Milli-Q-water was prepared in a Petri dish. Then, gold slides were immersed and boiled on a 95°C hotplate for 10 minutes. The slides were rinsed thoroughly with Milli-Q-water and dried with nitrogen stream.[11]

Preparation of "protein A" chip for antibody immobilization

The *Staphylococcus aureus* protein A (SpA) contains immunoglobulin-binding domains which can efficiently attach to the Fc regions of a variety of IgG molecules such as murine IgG2a and human IgG1 subclasses.[12] In the current study, a 0.5 mg per ml concentration of SpA was prepared in 10X PBS (pH7). 150 µl of SpA solution and 150 µl of Acetate buffer (800 mg of sodium acetate and 572 µl of acetic acid at pH 5.5) were coated on the Au surface of the cleaned chip.[13] After 1h of incubation at 25°C, the chip was thoroughly washed with 1X PBS (pH 7) and dried with nitrogen stream. Subsequently, 200µl of anti-CD20 MAb (1mg/ml) was added on the surface and incubated for 1h. Afterward, 2ml of BSA (1% in 10X PBS) was passed through a millipore syringe filter with a pore size of 0.22 µm and 200µl of the

filtered BSA was used for surface blocking. After 15 min of blocking, the chip was washed with PBS and utilized as cell binding platform (Figure 1).

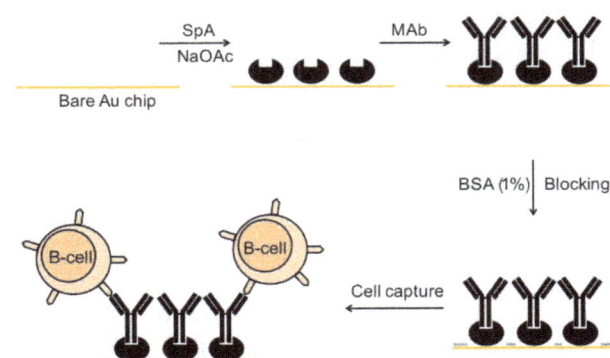

Figure 1. SpA mediated MAb immobilization on Au chip for cell detection

Preparation of MUA activated chip for antibody immobilization

A 5mM concentration of MUA (in absolute ethanol) was used for creation of functional carboxyl groups for MAb binding.[14] For this purpose, a bare Au slide was immersed in a solution containing MUA and Milli-Q-water in a ratio of 7:3. The slide was incubated at room temperature (~25°C) for 20 h and washed thrice with ethanol and then rinsed with phosphate buffered saline (PBS).[15] The functionalized gold slide was activated by NHS (0.05M) and EDC (0.2M). The Au chip was then treated with 200 µl of anti-CD20 MAb (1mg/ml). After 1 h incubation and complete washing/drying process, the chip surface was blocked with 200 µ of filtered BSA (1% in 10X PBS). After 15 min, the chip was washed and used for immuno-sensing of the target cells (Figure 2).

Cell capturing by the immobilized antibodies and SPR Measurements

A multi-parameter SPR device (MP-SPR Navi 210A, BioNavis Ltd, Tampere, Finland) was employed to investigate the antibody/cell interactions. This equipment utilizes the Kretscheman prism configuration with gold chips (BioNavis Ltd, Finland).[14] Prior to cell injection, Raji and MOLT-4 cell were harvested from culture media. After counting with a hemocytometer, 5×10^4 cells were washed and resuspended in 1ml of PBS. All cell injections were accomplished at 30°C in PBS (pH 7.4) as running buffer. Cell injection was performed in a 5 min period with a flow rate of 40 µl/min. After cell injection, the chips were rinsed with running buffer to remove the unbound cells. Data were analyzed using data viewer 210A SPR Bionavis software. In the current study, assessments were performed in fixed angle mode and a 670 nm laser was employed to excite the surface plasmon.

Experiment normalization for non-specific binding

An unblocked Au chip was placed in the slide-holder of the SPR equipment. Suspended Raji and MOLT-4 cells were injected via separate channels as mobile phase. The non-specific adhesion of the mentioned cells onto the bare Au surface was detected and automatically quantified (Figure 3). Using the same condition, a BSA blocked chip (bare Au chip with no MAb immobilization but BSA blocked) was considered for the experiment normalization (Figure 3).

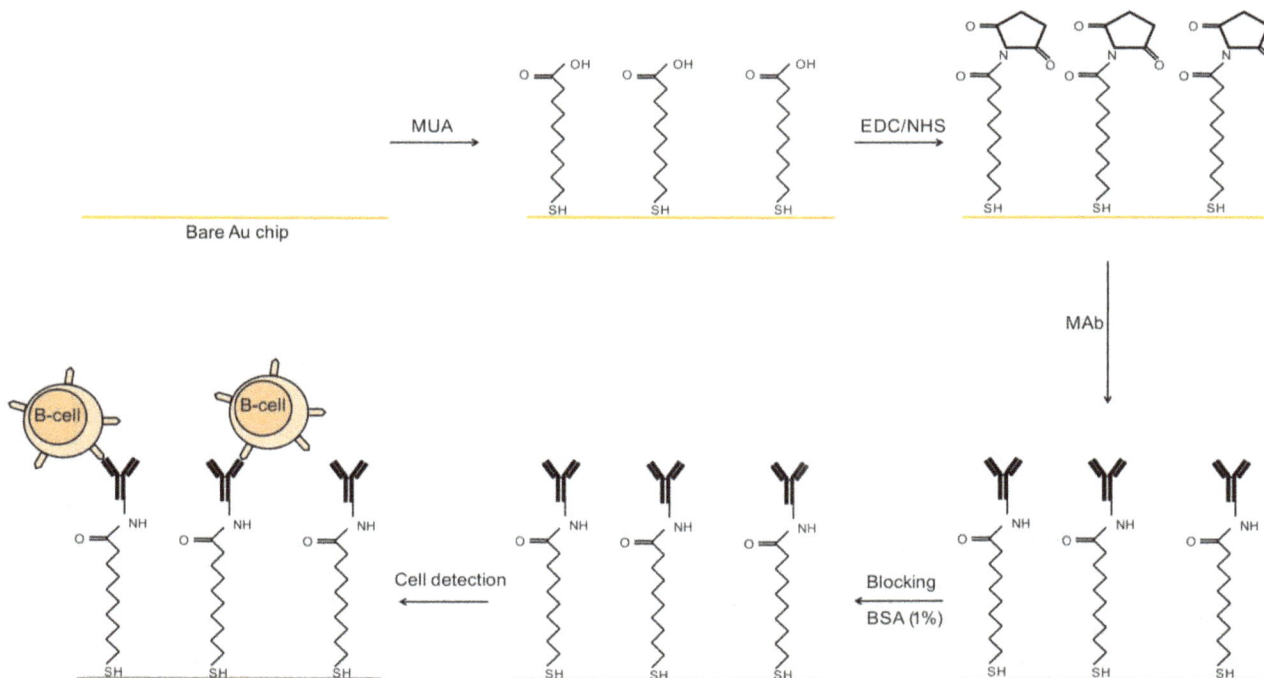

Figure 2. MAb immobilization on Au chip via MUA self assembled monolayer for cell detection

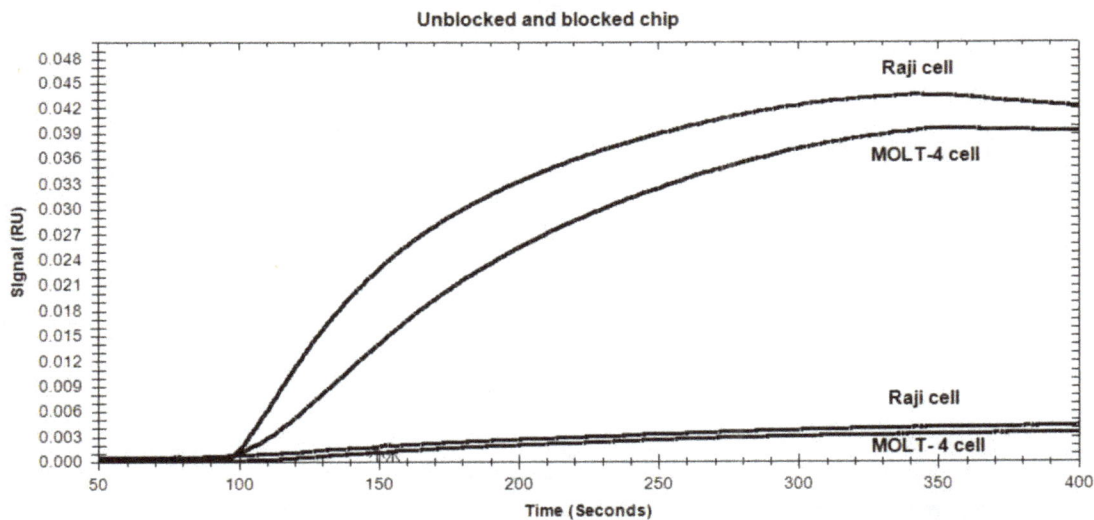

Figure 3. Sensorgrams of unblocked chip (above) and BSA blocked chip (below) for detection of nonspecific cell binding and selectivity of the biochip. Both Raji and MOLT-4 cells have bound to the unblocked chip, whereas their bindings to the BSA treated bare gold is negligible.

Results

Normalization of the non-specific binding

Sensorgrams of BSA blocked chip and unblocked chip were acquired for detection of "selectivity of the biochip" and "nonspecific cell binding", respectively. As shown in Figure 3, the response unit values (RU) for unblocked chip for MOLT-4 and Raji cells were ~ 0.040 and ~ 0.043, respectively. Compared to the unblocked chip, the

BSA blocked chip showed very low RU values for nonspecific binding of MOLT-4 and Raji cells (~0.003).

Immuno-detection by SpA mediated antibody immobilization method

Sensorgram of SpA mediated approach showed RU values of 0.003 and 0.009 for MOLT-4 and Raji cells, respectively (Figure 4). Considering the measured value for the BSA blocked normalizer chip (~0.003) (Figure 3), MOLT-4 cells indicated a similar RU value. This means that, MOLT-4 cell line had no sensible binding to the SpA immobilized anti-CD20 MAbs, whereas a time dependent increase in target binding was evident for

CD20-positive Raji cells. However, the quantified value was significantly lower than the value measured for the unblocked bare Au chip (Figure 3). It could be deduced that, binding onto the SpA sensor chip has been specific.

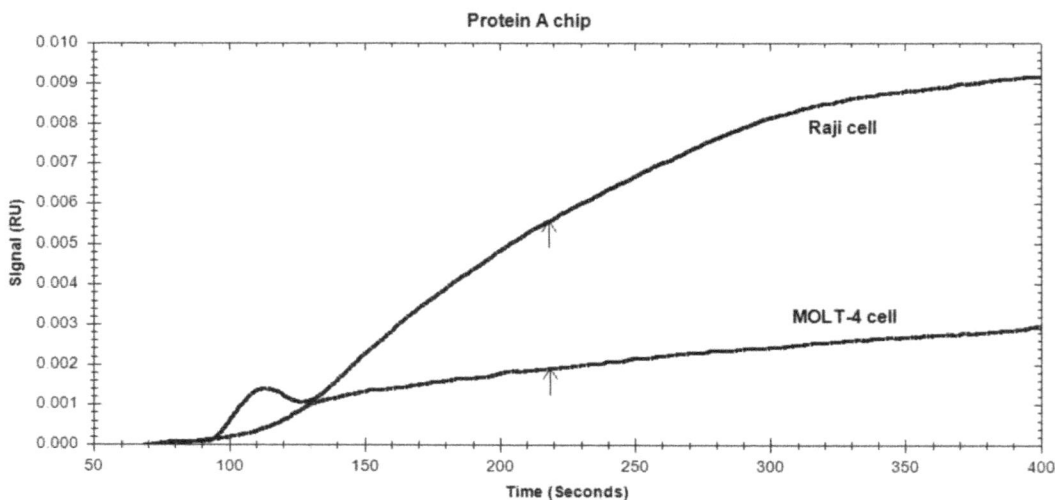

Figure 4. Sensorgrams of Raji and MOLT-4 cells detection by SpA immobilization method

Immuno-sensing using MUA mediated antibody immobilization method
Considering the corresponding sensorgram (Figure 5), the binding value of CD20-negative MOLT-4 cells was ~ 0.003 RU which is equal to the negative (BSA blocked)

normalizer chip. On the contrary, a time-dependent MAb/cell binding was measured for Raji cells (~ 0.022). This amount is significantly lower than the quantified value for the unblocked bare Au chip (Figure 3) indicating the selective binding of CD20-positive cells onto Au chip.

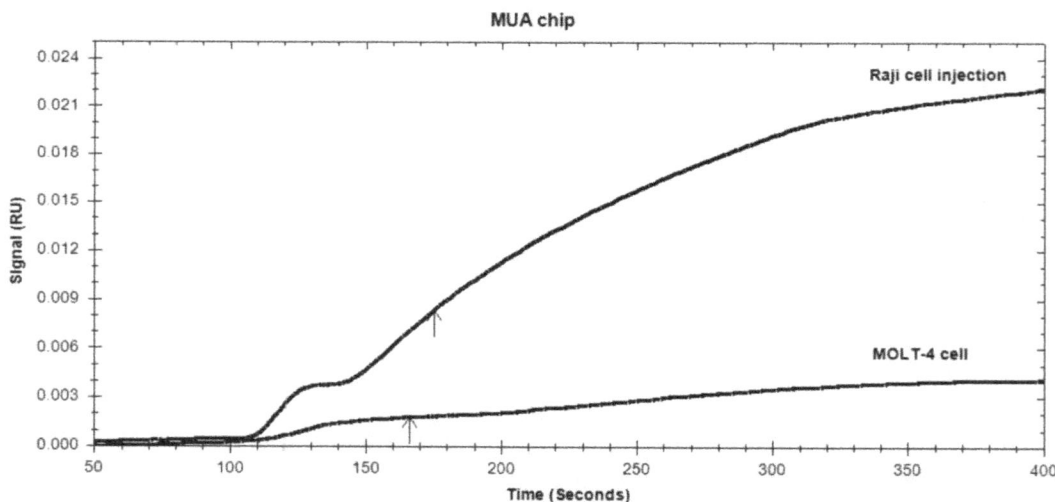

Figure 5. Sensorgrams of Raji and MOLT-4 cells detection by MUA mediated immobilization

Discussion
Several SPR-based experiments are designed for detection of isolated or recombinant antigens. However, detached antigens or recombinant proteins may fail to reflect the exact interactions of the *in vivo* interactions. CD20 is a surface protein which spans the cell membrane 4 times. Most of anti-CD20 MAbs bind to discontinuous epitopes on this molecule.[9] It is expected that, the antigens on the cell surfaces which retain their natural three dimensional (3D) conformations, produce more

factual binding values. In this regard, we tried to assess the interaction of a MAb with CD20 antigen on the intact cells. A number of studies have employed SPR for investigating ligand interactions with bacteria and mammalian intact cells.[16-19] It should be noticed that, because of having evanescent filed near 400 nm on the Au surface, the size of the ligands to be immobilized is limited in SPR method.[18] Alternatively, the interaction partner with applicable dimensions should be fixed on the sensor chip. In the present study, the antibody of interest was fixed on the Au chips and the investigated cells were injected as analyte.[1] By running the apparatus, sensorgrams indicating the cell binding/detection rates were obtained for the two studied strategies. In the first approach, SpA was used for antibody fixation on Au chips. SpA, a surface protein of *Staphylococcus aureus*, is widely used for antibody purification in laboratory. This molecule has five Fc-binding domains and shows acceptable binding affinities to different immunoglobulins, especially human IgG1 and mouse IgG2a molecules.[12]

In the second method, MUA was used for the creation of a self-assembled monolayer on Au chip. The chemical functionalization of SPR chip with the aforementioned protocol resulted in the creation of free carboxyl groups on MUA molecules which in turn provided platforms for MAb immobilization.[20]

MAbs are naturally composed of two main parts: The Fab region which is the fragment for antigen-binding, and the Fc region that is responsible for effector functions via binding to specific receptors on the cells of the immune system.[5] Hence, accessibility of the Fab region is necessary for antigen binding. Since SpA binds to the Fc regions, the epitope binding sites of the MAbs are arranged in the opposite direction of the Au chip, available for antigen binding (Figure 6a). On the contrary, binding to amine groups of the MAbs in MUA method is completely random and some antigen binding sites become inaccessible (Figure 6b).[21] Hence, due to the oriented fixation of the MAbs, the SpA mediated immobilization is expected to be more efficient.[13] However, according to the results of this study MUA mediated immobilization demonstrated higher response units compared to the SpA method.

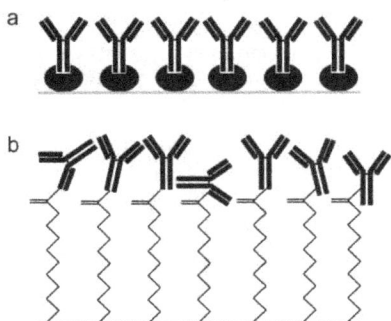

Figure 6. Schematic presentation of MAb immobilization approaches; a: oriented (with SpA) and b: random (with MUA)

Hypothetically, MUA because of its filamentous structure may occupy smaller area compared to macromolecule SpA. Consequently, MUA can create greater density on the chip surface and this larger quantity compensate for the effects of irregular orientation (Figure 7).

Regardless of the strategy used, target specific interactions were evident in this study and nonspecific MAb/cell bindings were not reflected in the outcomes. According to the results of the both immobilization

methods, the investigated antibody had an acceptable affinity and specificity to CD20 molecule.

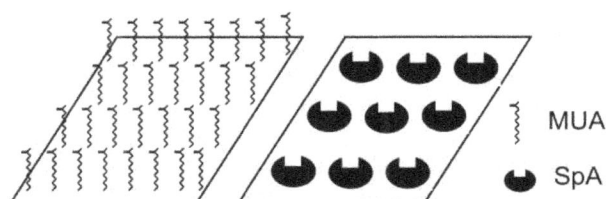

Figure 7. Hypothetic model for chip area occupation with SpA and MUA molecules

Conclusion

In this study, "11-mercaptoundecanoic acid" and *"Staphylococcus aureus* protein A" were utilized for immobilization of an anti-CD20 antibody on gold surface of SPR chips. According to the results, both strategies were applicable for this purpose and the created sensors were able to detect target cells. Furthermore, the investigated monoclonal antibody had acceptable binding specificity to CD20-positive Raji cells, whereas its interaction with CD20-negative MOLT-4 cells was negligible. Therefore, the introduced systems could be employed for immuno-detection of intact CD20-positive cells by SPR.

Acknowledgments

This work was supported by a grant from Immunology Research Center, Tabriz University of Medical Sciences, Tabriz, Iran. Here, we wish to express our sincere gratitude and appreciation to Dr. Gholamreza Ahmadian and Dr. Garshasb Rigi for providing recombinant protein A.

Ethical Issues
Not applicable.

Conflict of Interest
The authors declare no conflict of interests.

References

1. Mauriz E, García-Fernández MC, Lechuga LM. Towards the design of universal immunosurfaces for spr-based assays: A review. *TrAC Trends Anal Chem* 2016;79:191-8. doi: 10.1016/j.trac.2016.02.006
2. Liu R, Wang Q, Li Q, Yang X, Wang K, Nie W. Surface plasmon resonance biosensor for sensitive detection of microRNA and cancer cell using multiple signal amplification strategy. *Biosens Bioelectron* 2017;87:433-8. doi: 10.1016/j.bios.2016.08.090
3. Abadian PN, Kelley CP, Goluch ED. Cellular analysis and detection using surface plasmon resonance techniques. *Anal Chem* 2014;86(6):2799-812. doi: 10.1021/ac500135s
4. Patching SG. Surface plasmon resonance spectroscopy for characterisation of membrane protein-ligand interactions and its potential for drug discovery.

Biochim Biophys Acta 2014;1838(1 Pt A):43-55. doi: 10.1016/j.bbamem.2013.04.028

5. Shanehbandi D, Majidi J, Kazemi T, Baradaran B, Aghebati-Maleki L. CD20-based immunotherapy of B-cell derived hematologic malignancies. *Curr Cancer Drug Targets* 2017.

6. Robak T. Alemtuzumab for B-cell chronic lymphocytic leukemia. *Expert Rev Anticancer Ther* 2008;8(7):1033-51. doi: 10.1586/14737140.8.7.1033

7. Bonavida B. Postulated mechanisms of resistance of B-cell non-hodgkin lymphoma to rituximab treatment regimens: Strategies to overcome resistance. *Semin Oncol* 2014;41(5):667-77. doi: 10.1053/j.seminoncol.2014.08.006

8. Baleydier F, Domenech C, Thomas X. Novel conventional therapies in onco-hemathology. *Bull Cancer* 2011;98(8):901-13. doi: 10.1684/bdc.2011.1412

9. Shanehbandi D, Majidi J, Kazemi T, Baradaran B, Aghebati-Maleki L. Cloning and molecular characterization of the cDNAs encoding the variable regions of an anti-CD20 monoclonal antibody. *Hum Antibodies* 2017. doi: 10.3233/HAB-170314

10. Sineh sepehr K, Baradaran B, Majidi J, Abdolalizadeh J, Aghebati l, Zare Shahneh F. Mass-production and characterization of anti-CD20 monoclonal antibody in peritoneum of balb/c mice. *Adv Pharm Bull* 2013;3(1):109-13. doi: 10.5681/apb.2013.018

11. Yilmaz E, Majidi D, Ozgur E, Denizli A. Whole cell imprinting based escherichia coli sensors: A study for SPR and QCM. *Sensor Actuators B: Chem* 2015;209:714-21. doi: 10.1016/j.snb.2014.12.032

12. Rigi G, Mohammadi SG, Arjomand MR, Ahmadian G, Noghabi KA. Optimization of extracellular truncated staphylococcal protein A expression in escherichia coli BL21 (DE3). *Biotechnol Appl Biochem* 2014;61(2):217-25. doi: 10.1002/bab.1157

13. Chou SF, Hsu WL, Hwang JM, Chen CY. Development of an immunosensor for human ferritin, a nonspecific tumor marker, based on surface plasmon resonance. *Biosens Bioelectron* 2004;19(9):999-1005. doi: 10.1016/j.bios.2003.09.004

14. Fathi F, Ezzati Nazhad Dolatanbadi J, Rashidi MR, Omidi Y. Kinetic studies of bovine serum albumin interaction with PG and TBHQ using surface plasmon resonance. *Int J Biol Macromol* 2016;91:1045-50. doi: 10.1016/j.ijbiomac.2016.06.054

15. Law WC, Yong KT, Baev A, Hu R, Prasad PN. Nanoparticle enhanced surface plasmon resonance biosensing: Application of gold nanorods. *Opt Express* 2009;17(21):19041-6. doi: 10.1364/oe.17.019041

16. Wang S, Xie J, Jiang M, Chang K, Chen R, Ma L, et al. The development of a portable SPR bioanalyzer for sensitive detection of escherichia coli O157:H7. *Sensors (Basel)* 2016;16(11). doi: 10.3390/s16111856

17. Huynh HT, Gotthard G, Terras J, Aboudharam G, Drancourt M, Chabrière E. Surface plasmon resonance imaging of pathogens: The Yersinia pestis paradigm. *BMC Res Notes* 2015;8:259. doi: 10.1186/s13104-015-1236-3

18. Cortès S, Villiers CL, Colpo P, Couderc R, Brakha C, Rossi F, et al. Biosensor for direct cell detection, quantification and analysis. *Biosens Bioelectron* 2011;26(10):4162-8. doi: 10.1016/j.bios.2011.04.016

19. Quinn JG, O'Neill S, Doyle A, McAtamney C, Diamond D, MacCraith BD, et al. Development and application of surface plasmon resonance-based biosensors for the detection of cell-ligand interactions. *Anal Biochem* 2000;281(2):135-43. doi: 10.1006/abio.2000.4564

20. Tachibana M, Yoshizawa K, Ogawa A, Fujimoto H, Hoffmann R. Sulfur-gold orbital interactions which determine the structure of alkanethiolate/Au(111) self-assembled monolayer systems. *J Phys Chem B* 2002;106(49):12727-36. doi: 10.1021/jp020993i

21. Vashist SK, Dixit CK, MacCraith BD, O'Kennedy R. Effect of antibody immobilization strategies on the analytical performance of a surface plasmon resonance-based immunoassay. *Analyst* 2011;136(21):4431-6. doi: 10.1039/c1an15325k

17

Effect of Daily Caper Fruit Pickle Consumption on Disease Regression in Patients with Non-Alcoholic Fatty Liver Disease: a Double-Blinded Randomized Clinical Trial

Narjes Khavasi[1], Mohammad Hosein Somi[2], Ebrahim Khadem[3], Elnaz Faramarzi[2], Mohammad Hossein Ayati[3], Seyyed Muhammad Bagher Fazljou[1], Mohammadali Torbati[4]*

[1] Department of Traditional Medicine, Faculty of Traditional Medicine, Tabriz University of Medical Sciences, Tabriz, Iran.
[2] Department of liver and Gastrointestinal Diseases Research Center, Tabriz University of Medical sciences, Tabriz, Iran.
[3] Department of Traditional Medicine, School of Traditional Medicine, Tehran University of Medical Sciences, Tehran, Iran.
[4] Department of Food Science and Technology, Faculty of nutrition, Tabriz University of Medical Sciences, Tabriz, Iran.

Keywords:
· Iranian traditional medicine
· Non-alcoholic fatty liver
· Caper fruit
· Lipid profile

Abstract

Purpose: Despite numerous studies on the effects of complementary medicine, to our knowledge, there is no study on the effects of *Capparis spinosa* on disease regression in non-alcoholic fatty liver disease (NAFLD) patients. We compared the effects of caper fruit pickle consumption, as an Iranian traditional medicine product, on the anthropometric measures and biochemical parameters in different NAFLD patients.

Methods: A 12-weeks randomized, controlled, double-blind trial was designed in 44 NAFLD patients randomly categorized for the control (n=22) or caper (n=22). The caper group received 40-50 gr of caper fruit pickles with meals daily. Before and after treatment, we assessed anthropometric measures, grade of fatty liver, serum lipoproteins and liver enzymes.

Results: Weight and BMI were significantly decreased in the caper (p<0.001 and p<0.001) and control group (p=0.001 and p=0.001), respectively. Serum TG, TC and LDL.C just were significantly decreased in the control group (p=0.01, p<0.001 and p<0.001, respectively). Adjusted to the baseline measures, serum ALT and AST reduction were significantly higher in the caper than control group from baseline up to the end of the study (p<0.001 and p=0.02, respectively). After weeks 12, disease severity was significantly decreased in the caper group (p <0.001).

Conclusion: Our results suggest that daily caper fruit pickle consumption for 12 weeks may be potentially effective on improving the biochemical parameters in NAFLD patients. Further, additional larger controlled trials are needed for the verification of these results.

Introduction

Non-alcoholic fatty liver disease (NAFLD) is one of the increasing metabolic disorders which has a direct link with obesity, glucose intolerance, inflammatory pathways and dyslipidemia.[1] Fatty liver disease refers to a wide range of liver damages, ranging from plain steatosis to steatohepatitis, advanced fibrosis, and finally cirrhosis.[2,3] Drugs used to decrease NAFLD progression had inconclusive results.[4-9] Because lifestyle modifications and drugs cannot be implemented effectively, new pharmacological and/or complementary foods are needed to be studied for reducing NAFLD progression. Currently, plants and/or functional foods have been noticed for the disease control or treatment due to the ease of access and in some cases, due to fewer side effects.[10] Several traditional medicinal plants are used in different areas of the world to treat metabolic disorders.[11,12] *Capparis spinosa* (caper) belongs to the

family of Capparidaceae and is widely found in the southern area of Iran and the western or central regions of Asia.[13,14] Caper's root includes flavonoids, pectin, saponins, essential oils, tannins and particularly glycosinolate and glycosides as valuable biochemical compounds.[15,16] Aqueous extract of C. *spinosa* showed blood glucose and lipid profile lowering effects in diabetic patients.[17,18] Different parts of the plant, including fruits, leaves, seeds, etc., may have different effects due to various active ingredients. To our knowledge, human and animal studies have verified the positive effects of caper fruit on blood glucose in type 2 diabetic patients, and it has been used traditionally as an anti-hyperglycemic food by Iranian diabetic patients.[17-19] Despite numerous studies about the beneficial effects of caper aqueous extract consumption on disease control in type 2 diabetic patients, no study, to our knowledge, has

*Corresponding author: Mohammadali Torbati, Email: torbatim@tbzmed.ac.ir

evaluated whether daily caper fruit consumption as a food additive can be effective in disease regression or not. Moreover, there is no human trial in this field.

The purpose of this study was to assess the effects of caper fruit consumption, as an Iranian Traditional Medicine product, change in biochemical parameters include serum lipids, liver enzymes and disease severity as primary outcome, and change in anthropometric or nutritional parameters as secondary outcome in NAFLD patients after 12 weeks. We hypothesized that daily caper fruit pickle consumption leads to the improvement in anthropometric measures, liver function tests, lipid profile and grade of fatty liver in patients with NAFLD.

Materials and Methods
Study participants and recruitment
In total, 44 NAFLD patients were selected between March 2016 and April 2017 from among patients with NAFLD diagnosis who were attending the Metabolic Disease Research Center and Valie-Asr Hospital, Zanjan University of Medical Sciences, Zanjan, Iran. The inclusion criteria were as follows: patients aged 12-80 y, BMI (in kg/m^2) of 25- 35, and willingness to consume caper fruit pickle as food additive. The exclusion criteria were any known allergies to caper, cigarette smoking, pregnancy or pregnancy planning in the next 6 months, breastfeeding, history of stroke, cirrhosis, viral hepatitis, liver obstructive diseases, heart disease or thyroid disorders, diabetes, dyslipidemia, intake of anti-diabetic or lipid lowering drugs, as well as anticoagulants, intake

of medications that could affect body weight and/or energy expenditure, following vegetarian or weight-loss diets up to 2 months before the beginning of the study. Caper has interaction with coagulopathies due to involvement in the coagulation pathways. Then, we excluded all the patients with coagulopathy diseases.[20]

Study design and intervention
A randomized, double-blind, controlled trial was designed that aimed to assess the effects of caper fruit consumption on liver enzymes, lipid profile and grade of fatty liver in NAFLD patients. At the beginning of the study, baseline measures were recorded and qualified participants were randomly categorized by using block randomization method according to BMI. Forty four patients were randomly assigned to caper group (n=22) or control group (n=22) (Figure 1). Caper fruit was collected from Moghan, Pars Abad, Iran. The whole part of the plant was sent to the laboratory of the Herbarium Research Center, Shahid Beheshti University of Medical Sciences, Tehran, Iran (Herbarium Code: 3969). After being boiled, the fruits were soaked in home-made grape vinegar. Microbial and fungal tests were carried out before pickle distribution. The patients were advised to receive 40-50 gr of caper fruit pickles with their meals. All participants were instructed by a specialized nutritionist for lifestyle changes, similarly. Compliance of the participants was assessed by telephone interview every week. Side effects were explained to all participants and followed up each interview.

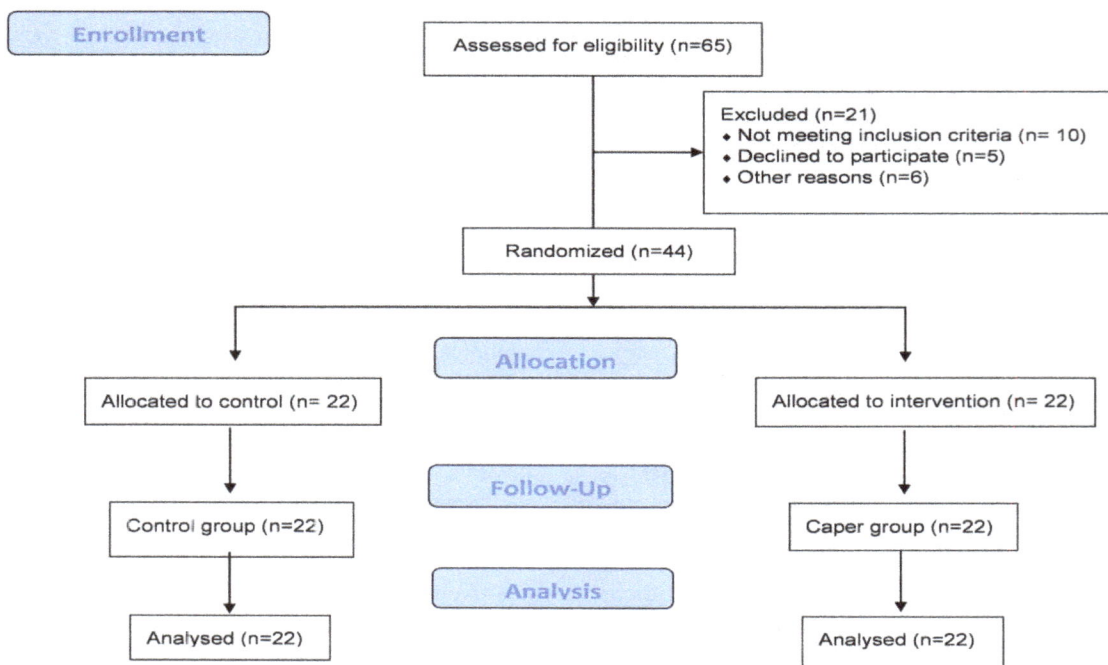

Figure 1. Screening, enrollment, random assignment, and follow-up of study participants

Measures
In the beginning, 24-hour dietary recall forms were completed and analyzed by the N4 software (Nutritionist 4, First Databank Division, Hearts Corporation).

Anthropometric measures were recorded at the beginning and end of the intervention in both groups.

Blood samples of all patients were taken from the antecubital vein after 10-12 h fasting, at baseline and at

12 weeks for biochemical measurements. After centrifugation for 15 min (2500 g), the serum samples were frozen simultaneously and stored at -80 °C until analyzed. Lipid profile and liver enzyme tests were measured by an enzymatic method (Pars Azmoon Co. Kit, Tehran, Iran) using Liasys autoanalyzer.

Grades of fatty liver classification
Liver ultra-sonography (US) was performed by Siemens brand Sonoline G50 series - 3.5e5 MHz probe made in Germany. Liver steatosis was classified through sonographic echogenicity of liver as: 1) normal: echogenicity, the same as renal cortex; 2) grade I: mild steatosis that increased liver echogenicity with visible diaphragmatic and periportal echogenicity; 3) grade II: moderate steatosis, increased liver echogenicity with imperceptible periportal echogenicity, without obscuration of diaphragm; 4) grade III: severe, steatosis; increased liver echogenicity with imperceptible periportal echogenicity and obscuration of diaphragm.[21]

Sample size and statistical analysis
In the present study, power of 80% with a two-sided test with $\alpha=0.05$ (type I error) and mean difference of 25 IU/L for changes in ALT levels were considered to determine the sample size. On the basis of means, as stated in the previous studies,[22] the number of participants needed to detect this difference was 22 in each group. By considering the dropout rate of 10 percent, we set the enrollment target of 25 subjects.
Numeric variables were expressed by means ± SD. The level of significance was set at $P < 0.05$. Statistical analyses were accomplished with IBM SPSS Statistics software (version 22; SPSS, Inc). We used Kolmogorov-Smirnov Test to assess the normal distribution of the data. Independent sample t-test was used to assess the differences in mean values of the variables between the two groups. The comparison of mean values of variables before and after the intervention in each group was examined by paired t-tests. For non-normally distributed data, appropriate non-parametric test was used. The comparison of mean change in each parameter during the trial was assessed by ANCOVA test, adjusted for baseline measures as covariates.

Results and Discussion
Dietary intake and physical activity had no significant difference between the two studied groups (p>0.05). Baseline levels of AST, HDL.C and LDL.C were significantly different between the two groups (p<0.001). 72.7% of the participants in the caper and 59.1% of them in the control group were female. Gender distribution between the two groups were not significantly different (p=0.4). Mean age of the participants was 40.32±10.04 y in the caper and 45±10.03 y in the control group, with no significant difference between the two groups. Weight and BMI were significantly decreased in the caper (p<0.001 and p<0.001) and control groups (p=0.001 and p=0.001), respectively.

Serum ALT levels were significantly decreased at the end of the study in the caper and control groups (p<0.001 and p<0.001, respectively). Also, serum AST levels decreased in both of the studied groups (p<0.001 and p<0.001, respectively). Serum TG, TC and LDL.C were significantly decreased only in the control group (p=0.01, p<0.001 and p<0.001, respectively) (Table 1).
Adjusted to the baseline measures, the mean change in serum ALT and AST concentrations was significantly higher in the caper than the control group (p<0.001 and p=0.02, respectively). The mean change in serum of LDL.C levels was significantly higher in the control than the caper group, adjusted for the baseline measures (p=0.03) (Table 1).
At the end of the study, grade of fatty liver was significantly different between the two studied groups (p <0.001). Improve on the stage of NAFLD was significantly higher in the caper group than the control group, adjusted for the baseline measures (Table 2).
Although the standard method for NAFLD treatment is weight loss, drug and supplement trials have shown inconclusive results.[6-10] To our knowledge, there is no concise therapy for NAFLD treatment. Thus more studies on dietary supplements and/or functional foods are needed for prevention or regression of NAFLD. Dietary supplements or functional foods which have beneficial effects on insulin resistance and blood glucose control, as well as antioxidant and anti-inflammatory activity, may be effective in the NAFLD treatment. On the other hand, many patients tend to use traditional medicine and its products for disease treatment. The present study has shown that weight loss, as the routine method for NAFLD treatment, was more pronounced in the caper than in the control L. Furthermore, a mean difference of change in serum ALT and AST concentrations was higher pronounced in the caper than the control group. Also, disease severity was significantly decreased in the caper group, adjusting for the baseline measures. Results showed that caper fruit pickle consumption in the diet can show fatty liver progression. Our results are in agreement with the previous study showing the weight-reducing effect of caper.[23]
Caper fruit, as an ITM herb, has a bitter taste which is not favored by consumers. Therefore, we prepared its pickle for patients' convenience. Numerous studies are available assessing the effect of caper components, including fruit, seed, stem, leaf and the whole of the plant in the treatment of several other diseases such as metabolic syndrome and type II diabetes.[18,19,24] The anti-hyperglycemic property of caper is due to the reduced absorption of carbohydrates from the small intestine, increased glucose uptake in the tissue, glucose-depletion in the liver, and the regeneration or protection of the beta cells of the pancreas.[21] Caper is known as an herb with antioxidant properties.[16] In addition to the effect of alcoholic and aqueous extract of caper on lipid profile, it is shown that it has hepato- and nephroprotctive effects

against toxins.[24,25] The most useful effects of caper fruit pickle on health are due to high bioactive compounds, especially polyphenols.[25,26] According to the ITM opinion, caper has an important role in spleen performance, excretion of toxins, as well as excess "Soda" and "Balgham", from the liver.[27] One study reported that "Balgham", as a component of quadruple humors, has a relationship with lipid profile.[28]

Table 1. Anthropometric and biochemical measurement characteristics at baseline and weeks 12 between the groups[a]

| Variables | Caper (n=22) | | Control (n=22) | | p value[†] |
	Baseline	Weeks 12	Before	After	
Weight (kg)	81.32±9.93	78.93±9.95	81.32±13.92	79.77±13.21	0.08
p value[‡]		<0.C01		0.001	
BMI (kg/m2)	27.76±3.22	26.94±3.21	31.5±2.24	30.93±2.29	0.2
p value		<0.001		0.001	
ALT(U/L)	71.09±31.4	42.18±24.10	70.95±9.94	63.59±12.06	<0.001
p value		<0.001		<0.001	
AST(U/L)	38.91±13.16	27.50±10.91	67.73±10.18	59.95±14.1	0.02
p value		<0.001		<0.001	
TC (mg/dl)	191.28±47.19	183.87±44.79	166.77±37.09	152.54±35.88	0.09
p value		0.25		<0.001	
TG (mg/dl)	189.19±55.98	190.76±79.85	225±90.5	215.68±93.54	0.053
p value		C.9		0.01	
LDL(mg/dl)	112.05±35.82	103.1±280.08	77.27±44.55	64.86±40.76	0.03
p value		0.1		<0.001	
HDL (mg/dl)	38.42±8.16	39.05±7.82	44.04±5.22	44.13±6.04	0.3
p value		0.7		0.93	

[a] Values are means ± SE. p < 0.05 was considered as significant
BMI: body mass index; ALT: alanine transaminase; AST: aspartate transaminase; TC: total cholesterol; TG: triglycerides
[†] p values are related to the differences between the groups after 12 wk of treatment; evaluated by using an ANCOVA with baseline values as covariate
[‡] p values are related to the differences within the groups from baseline to the end; evaluated by paired sample t-test

Table 2. Grade of fatty liver in the groups before and after the 12-wk intervention

Group	Grade of fatty liver	Baseline N (%)	Weeks 12 N (%)	Changes[†], N	p value
Control	Normal	0	1 (4.5)	Without change: 18	<0.001
	Stage 1	12(54.5)	12(54.5)	1 degree reduction: 4	
	Stage 2	9 (40.9)	8 (36.4)	2 degree reduction: 0	
	Stage 3	1 (4.5)	1 (4.5)		
Caper	Normal	0	2 (9.1)	Without change: 15	
	Stage 1	13 (59.1)	13 (59.1)	1 degree reduction: 5	
	Stage 2	7 (31.8)	6 (27.3)	2 degree reduction: 1	
	Stage 3	2 (9.1)	0		

*P value by using chi-square test; [†] Reduction in the grade of NAFLD after 12 weeks of the study

After 12 weeks of daily caper fruit consumption, ALT and AST reduction were higher compared with the control group. One study showed the same results. Streptozotocin induced diabetic rats were treated with the caper root extract for four weeks. Serum glucose level was decreased without any change in serum insulin level. Also, liver enzyme tests were significantly decreased in the caper extract-fed group.[29] One study has shown that Capparis spinosa as an antidiabetic plant is capable to reduce blood glucose in streptozotocin-induced diabetic mice.[30] In another study with the aim of evaluating the hepatoprotective effect of C.spinosa, ethanolic root bark extract of this medicinal plant was evaluated in a mouse model of CCl4-induced hepatotoxicity. Serum liver enzymes were reduced in the C-spinosa supplemented group with ethanolic extract of C.spinosa.[31] In contrast, another study showed no significant effect of aqueous extract of caper fruit on liver enzyme tests in patients with type II diabetes.[19] Serum liver enzymes were in normal range in the mentioned study, which may be one of probable reasons for this result. On the other hand, the effect of caper on reducing serum glucose and lipid profile is dose-dependent manner. Therefore, inconclusive results of the previous studies may be due to the effective dose. Also, caper fruit may have various components and/or amounts of polyphenols in different regions depending on the cultivation soil. Serum levels of lipid profile and/or liver enzymes shown inconsistency in various studies. These differences lead to various results.

One study assessed the effects of the caper fruit extract on the serum levels of ALT, AST, ALP, bilirubin, creatinine, urea and uric acid, as well as histo-pathologic properties of the liver, kidneys, pancreas and stomach in a rat model of type 1 diabetes.[32] Cellular necrosis occurred in the liver, pancreas and kidneys of diabetic rats, but changes in the diabetic treated group with caper fruit extract were lower than the control group. Similarly, the serum levels of creatinine, liver enzymes, and other factors decreased. Another study assessed the anti-inflammatory properties of caper in the cell line. They showed that caper fruit inhibits cytokine gene expression, including IFNγ, IL-17 and IL-4. They concluded that the beneficial effects of caper fruit are due to saponins, flavonoids and alkaloids.[33]

To our knowledge, this is the preliminary RCT aimed to assess the effect of caper fruit pickle consumption on the hepatic lipid accumulation, serum lipid profile and liver enzyme tests in the patients with NAFLD. Caper has more benefits on lipid accumulation in the liver and grade of fatty liver. However, a study with more sample size and longer duration is needed before reaching conclusive results. There are some limitations to our results; firstly that NAFLD was diagnosed by biochemical and ultra-sonographic findings in our patients, which is not able to distinguish between simple fatty liver and NASH. Fibroscan, as a precise method for detection and staging of the liver diseases, is more expensive. Liver biopsy is the gold standard for NAFLD diagnosis, but it is an invasive and expensive method. Secondly, we did not match the patients according to their NAFLD at enrollementwe. We suggest that patients could be matched according to the grade of the fatty liver disease in the oncoming studies. In future studies, precise control of dietary intake and physical activity level is suggested. Also, caper components should be analyzed in future. Another study with the higher levels of these enzymes is needed to assess the effects of caper fruit on NAFLD progression. Insulin resistance, inflammatory and oxidative pathways should be assessed to determine the involved signaling pathways.

Conclusion
The present study showed that caper fruit as an herbal drug may be effective in reducing the NAFLD progression because of natural compounds such as comarin and flavonoids. Thus, this fruit has medicinal properties. However, more studies are needed to obtain concise results.

Acknowledgments
Authors are very thankful to all participated patients. Fund of the present study was provided by Vice chancellor for research, Tabriz University of Medical Sciences, Tabriz, Iran.

Ethical Issues
The present study was approved by the Ethical Committee of Tabriz University of Medical Sciences, Tabriz, Iran (TBZMED.REC.1394.650).

Conflict of Interest
The authors declare that there is no conflict of interest.

References
1. Berlanga A, Guiu-Jurado E, Porras JA, Auguet T. Molecular pathways in non-alcoholic fatty liver disease. *Clin Exp Gastroenterol* 2014;7:221-39. doi: 10.2147/CEG.S62831
2. Angulo P. Nonalcoholic fatty liver disease. *N Engl J Med* 2002;346(16):1221-31. doi: 10.1056/NEJMra011775
3. Esposito E, Iacono A, Bianco G, Autore G, Cuzzocrea S, Vajro P, et al. Probiotics reduce the inflammatory response induced by a high-fat diet in the liver of young rats. *J Nutr* 2009;139(5):905-11. doi: 10.3945/jn.108.101808
4. Adams LA, Zein CO, Angulo P, Lindor KD. A pilot trial of pentoxifylline in nonalcoholic steatohepatitis. *Am J Gastroenterol* 2004;99(12):2365-8. doi: 10.1111/j.1572-0241.2004.40064.x
5. Harrison SA, Fincke C, Helinski D, Torgerson S, Hayashi P. A pilot study of orlistat treatment in obese, non-alcoholic steatohepatitis patients. *Aliment Pharmacol Ther* 2004;20(6):623-8. doi: 10.1111/j.1365-2036.2004.02153.x
6. Belfort R, Harrison SA, Brown K, Darland C, Finch J, Hardies J, et al. A placebo-controlled trial of pioglitazone in subjects with nonalcoholic steatohepatitis. *N Engl J Med* 2006;355(22):2297-307. doi: 10.1056/NEJMoa060326
7. Lorvand Amiri H, Agah S, Tolouei Azar J, Hosseini S, Shidfar F, Mousavi SN. Effect of daily calcitriol supplementation with and without calcium on disease regression in non-alcoholic fatty liver patients following an energy-restricted diet: Randomized, controlled, double-blind trial. *Clin Nutr* 2017;36(6):1490-7. doi: 10.1016/j.clnu.2016.09.020
8. Lorvand Amiri H, Agah S, Mousavi SN, Hosseini AF, Shidfar F. Regression of Non-Alcoholic Fatty Liver by Vitamin D Supplement: A Double-Blind Randomized Controlled Clinical Trial. *Arch Iran Med* 2016;19(9):631-8.
9. Mousavi SN, Faghihi A, Motaghinejad M, Shiasi M, Imanparast F, Amiri HL, et al. Zinc and Selenium Co-supplementation Reduces Some Lipid Peroxidation and Angiogenesis Markers in a Rat Model of NAFLD-Fed High Fat Diet. *Biol Trace Elem Res* 2017. doi: 10.1007/s12011-017-1059-2
10. Shidfar F, Jazayeri S, Mousavi SN, Malek M, Hosseini AF, Khoshpey B. Does Supplementation with Royal Jelly Improve oxidative Stress and Insulin Resistance in Type 2 Diabetic Patients? *Iran J Public Health* 2015;44(6):797-803.

11. Patel DK, Kumar R, Laloo D, Hemalatha S. Diabetes mellitus: an overview on its pharmacological aspects and reported medicinal plants having antidiabetic activity. *Asian Pac J Trop Biomed* 2012;2(5):411-20. doi: 10.1016/S2221-1691(12)60067-7

12. Patel DK, Prasad SK, Kumar R, Hemalatha S. An overview on antidiabetic medicinal plants having insulin mimetic propert. *Asian Pac J Trop Biomed* 2012;2(4):320-30. doi: 10.1016/S2221-1691(12)60032-X

13. Azaizeh H, Fulder S, Khalil K, Said O. Ethnobotanical knowledge of local Arab practitioners in the Middle Eastern region. *Fitoterapia* 2003;74(1-2):98-108. doi: 10.1016/s0367-326x(02)00285-x

14. Jiang HE, Li X, Ferguson DK, Wang YF, Liu CJ, Li CS. The discovery of Capparis spinosa L. (Capparidaceae) in the Yanghai Tombs (2800 years b.p.), NW China, and its medicinal implications. *J Ethnopharmacol* 2007;113(3):409-20. doi: 10.1016/j.jep.2007.06.020

15. Khanfar MA, Sabri SS. Zarga MH, Zeller KP. The chemical constituents of Capparis spinosa of Jordanian origin. *Nat Prod Res* 2003;17(1):9-14. doi: 10.1080/10575630290034302

16. Yang T, Liu YQ, Wang CH, Wang ZT. Advances on investigation of chemical constituents, pharmacological activities and clinical applications of Capparis spinosa. *Zhongguo Zhong Yao Za Zhi* 2008;33(21):2453-8.

17. Matthaus B, Ozcan M. Glucosinolates and fatty acid, sterol, and tocopherol composition of seed oils from Capparis spinosa Var. spinosa and Capparis ovata Desf. Var. canescens (Coss.) Heywood. *J Agric Food Chem* 2005;53(18):7136-41. doi: 10.1021/jf051019u

18. Eddouks M, Lemhadri A, Michel JB. Hypolipidemic activity of aqueous extract of Capparis spinosa L. in normal and diabetic rats. *J Ethnopharmacol* 2005;98(3):345-50. doi: 10.1016/j.jep.2005.01.053

19. Huseini HF, Hasani-Rnjbar S, Nayebi N, Heshmat R, Sigaroodi FK, Ahvazi M, et al. Capparis spinosa L. (Caper) fruit extract in treatment of type 2 diabetic patients: A randomized double-blind placebo-controlled clinical trial. *Complement Ther Med* 2013;21(5):447-52. doi: 10.1016/j.ctim.2013.07.003

20. Wang H, Wang H, Shi S, Duan J, Wang S. Structural characterization of a homogalacturonan from Capparis spinosa L. fruits and anti-complement activity of its sulfated derivative. *Glycoconj J* 2012;29(5-6):379-87. doi: 10.1007/s10719-012-9418-x

21. Goodman E, Daniels SR, Morrison JA, Huang B, Dolan LM. Contrasting prevalence of and demographic disparities in the World Health Organization and National Cholesterol Education Program Adult Treatment Panel III definitions of metabolic syndrome among adolescents. *J Pediatr* 2004;145(4):445-51. doi: 10.1016/j.jpeds.2004.04.059

22. Soza A, Riquelme A, Gonzalez R, Alvarez M, Perez-ayuso RM, Glasinovic JC, et al. Increased orocecal transit time in patients with nonalcoholic fatty liver disease. *Dig Dis Sci* 2005;50(6):1136-40. doi: 10.1007/s10620-005-2720-8

23. Rahnavard R, Razavi N. A review on the medical effects of Capparis spinosa L. *Adv Herb Med* 2016;2(1):44-53.

24. Tlili N, Feriani A, Saadoui E, Nasri N, Khaldi A. Capparis spinosa leaves extract: Source of bioantioxidants with nephroprotective and hepatoprotective effects. *Biomed Pharmacother* 2017;87:171-9. doi: 10.1016/j.biopha.2016.12.052

25. Nabavi SF, Maggi F, Daglia M, Habtemariam S, Rastrelli L, Nabavi SM. Pharmacological Effects of Capparis spinosa L. *Phytother Res* 2016;30(11):1733-44. doi: 10.1002/ptr.5684

26. Mansour RB, Jilani IB, Bouaziz M, Gargouri B, Elloumi N, Attia H, et al. Phenolic contents and antioxidant activity of ethanolic extract of Capparis spinosa. *Cytotechnology* 2016;68(1):135-42. doi: 10.1007/s10616-014-9764-6

27. Nazem Jahan MA. Eksir -e- Aazam [Great Elixir]: (Diseases). Tehran: Sarir -e- Ardehal; 2008. [In Persian].

28. Emtiazy M, Keshavarz M, Khodadoost M, Kamalinejad M, Gooshahgir SA, Shahrad Bajestani H, et al. Relation between body humors and hypercholesterolemia: An Iranian traditional medicine perspective based on the teaching of Avicenna. *Iran Red Crescent Med J* 2012;14(3):133-8.

29. Kazemian M, Abad M, Haeri MR, Ebrahimi M, Heidari R. Anti-diabetic effect of Capparis spinosa L. root extract in diabetic rats. *Avicenna J Phytomed* 2015;5(4):325-32.

30. Eddouks M, Lemhadri A, Hebi M, El Hidani A, Zeggwagh NA, El Bouhali B, et al. Capparis spinosa L. aqueous extract evokes antidiabetic effect in streptozotocin-induced diabetic mice. *Avicenna J Phytomed* 2017;7(2):191-8.

31. Aghel N, Rashidi I, Mombeini A. Hepatoprotective Activity of Capparis spinosa Root Bark against CCl4 Induced Hepatic Damage in Mice. *Iran J Pharm Res* 2007;6(4):285-90.

32. Taghavi MM, Nazari M, Rahmani R, Sayadi AR, Hajizadeh MR, Mirzaei MR, et al. Outcome of Capparis Spinosa Fruit Extracts Treatment on Liver, Kidney, Pancreas and Stomach Tissues in Normal and Diabetic Rats. *Med Chem* 2014;4:717-21.

33. El Azhary K, Tahiri Jouti N, El Khachibi M, Moutia M, Tabyaoui I, El Hou A, et al. Anti-inflammatory potential of *Capparis spinosa* L. in vivo in mice through inhibition of cell infiltration and cytokine gene expression. *BMC Complement Altern Med* 2017;17(1):81. doi: 10.1186/s12906-017-1569-7

18

Targeted Co-Delivery of Docetaxel and cMET siRNA for Treatment of Mucin1 Overexpressing Breast Cancer Cells

Naime Majidi Zolbanin[1,2] ⓘD, **Reza Jafari**[3,4] ⓘD, **Jafar Majidi**[5,6] ⓘD, **Fatemeh Atyabi**[7,8] ⓘD, **Mehdi Yousefi**[5,6] ⓘD, **Farhad Jadidi-Niaragh**[5,6] ⓘD, **Leili Aghebati-Maleki**[5] ⓘD, **Dariush Shanehbandi**[5] ⓘD, **Mohammad-Sadegh Soltani Zangbar**[6], **Alireza Mohajjel Nayebi**[1,2]* ⓘD

[1] *Drug Applied Research Center, Tabriz University of Medical Sciences, Tabriz, Iran.*

[2] *Pharmacology and Toxicology Department, School of Pharmacy, Tabriz University of Medical Sciences, Tabriz, Iran.*

[3] *Department of Immunology, Faculty of Medicine, Mashhad University of Medical Sciences, Mashhad, Iran.*

[4] *Immunology Research Center, Inflammation and Inflammatory Diseases Division, School of Medicine, Mashhad University of Medical Sciences, Mashhad, Iran.*

[5] *Immunology Research Center, Tabriz University of Medical Sciences, Tabriz, Iran.*

[6] *Department of Immunology, School of Medicine, Tabriz University of Medical Sciences, Tabriz, Iran.*

[7] *Department of Pharmaceutics, Faculty of Pharmacy, Tehran University of Medical Sciences, Tehran, Iran.*

[8] *Nanotechnology Research Centre, Faculty of Pharmacy, Tehran University of Medical Sciences, Tehran, Iran.*

Keywords:
· Aptamer
· Chitosan
· cMET siRNA
· Docetaxel
· Metastatic breast cancer

Abstract

Purpose: Targeted treatment of breast cancer through combination of chemotherapeutic agents and siRNA had been drawing much attention in recent researches. This study was carried out to evaluate mucin1 aptamer-conjugated chitosan nanoparticles containing docetaxel and cMET siRNA on SKBR3 cells.

Methods: Nano-drugs were characterized by transmission electron microscope, Zetasizer and loading efficiency calculation. siRNA entrapment onto nanoparticles, stability of siRNA-loaded nanoparticles and conjugation of mucin1 aptamer to nanoparticles were evaluated via separate electrophoresis. Cellular uptake of the targeted nanoparticles was evaluated through GFP-plasmid expression in mucin1$^+$ SKBR3 *vs.* mucin1$^-$ CHO cells. Protein expression, cell viability and gene expression were assessed by Western Blotting, MTT assay, and Quantitative Real Time-PCR, respectively.

Results: Characterization of nano-drugs represented the ideal size (110.5± 3.9 nm), zeta potential (11.6± 0.8 mV), and loading efficiency of 90.7% and 88.3% for siRNA and docetaxel, respectively. Different gel electrophoresis affirmed the conjugation of aptamers to nanoparticles and entrapment of siRNA onto nanoparticles. Increased cellular uptake of aptamer-conjugated nanoparticles was confirmed by GFP expression. cMET gene silencing was confirmed by Western Blotting. The significant ($p \leq 0.0001$) impact of combination targeted therapy *vs.* control on cell viability was shown. Results of Quantitative Real Time-PCR represented a remarkably decreased ($p \leq 0.0001$) expression of the studied genes involving in tumorigenicity, metastasis, invasion, and angiogenesis (STAT3, IL8, MMP2, MMP9, and VEGF) by targeted combination treatment *vs.* control.

Conclusion: The mucin1 aptamer-conjugated chitosan nanoparticles, containing docetaxel and cMET siRNA, is suggested for treatment of mucin1$^+$ metastatic breast cancer cells. However, further studies should be conducted on animal models.

Introduction

Breast cancer treatment has become a complicated issue worldwide since the adverse reactions of the used medications decrease the patient compliance and the new drug resistance mechanisms are appeared.

cMET, the essential receptor tyrosine kinase for embryonic development of epithelial and endothelial cells, is normally activated by its ligand, Hepatocyte Growth Factor (HGF). The formed complex activates many signaling pathways such as Signal Transducer and Activator of Transcription 3 (STAT3). This causes an increase in inflammation, migration/ invasion, and angiogenesis via up-regulation of IL8, Matrix Metalloproteinases 2 and 9 (MMP2, MMP9), and Vascular Endothelial Growth Factor (VEGF), respectively. In many cancers, overexpression/ activation of cMET occur, which may be responsible for tumorigenicity, metastasis, and immunosuppression.[1,2] HGF/ cMET signaling is increased in breast cancer cells,

---

*Corresponding author: Alireza Mohajjel Nayebi, Email: nayebia@tbzmed.ac.ir

especially in the Her2[+] subtype. This is related with drug resistances and reduced survival, and thus, cMET has become a therapeutic target.[3] Standard approved therapeutic protocol for Her2[+] metastatic breast cancer includes Trastuzumab, accompanied with the preferable chemotherapeutic agents, Docetaxel or Paclitaxel.[4] Apart from these two mentioned common therapies, gene silencing has become a research interest. This can be put to use by applying micro RNA (miRNA) and small-interfering RNA (siRNA).[5] Among the mentioned chemotherapeutic agents, docetaxel has been used successfully. However, its adverse hematological (febrile neutropenia) and non-hematological (hypersensitivity reactions, fluid retention, nail toxicities, etc.) reactions have reduced patients' compliance.[6] The application of safe biodegradable nano-carriers, such as chitosan nanoparticles (NPs), is one of the novel solutions of pharmaceutical technology in reducing the adverse drug reactions. This is done for the delivery of chemotherapeutic agents, which results in dose reduction of loaded agent.[7] On the other hand, using positively charged chitosan for loading the desired drug gives chance to load negatively charged easily degradable siRNA molecules simultaneously.[8] Moreover, the mentioned co-delivery of chemotherapeutic drug and siRNA can be better targeted and specific to cancer cells through the novel DNA/RNA molecules, Aptamers (APT).[9] The anti-mucin1 aptamer is used because mucin1 is one of the distinctly over expressed glycoproteins on breast cancer cells.[10]

The aim of this study was designing of the co-delivery system of docetaxel and cMET siRNA in the form of targeted chitosan NPs conjugated to the mucin1 APT. Cellular evaluations of the designed system were done on metastatic breast cancer cell line, SKBR3.

Materials and Methods
Materials
Carboxymethyl dextran (CMD), 1-Ethyl-3-(3-dimethylaminopropyl) carbodiimide (EDC), N-Hydroxysuccinimide (NHS) and 3-(4,5-dimethylthiazol-2-yl)-2,5-diphenyltetrazolium bromide (MTT) powder were all supplied from Merck® (Darmstadt, Germany). Mucin1 aptamer (APT) with the following sequence (5'-Amino-C6-GGG AGA CAA GAA TAA ACG CTC AAG AAG TGA AAA TGA CAG AAC ACA ACA TTC GAC AGG AGG CTC ACA ACA GGC- 3') was purchased from TAG Copenhagen® (Frederiksberg, Denmark). Docetaxel (DTX) was ordered from AqVida® (Hamburg, Germany). Human-specific cMET-siRNA (catalog number: sc-29397) and non-targeting (scrambled) siRNA (catalog number: sc-37007, Sense: UUCUCCGAACGUGUCACGUTT, Antisense: ACGUGACACGUUCGGAGAATT) were purchased from Santa Cruz Biotechnology® (Santa Cruz, CA, USA). The SKBR3 and CHO cell lines were obtained from the National Cell Bank of Iran (Pasteur Institute of Iran, Tehran, Iran). Roswell Park Memorial Institute (RPMI) 1640 medium, Fetal Bovine Serum (FBS),

Trypsin, and Penicillin-Streptomycin were all purchased from Gibco® (Waltham, MA USA). RNA extraction solution was purchased from SinaClon® (Tehran, Iran). GFP containing plasmid was obtained from Clontech Laboratories (Mountain View, CA, USA). cMET primary monoclonal antibody (catalog number: sc-514148), horseradish conjugated anti-IgG secondary polyclonal antibody (catalog number: sc-2005), and beta-actin primary monoclonal antibody (catalog number: sc-47778) were all purchased from Santa Cruz Biotechnology® (Santa Cruz, CA, USA).

Depolymerization of 50 kDa chitosan
In order to prepare chitosan with MW of 50 kDa, the chitosan with medium MW of 400 kDa was depolymerized according to the protocol described previously.[11] Briefly, 2 g of chitosan was dissolved in 10 ml of acetic acid (6% v/v) to gain 2% v/v solution of chitosan in acetic acid. Thereafter, 10 ml of sodium nitrite (NaNO$_2$, 2.5 mg/ml) was added to the dissolved chitosan under magnetic stirring at 25 °C for 2 h in order to obtain 50 kDa chitosan. In order to precipitate the depolymerized chitosan (dCS), the pH was gained to 9 by adding of NaOH (4M). The precipitated depolymerized chitosan (white/ yellow in color) was then filtrated and washed for three times with acetone. The yield product was dissolved in 40 ml of acetic acid (0.1 N). The dialysis of the dissolved chitosan in acetic acid against demineralized water was done to obtain the purified depolymerized chitosan (Sigma dialysis tubes, cutoff 12 kDa). It was then lyophilized by Alpha 2-4 LD plus freeze dryer (Martin Christ, Osterode am Harz, Germany). The MW of the yield product was assessed via gel permeation chromatography (Agilent Technologies, Santa Clara, CA, USA), as described previously.[12]

Preparation of loaded nanoparticles
Nanodrugs were prepared through ionotropic gelation method. dCS (0.1% w/v) was dissolved in diethylpyrocarbonate (DEPC) treated water under magnetic stirring (140 rpm) for two hours. 3 µl of siRNA (19 µg/µl, 3×10^{-6} µmol) and 5 µl of DTX (50 µg/ml, 61.9 µM) were added to 1.2 ml of CMD (0.1% w/v). Then the obtained mixture was added dropwise (with time intervals of 5 seconds between drops) to 1 ml of dCS solution under gentle stirring (140 rpm) for 10 minutes and then incubated in the dark place for 30 minutes at 25 °C. In order to remove the unloaded drugs, membrane dialysis bag (12 kDa cutoff, Merck®, Darmstadt, Germany) was used twice in DEPC-treated water for 90 minutes and once overnight.

In vitro evaluations of nanoparticles
Investigation of shape and surface morphology of freshly prepared NPs were assessed by transmission electron microscope (TEM, LE-O906, Zeiss®, Jena, Germany). Particle size, Polydispersity Index (PDI), and zeta potential were determined by Photon Correlation

Spectroscopy using Zetasizer Nano-ZS (Malvern Instruments, Malvern, UK) at a wavelength of 633 nm.

In order to confirm siRNA entrapment onto nanoparticles, the electrophoresis on a 4% agarose gel was done with siRNA loaded NPs, blank NPs, and plain siRNA.

The UV-vis spectrophotometer (Nanodrop® 2000, Thermo Fisher Scientific, Waltham, MA, USA) was used for measuring loading efficiency % (LE%) of cMET siRNA (at 260 nm) and DTX (at 230 nm). Ultimately, the LE% was calculated with the help of the following equation:

$$LE(\%) = \left[1 - \left(\frac{\text{OD of sample in supernatant}}{\text{OD of initial feeding amount of sample}} \right) \right] \times 100$$

Serum and heparin stability of siRNA loaded nanoparticles

400 µl of the siRNA-loaded NPs (0.15 µg/µl) was added to 200 µl of FBS (10%) and the mixture was incubated at 37 °C shaker for sequential sampling at time intervals of 0, 2, 8, 12, 24, and 48 hours. The collected samples were kept at -20 °C. Furthermore, 60 µl of siRNA-loaded NPs was added to heparin solution (2 µg/µl) in volumes of 0, 0.6, 1.5, and 3 µl and they all were incubated at 37 °C shaker for 1 h. Moreover, 4% agarose gel electrophoresis was run with the mentioned samples and the plain siRNA as control.

In vitro DTX and siRNA release

The release of siRNA loaded and DTX loaded NPs was evaluated by incubation of the mentioned samples inside the membrane dialysis bag (12 kD cut off, Merck) in 50 ml of phosphate buffer solutions (PBS, pH = 7.4 and pH = 5.5) at 37 °C for 120 h. Subsequently, 2 ml of solutions was withdrawn and replaced with the same volume of fresh PBS under same condition at several intervals. Finally, siRNA and DTX released contents were assessed by UV-vis spectrophotometer at 260 and 230 nm, respectively. Furthermore, the released medium collected from blank NPs was used as the blank sample. In vitro siRNA and DTX release (%) were calculated with the help of the following equation:

$$\text{Released DTX or siRNA (\%)} = \left(\frac{\text{OD of DTX or siRNA in the PBS}}{\text{OD of initial total content of DTX or siRNA}} \right) \times 100$$

Conjugation of mucin1 aptamer to chitosan nanoparticles

NPs were suspended in 200 µl of DNase/RNase-free water and activated with EDC (10 mg) and NHS (8 mg) and stirred at 25 °C for 2 h in order to conjugate APT to NPs, according to the previously described EDC/NHS method.[13] The unreacted EDC and NHS were removed through membrane dialysis bag (12 kDa cutoff, Merck®, Darmstadt, Germany). Then, 5'-NH₂-modified Mucin1 APT (1% w/ w) was reacted with activated NPs for 8 h at 25 °C. Eventually, in order to remove un-conjugated APT, the sample was centrifuged (2 × 10 min, 16,000 g,

5 °C) and washed with DEPC-treated water. Agarose gel (4%) electrophoresis was run in Tris-acetate-EDTA (1M) solution to confirm APT conjugation to NPs. To calculate APT conjugation efficiency, the Optical Density (OD) of the final sample was measured at 260 nm via UV-vis spectrophotometer (Nanodrop® 2000).

Evaluation of cellular uptake

In order to compare efficiency of mucin1 APT on cellular uptake of NPs, SKBR₃ cells (mucin1⁺) and CHO cells (mucin1⁻) were seeded in 6-well culture plates (1.5 × 10⁵ cells/ well) with RPMI-1640 medium supplemented with FBS 10%, penicillin 100 units/ mL and streptomycin 100 µg/ mL, kept at 37 °C in 5% CO_2 incubator. To prepare the pharmaceutical groups, briefly, CMD solution (0.1% w/ v) was prepared by dissolving CMD in DEPC-treated water (pH = 7). Subsequently, 3 µl of GFP plasmid (1 µg/ µl) was added into 1.2 ml of CMD. Eventually, the yielded aqueous solution was added dropwise into 1 ml of dCS solution under gentle stirring (140 rpm) for 10 minutes. The nanodrugs were then incubated in the dark at room temperature for 30 minutes. Aptamer conjugation was done according to the EDC/ NHS method described at the previous section. Then the cells were treated with "NPs + GFP" and "NPs + APT + GFP" for 24 h and incubated at 37 °C in 5% CO_2. Thereafter, the cells were washed with PBS (pH = 7.4) and fixed with 4% formaldehyde for 30 minutes at 25 °C. The fixed cells were incubated with DAPI (nucleic acid stain) for 5 minutes. Cellular uptake was assessed by cell imaging system, Cytation™ 5 (BioTek Instruments, Winooski, Vermont, USA).

Protein extraction and western blotting

5 × 10⁶ SKBR3 cells were treated by "NPs + siRNA" for 48 h. The protein extraction by RIPA lysis buffer system (Santa Cruz Biotechnology®, Santa Cruz, CA, USA) and the protein concentration assay via Bradford method (Protein assay Kit, Razibiotech, Tehran, Iran) were done. The supernatant was stored at -80 °C. Thereafter, the electrophoresis was run on 8% SDS-PAGE gel and the wet transfer system (Bio Rad Laboratories, Hercules, CA, USA) was used for transfection of proteins onto PVDF membrane. The membrane was blocked via incubation at 4 °C for overnight in Tris-Buffered Saline Tween 20 (TBST) buffer supplemented by 3% Bovine Serum Albumin (BSA). Subsequently, incubation at 25 °C for 1 h with 1:500 dilution of cMET primary antibody was done. The 1:2000 dilution of horseradish conjugated anti-IgG secondary antibody was added for membrane washing and was incubated for 2 h at 25 °C. The monoclonal beta-actin primary antibody at a dilution of 1:500 was used as the control. Super Signal West Pico Chemiluminescent Substrate (Thermo fisher scientific, Waltham, MA, USA) was used to detect the created bands. Protein bands' intensity were quantified by ImageJ software (National institutes of health,

Maryland, USA) and normalized to the corresponding beta-actin.

MTT bioassay
The cytotoxicity and IC50-values of free DTX and NPs loaded by DTX were assessed previously.[14,15] To evaluate cell viability, the SKBR3 cells were seeded in 96-well plates (1×10^4 cells/well) in triplicate mode and treated for 24 and 48 hours. Then, 100 µl of fresh medium and 100 µl of MTT solution (5mg/ ml) were added to each well and incubated at 37 °C for 4 h. After removing the medium, 200 µl of dimethyl sulfoxide (DMSO) and 25 µl of Sorenson's buffer were added and incubated (20 minutes, 25 °C). Optical density was read at 570 nm versus 630 nm reference wavelength by ELISA reader (Stat Fax 2100, Awareness Technology, Palm City, FL, USA). Ultimately the cell viability (%) was calculated with the help of the following equation:

$$\text{Cell viability (\%)} = \left(\frac{\text{OD of sample}}{\text{OD of control}} \right) \times 100$$

RNA extraction, cDNA synthesis and Quantitative Real Time-PCR analysis
5×10^5 SKBR3 cells/well were cultured and treated for 24 and 48 hours. RNA extraction was done by RNX-Plus® solution according to manufacturer's instructions. The high-quality RNA samples which were assessed by UV-vis spectrophotometer at 260 nm, were stored at -70 °C. Thereafter 1 µl of the random hexamer, 1 µl of oligo dT, 4 µl of RT buffer (5X), 0.5 µl of RT and 2 µl of dNTP mix were added to 1 µl of total RNA (5 ng). In order to synthesis complementary DNA (cDNA), the reaction was carried out in a Bio-Rad thermal cycler (Hercules, CA, USA) at 25 °C for 5 min, 42 °C for 60 min and 85 °C for 5 min. The QRT-PCR method was then conducted by using the SYBR Green Real-time PCR master mix (Ampliqon®, Odense, Denmark) with the total volume of 10 µL on the LightCycler® 96 System (Roche, Basel, Switzerland). The primers were designed by OLIGO 7 software (Table 1). The system was setup according to the following: denaturation (94 °C, 10 minutes), amplification (94 °C, 45 cycles of 10 seconds), annealing temperature (30 seconds) and extension (72 °C, 10 seconds). Melting curve analysis was used for gene-specific amplification. Determination of relative mRNA level was done through the $2^{-\Delta\Delta Ct}$ (Livak) method on the basis of relative expression of target mRNA to 18S rRNA mRNA level as the housekeeping gene.

Statistics
Statistical analysis was performed via GraphPad Prism 6.0. The results were evaluated by one-way ANOVA test and Tukey post-test as necessity. Probability values of less than 0.05 were considered significant. The results presented in text and tables represent mean± standard deviation (SD).

Table 1. Sequences of primers

Primer	Sequence (5'→ 3')	Gene accession number
18S rRNA	F: GATCAGATACCGTCGTAGTTCC	NR_146144.1
	R: CTGTCAATCCTGTCCGTGTC	
STAT3	F: AGTTTCTGGCCCCTTGGATTG	NM_139276.2
	R: CAGGAAGCGGCTATACTGCTG	
IL8	F: CGGAGCACTCCATAAGGCA	NM_000584.3
	R: TGGTCCACTCTCAATCACTC	
MMP2	F: GCCCTCCTGGGAATGAAGCAC	NM_001127891.2
	R: GCATTGCCTCTGGACAACACA	
MMP9	F: ATTCATCTTCCAAGGCCAATCC	NM_004994.2
	R: CTTGTCGCTGTCAAAGTTCG	
VEGF	F: TCACCAAGGCCAGCACATAG	NM_001025366.2
	R: GACAGCAGCGGGCACCAAC	

18S rRNA: 18S ribosomal ribonucleic acid, STAT3: Signal transducer and activator of transcription 3, IL8: Interleukin 8, MMP: Matrix metalloproteinase, VEGF: Vascular endothelial growth factor

Results and Discussion
Physicochemical characteristics of nanoparticles
The results of mean diameter size, zeta potential, and PDI are represented in Figure 1 and Table 2. The morphological property of the NPs containing DTX and siRNA, which was obtained through TEM, is shown in Figure 1. This represented the smooth and spherical shaped NPs. Figure 2-A indicated the electrophoresis of siRNA loaded NPs, which confirmed the complete entrapment of siRNA onto the NPs. The loading efficiency of siRNA loaded NPs and DTX loaded NPs was 90.7% and 88.3%, respectively. As results of characterizations of the NPs represented, all nano-drugs had a smooth spherical surface with a positive charge and the diameter less than 150 nm. According to other studies, the positive charge on NPs causes increased uptake and cytotoxicity in tumor cells.[16] On the other hand, the larger size of NPs (that is more than 200 nm) would lead to more degradation by phagocytes.[17] Moreover, as the positive charge increases, the possibility of nonspecific interactions with non-tumor cells increases too. Therefore, the importance of NP modification through specific APT utilization becomes more obvious. This consequently causes targeted delivery of drug to the specific site of action.[18] Results of our study determined that the size, zeta potential, and pharmacokinetic properties of nano-drugs were not affected by APT conjugation. These results are consistent with the findings of Sayari et al.[13] and Dhar et al.,[19] which affirm the advantage of the APT to antibodies that have high impacts on the size and zeta potential. Another advantage of the appropriate positive charge of chitosan NPs is its usefulness for more efficient loading of therapeutic oligonucleotides such as siRNA.[20] Furthermore, other investigations have reported that the molecular weight of chitosan plays a very important role on nanoparticles' size and loading

efficiency of siRNA.[21] On the basis of the study by Jadidi et al.,[22] the most appropriate molecular weight of chitosan with the highest loading efficiency of oligonucleotides, is approximately 50 KDa.

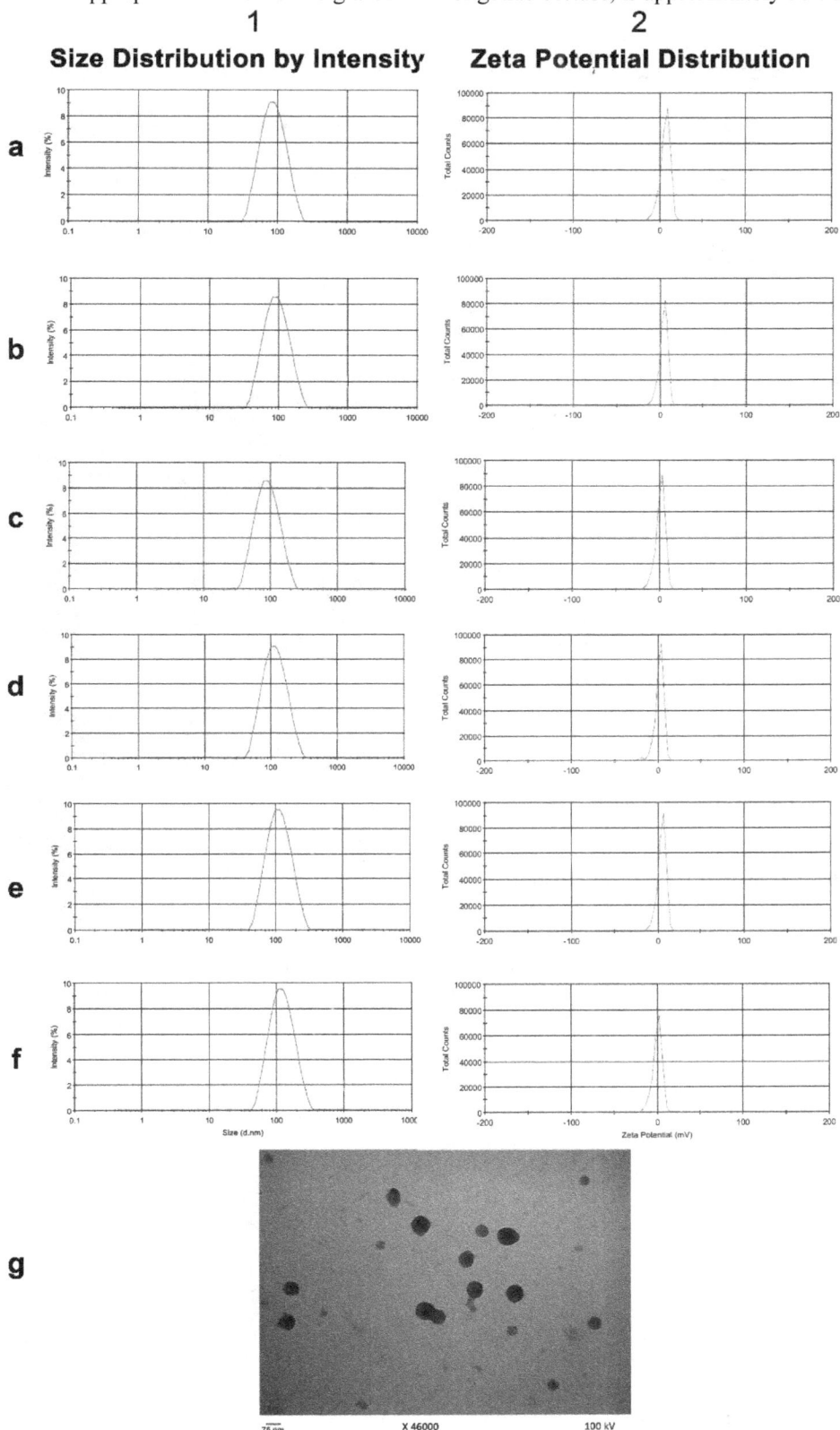

Figure 1. Particle size and Zeta potential distribution for (a) blank dCS, (b) dCS + APT, (c) dCS + siRNA, (d) dCS + APT + siRNA, (e) dCS + DTX+ siRNA and (f) dCS + APT + DTX + siRNA. g) Transition electron microscopy image of NPs. (dCS: depolymerized chitosan, APT: Aptamer, DTX: Docetaxel, NPs: Nanoparticles)

Table 2. Results of mean diameter size, zeta potential and polydispersity index (PDI)

Nano-drug	Characteristics		
	Mean diameter size (nm)	Zeta potential (mV)	PDI
Blank dCS	93.1±5.1	18.9±0.2	0.212
dCS+APT	98.7±4.5	12.9±0.5	0.238
dCS+siRNA	95.2±2.7	12.8±0.3	0.218
dCS+APT+siRNA	105.8±1.3	11.1±0.1	0.281
dCS+DTX+siRNA	102.3± 6.7	13.2± 0.3	0.227
dCS+APT+DTX+siRNA	110.5± 3.9	11.6± 0.8	0.292

dCS: depolymerized chitosan, DTX: docetaxel, APT: aptamer

Serum and heparin stability of siRNA loaded nanoparticles

As represented in Figure 2-B, releasing of siRNA from NPs was observed 12 h after incubation with FBS. Furthermore, the electrophoresis of siRNA-loaded NPs, which were incubated with different concentrations of heparin, represented the stable structure of NPs in this medium (Figure 2-C). Stability of the NPs in the *in vivo*-like environments, is one of the important factors which should be considered for drug delivery. Exposure of the NPs to the FBS and polyanions such as heparin is suitable for evaluation of stability of positively charged NPs in these negatively charged environments. In this regard, Jadidi et al.[22] stated that heparin had no impact on siRNA loaded chitosan NPs and the siRNA releasing started after 9 hours of exposure to serum solution and completed at the 48th hour. However, Raja et al.[23] reported that chitosan NPs, which were loaded with siRNA, were stable in serum environment up to 48 hours.

In vitro DTX and siRNA release

Figure 2-E indicated that siRNA was progressively released till 48 hours and the steady state phase started at the 60th hour. The pattern of DTX release in both mentioned pH indicated that the gradual releasing continued up to 60 hours and the steady state phase started at the 72nd hour. For the formulations in both pH, releasing of the encapsulated content of the NPs reached to 50% at the 36th hour. The pH 7.4 and 5.5 simulated the pH of normal and tumoric tissues, respectively. According to the study by Jadidi et al.,[22] releasing of the siRNA from chitosan-lactate NPs was gradually continued up to 72nd hour and then reached to the steady state phase.

Evaluations of mucin1 aptamer-conjugated nanoparticles

As represented in Figure 2-D, the agarose gel electrophoresis of intact APT was compared with the unpurified and purified conjugations of "NPs + APT". The obvious band shown with intact APT in comparison to other formulations confirmed the appropriate conjugation of APT to NPs. Results of Nanodrop® measurement represented that 92.3% of APT was conjugated to NPs. Conjugation of mucin1 APT to NPs was through activation of connection sites on NPs via EDC and NHS that caused these sites' interaction with

NH2 groups of the mucin1 APT. The agarose gel electrophoresis confirmed this conjugation. The mucin1 APT conjugated NPs created no distinct band on the agarose gel, neither before nor after purification. This finding showed that the activated NPs interacted with approximately all molecules of APT and no detectable free APT remained. Furthermore, utilization of mucin1 APT for targeted delivery increased the absorption of NPs to tumor cells. It seems that mucin1 APT plays an important role in uptake of the NPs by mucin1 expressing cells. However, the usage of mucin1 APT conjugated NPs on mucin1⁻ cells did not change the level of cellular uptake. The studies by Ghasemi et al.[24] and Sayari et al.[13] confirmed the results of our study.

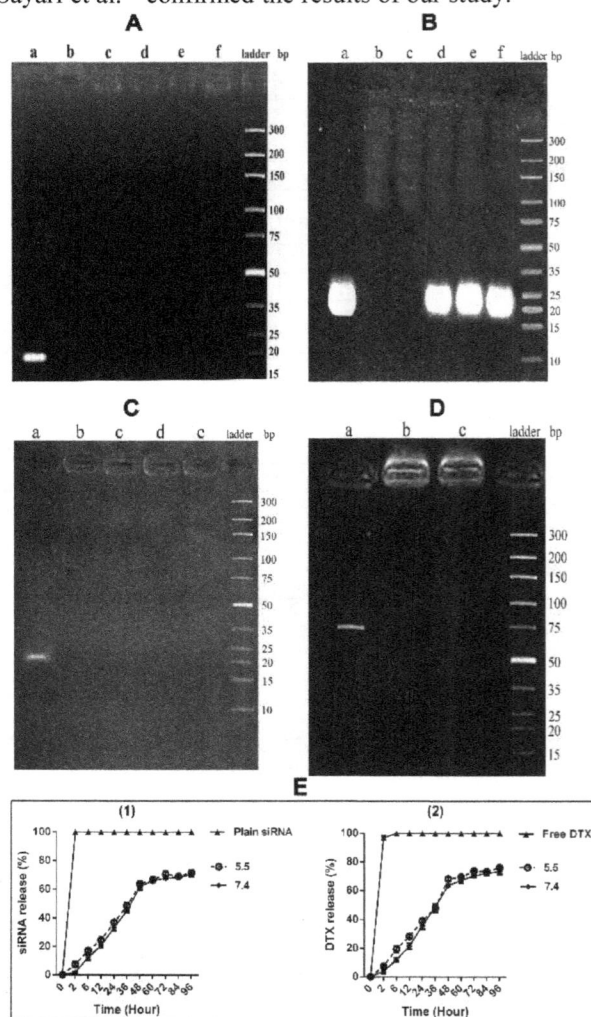

Figure 2. In vitro characterizations of nanodrugs. **A)** Electrophoresis of siRNA loaded NPs. a) Plain siRNA, b) NPs +siRNA (28.5 µg), c) NPs +siRNA (57 µg), d) NPs +siRNA (85.5 µg), e) Blank NPs, f) NPs+ APT+ siRNA (85.5 µg). **B)** FBS stability test. a) Plain siRNA, b) NPs +siRNA (2 h), c) (8 h), d) (12 h), e) (24 h), f) (48 h). **C)** Heparin stability test. a) Plain siRNA (57µg), b) NPs +siRNA, c) [NPs +siRNA] + 0.6 µl Heparin (2 µg/ml), d) [NPs +siRNA] + 1.5 µl Heparin, e) [NPs +siRNA] + 3 µl Heparin. **D)** Aptamer conjugation confirmation. a) Intact mucin1 APT, b) un-purified (NPs + APT), c) purified (NPs + APT). **E)** Drug release (%). a) siRNA release (%), b) DTX release (%) at PBS solutions with pH of 5.5 and 7.4; Equivalent free drugs (siRNA, DTX) were dispersed in PBS buffer as a control. (NPs: Nanoparticles, APT: Aptamer, DTX: Docetaxel)

Cellular uptake

The fluorescence intensity of GFP expression in cell was the qualitative indicator of cellular uptake of NPs. Figure 3 showed that the most fluorescence reaction occurred in SKBR3 cells that were treated with "NPs + GFP + APT" and the least was shown with CHO cells, treated by "NPs + GFP + APT". According to the study of Ghasemi et al.,[24] the significant uptake of the mucin1 APT conjugated NPs by HT-29 mucin1[+] cells was obvious in comparison to the non-targeted NPs. Actually, mucin1 APT acts like a linker between the NPs and the mucin1 expressing cells and facilitates cellular uptake of NPs.

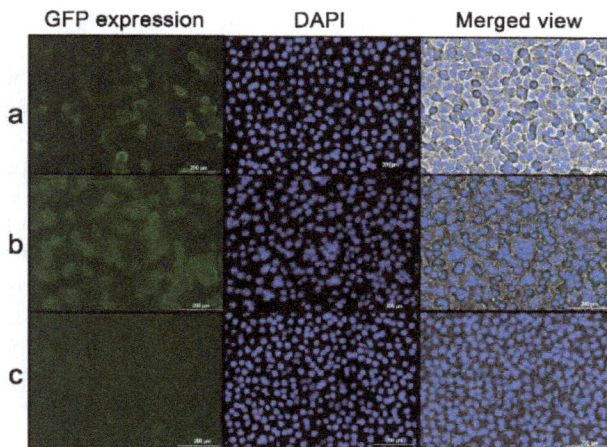

Figure 3. Cellular uptake evaluation. a) SKBR3 cells treated by NPs + GFP (1µg/µl); b) SKBR3 cells treated by NPs + GFP + APT and c) CHO cells treated by NPs + GFP + APT (GFP: Green Fluorescent Protein, NPs: Nanoparticles, APT: Aptamer)

Evaluation of cMET protein expression

For confirming cMET gene silencing via siRNA, western blotting assay was used. According to Figure 4, cMET protein was over expressed in untreated SKBR3 cells and its expression was silenced in the cells treated by "NPs + siRNA" for 48 h.

After cellular uptake of the NPs containing siRNA, the siRNA is released inside the cells. It targets the complementary mRNA in the cytoplasm and subsequently knock downs the targeted protein. Results of western blotting assay represented this knock downing of cMET protein after 48 h of treatment with siRNA-loaded NPs.

Cell viability assay

In order to investigate cell viability of SKBR3 cells in exposure to different treatment groups, MTT tetrazolium bioassay was done. As represented in Figure 5 (a and c), comparison of the treatment groups lacking mucin1 APT vs. control cells showed a significant decline in cell viability percentage in both 24 and 48 hours after treatment ($p \leq 0.0001$ for all mentioned comparisons; $p \leq 0.01$ for "NPs + siRNA" at 24 h). Also when comparing "NPs + siRNA" vs. "NPs + APT + siRNA" and "NPs + siRNA + DTX" vs. "NPs + APT + siRNA + DTX" at 24 h after treatment, the significant ($p \leq 0.0001$) difference was obvious which

showed the role of APT-conjugated NPs on cell viability (Figure 5-b). The significant ($p \leq 0.0001$) difference represented when comparing "NPs + APT + siRNA + DTX" vs. "NPs + siRNA + DTX" at 48 h (Figure 5-d). Several investigations have been done on nano-formulating of DTX and evaluation of its impact on cellular viability and toxicity in various cancerous cell lines.[7,25] According to our study, using of chitosan NPs for the delivery of DTX was safe since the intact NPs had no toxic effects on cell viability. Usage of the combination therapy system such as "DTX + siRNA" loaded NPs, as compared to monotherapy with "DTX"-loaded NPs, represented better results on inhibition of cell viability. Furthermore, providing the targeted therapy via APT resulted in improvement of the combination therapy. According to the results of cell viability after 48 h of treatments, when comparing "NPs + DTX" vs. "NPs + DTX + siRNA" and "NPs + APT + DTX" vs. "NPs + APT + DTX + siRNA", no significant difference was represented which showed that cMET siRNA did not have a significant effect on cell viability and also could not have a synergistic effect with DTX.

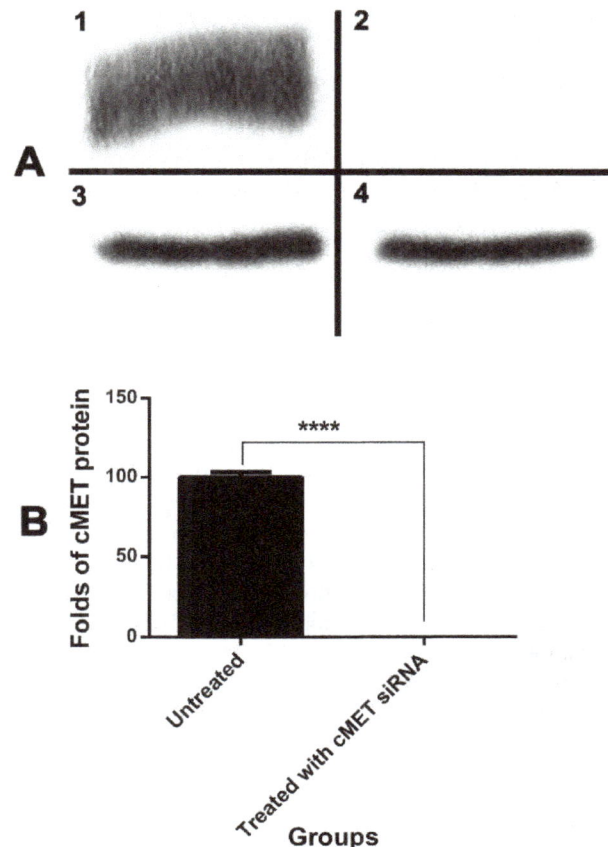

Figure 4. Protein expression assay. **A)** Western Blotting. 1) cMET protein expression in control SKBR3 cells; 2) cMET protein knock downing by siRNA in SKBR3 cells; 3) β-actin protein expression in control SKBR3 cells. 4) β-actin protein expression in SKBR3 cells treated with cMET siRNA. **B)** Quantification of cMET protein expression by ImageJ software; ****: $p \leq 0.0001$

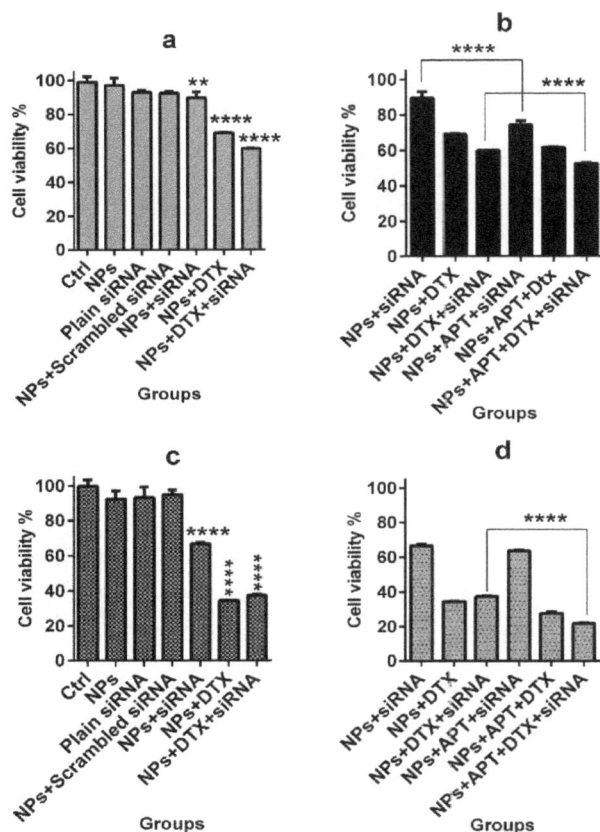

Figure 5. MTT assay. Control groups *vs.* groups lacking mucin1 APT (a: 24 h and c: 48 h); groups lacking mucin1 aptamer *vs.* groups containing mucin1 APT (b: 24 h and d: 48 h); **: *p*≤ 0.01, ****: *p*≤ 0.0001 (APT: Aptamer)

Gene expression assay

Quantitative Real Time-PCR was done to assess the effect of different treatment groups on the expression of five genes including IL8, STAT3, MMP2, MMP9, and VEGF. All data is normalized to the housekeeping gene (18S rRNA). Figure 6 shows the related results gene by gene in two time intervals of treatment (24 h and 48 h).

About IL8 gene, comparison of the "NPs+ siRNA" and "NPs+ DTX+ siRNA" groups with the control group showed significant reduction ($p \leq 0.0001$) of gene expression after 24 and 48 hours. However, "NPs+ DTX" group in compare to the control showed the significant reduction ($p \leq 0.0001$) at 48 h (Figure 6, a and c). When comparing "NPs+ APT+ siRNA" *vs.* "NPs+ siRNA" and also "NPs + APT + DTX + siRNA" *vs.* "NPs + DTX + siRNA" the significant reduction ($p \leq 0.0001$) in IL8 expression was obvious after 24 and 48 hours. The comparison of the "NPs+ APT+ DTX " group *vs.* "NPs + DTX" represented the significant reduction ($p \leq 0.0001$) of IL8 expression at 48 h (Figure 6, b and d).

About the STAT3 gene, the comparison of the "NPs + siRNA" and "NPs + siRNA + DTX" groups *vs.* control group represented significant reduction ($p \leq 0.0001$) of gene expression in both time intervals (Figure 6, e and g). Also, "NPs + DTX" *vs.* control significantly reduced gene expression at 24 h ($p \leq 0.01$) and 48 h ($p \leq 0.0001$). Comparison of the mucin1 APT containing groups with

the lacking ones in both 24 h and 48 h, represented significant reduction ($p \leq 0.0001$) of gene expression by "NPs + APT + siRNA" and "NPs + APT + DTX + siRNA" groups (Figure 6, f and h).

Gene expression patterns of MMP2 were as the following: all mucin1 APT lacking groups *vs.* control group (Figure 6, i and k) represented significant reduction ($p \leq 0.0001$) of gene expression after 24 and 48 hours. Also, all mucin1 APT containing groups *vs.* mucin1 APT lacking corresponding groups (Figure 6, j and l) represented significant reduction ($p \leq 0.0001$) of gene expression after 24 and 48 hours. However, comparison of the "NPs + APT + DTX + siRNA" group *vs.* "NPs + DTX + siRNA" group represented significant reduction ($p \leq 0.001$) of the gene expression after 48 h.

About MMP9, the comparison of all treatment groups *vs.* control group represented significant reduction ($p \leq 0.0001$) of gene expression at 24 and 48 hours (Figure 6, m and o). Furthermore, all mucin1 APT containing groups *vs.* mucin1 APT lacking corresponding groups (Figure 6, n and p) represented significant reduction ($p \leq 0.0001$) of gene expression after 24 and 48 hours. However, the "NPs + APT + siRNA" group *vs.* "NPs + siRNA" significantly decreased ($p \leq 0.001$) gene expression at 24 h.

About the VEGF gene, all mucin1 APT lacking groups *vs.* control group significantly decreased ($p \leq 0.0001$) gene expression at 24 and 48 hours (Figure 6, q and s). Also, "NPs + APT + siRNA" and "NPs + APT + DTX + siRNA" groups *vs.* APT lacking corresponding groups showed significant reduction ($p \leq 0.0001$) of gene expression at 24 and 48 hours. However, the "NP + APT+ DTX" group *vs.* "NP + DTX" represented the significant reduction ($p \leq 0.0001$) of gene expression after 48 h (Figure 6, r and t).

It has been proved that the cMET signaling is one of the most important pathways involving in tumorigenicity and metastasis of breast cancer cells[2] and the key factor in this process is STAT3.[26] The blocking of cMET expression caused the declining of STAT3 expression, although NPs loaded with DTX could somewhat be effective on decreasing the expression of STAT3 gene too. The dramatic declining of STAT3 gene expression occurred when combination therapy accompanied by targeted therapy. Similarly, regarding the other studied genes (MMP2, MMP9, VEGF, and IL8), targeted combination therapy as compared to passive combination therapy, had the highest impact on gene expression attenuation. Detailed comparisons represented that the combination therapy, either targeted or passive, had better effects on decreasing the gene expression of MMP2, MMP9 and VEGF vs. STAT3 and IL8. Moreover, gene expression of MMP9 was more affected by NPs loaded with DTX, while NPs loaded with cMET siRNA had more impacts on gene expression of IL8 and STAT3. Therefore, as each gene was especially affected by the different part of the combination therapy, it can be suggested that the application of both chemotherapeutic agent and siRNA may be beneficial for providing the maximum anti-cancerous effects.

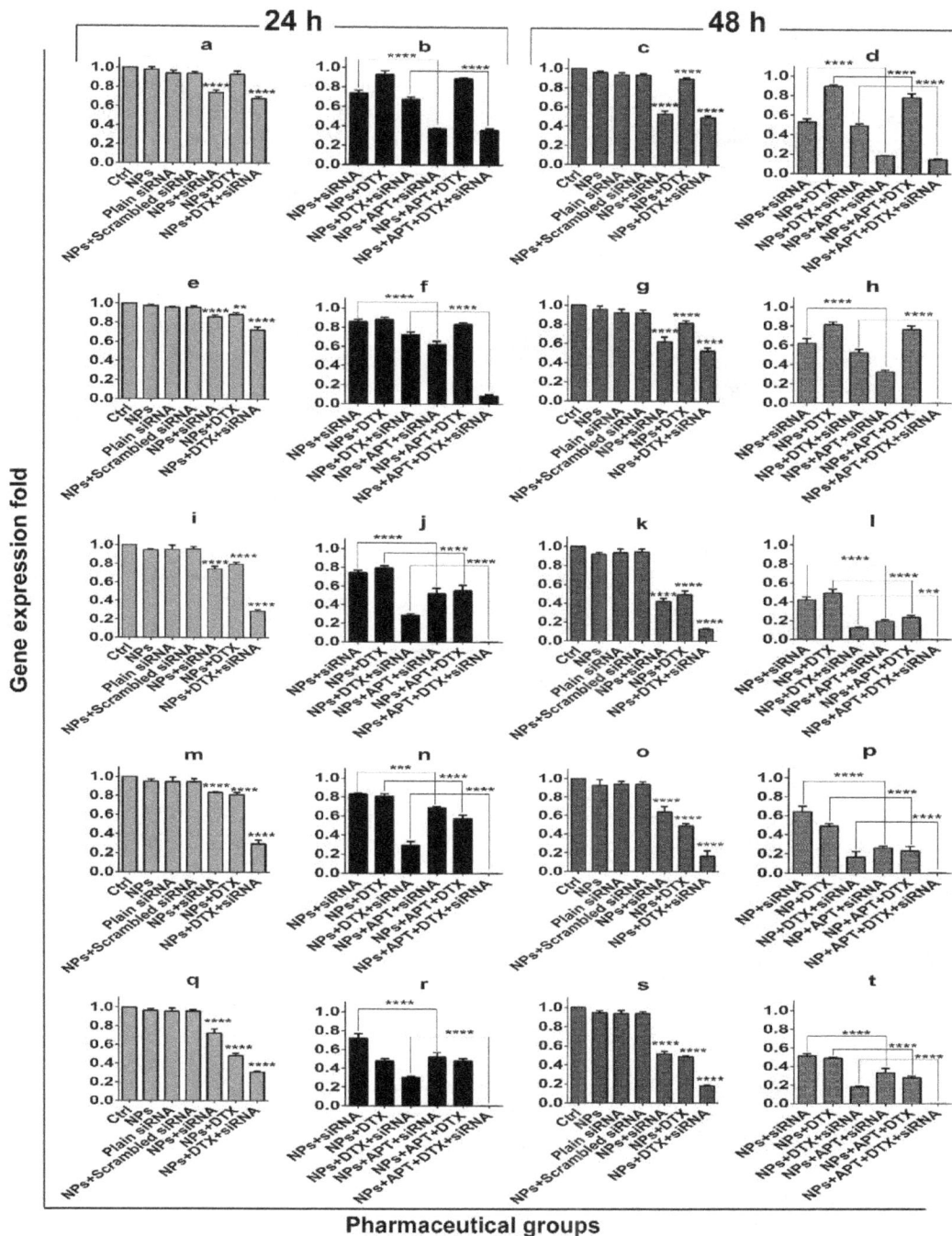

Figure 6. Gene expression folds at 24 h and 48 h for IL8 (a, b, c and d); STAT3 (e, f, g and h); MMP2 (I, j, k and l); MMP9 (m, n, o and p) and VEGF (q, r, s and t). **: $p \leq 0.01$, ***: $p \leq 0.001$ and ****: $p \leq 0.0001$.

Conclusion

Our study was focused on usage of targeted combination therapy involving chitosan NPs, mucin1 APT, the chemotherapeutic agent DTX, and cMET siRNA. This is suggested as an effective treatment of mucin1+ metastatic breast cancer on the cell line level. The advantage of this combination, which can lead to more investigations on animal models, is the targeted delivery of drugs. This may consequently cause dose reduction and fewer cell toxicities. Moreover, the dual effects of chemotherapy and gene therapy can be accompanied by application of this suggested delivery system.

Acknowledgments

This work was supported by the Drug Applied Research Center of Tabriz university of Medical Sciences [grant numbers 128/93].

Ethical Issues

This study was approved by ethics committee at Tabriz University of Medical Sciences. The ethical code is TBZMED.REC.1394.413.

Conflict of Interest

There is no conflict of interest to declare.

References

1. Al Zaid Siddiquee K, Turkson J. Stat3 as a target for inducing apoptosis in solid and hematological tumors. *Cell Res* 2008;18(2):254-67. doi: 10.1038/cr.2008.18
2. Sierra JR, Tsao MS. C-met as a potential therapeutic target and biomarker in cancer. *Ther Adv Med Oncol* 2011;3(1 Suppl):S21-35. doi: 10.1177/1758834011422557
3. Ho-Yen CM, Jones JL, Kermorgant S. The clinical and functional significance of c-met in breast cancer: A review. *Breast Cancer Res* 2015;17:52. doi: 10.1186/s13058-015-0547-6
4. Loibl S, Gianni L. Her2-positive breast cancer. *Lancet* 2017;389(10087):2415-29. doi: 10.1016/s0140-6736(16)32417-5
5. Ozpolat B, Sood AK, Lopez-Berestein G. Liposomal sirna nanocarriers for cancer therapy. *Adv Drug Deliv Rev* 2014;66:110-6. doi: 10.1016/j.addr.2013.12.008
6. Tavassolian F, Kamalinia G, Rouhani H, Amini M, Ostad SN, Khoshayand MR, et al. Targeted poly (l-gamma-glutamyl glutamine) nanoparticles of docetaxel against folate over-expressed breast cancer cells. *Int J Pharm* 2014;467(1-2):123-38. doi: 10.1016/j.ijpharm.2014.03.033
7. Hwang HY, Kim IS, Kwon IC, Kim YH. Tumor targetability and antitumor effect of docetaxel-loaded hydrophobically modified glycol chitosan nanoparticles. *J Control Release* 2008;128(1):23-31. doi: 10.1016/j.jconrel.2008.02.003
8. Zheng Y, Su C, Zhao L, Shi Y. Chitosan nanoparticle-mediated co-delivery of shatg-5 and gefitinib synergistically promoted the efficacy of chemotherapeutics through the modulation of autophagy. *J Nanobiotechnology* 2017;15(1):28. doi: 10.1186/s12951-017-0261-x
9. Esfandyari-Manesh M, Mohammadi A, Atyabi F, Nabavi SM, Ebrahimi SM, Shahmoradi E, et al. Specific targeting delivery to MUC1 overexpressing tumors by albumin-chitosan nanoparticles conjugated to DNA aptamer. *Int J Pharm* 2016;515(1-2):607-15. doi: 10.1016/j.ijpharm.2016.10.066
10. Ni X, Castanares M, Mukherjee A, Lupold SE. Nucleic acid aptamers: Clinical applications and promising new horizons. *Curr Med Chem* 2011;18(27):4206-14.
11. Moghaddam FA, Atyabi F, Dinarvand R. Preparation and in vitro evaluation of mucoadhesion and permeation enhancement of thiolated chitosan-phema core-shell nanoparticles. *Nanomedicine* 2009;5(2):208-15. doi: 10.1016/j.nano.2008.09.006
12. Akhlaghi SP, Saremi S, Ostad SN, Dinarvand R, Atyabi F. Discriminated effects of thiolated chitosan-coated pmma paclitaxel-loaded nanoparticles on different normal and cancer cell lines. *Nanomedicine* 2010;6(5):689-97. doi: 10.1016/j.nano.2010.01.011
13. Sayari E, Dinarvand M, Amini M, Azhdarzadeh M, Mollarazi E, Ghasemi Z, et al. MUC1 aptamer conjugated to chitosan nanoparticles, an efficient targeted carrier designed for anticancer SN38 delivery. *Int J Pharm* 2014;473(1-2):304-15. doi: 10.1016/j.ijpharm.2014.05.041
14. Koopaei MN, Dinarvand R, Amini M, Rabbani H, Emami S, Ostad SN, et al. Docetaxel immunonanocarriers as targeted delivery systems for her 2-positive tumor cells: Preparation, characterization, and cytotoxicity studies. *Int J Nanomedicine* 2011;6:1903-12. doi: 10.2147/ijn.s23211
15. Mirzaie ZH, Irani S, Mirfakhraie R, Atyabi SM, Dinarvand M, Dinarvand R, et al. Docetaxel-chitosan nanoparticles for breast cancer treatment: Cell viability and gene expression study. *Chem Biol Drug Des* 2016;88(6):850-8. doi: 10.1111/cbdd.12814
16. He C, Hu Y, Yin L, Tang C, Yin C. Effects of particle size and surface charge on cellular uptake and biodistribution of polymeric nanoparticles. *Biomaterials* 2010;31(13):3657-66. doi: 10.1016/j.biomaterials.2010.01.065
17. Smith DM, Simon JK, Baker JR, Jr. Applications of nanotechnology for immunology. *Nat Rev Immunol* 2013;13(8):592-605. doi: 10.1038/nri3488
18. Zhou J, Rossi JJ. Cell-specific aptamer-mediated targeted drug delivery. *Oligonucleotides* 2011;21(1):1-10. doi: 10.1089/oli.2010.0264
19. Dhar S, Gu FX, Langer R, Farokhzad OC, Lippard SJ. Targeted delivery of cisplatin to prostate cancer cells by aptamer functionalized pt(iv) prodrug-plga-peg nanoparticles. *Proc Natl Acad Sci U S A* 2008;105(45):17356-61. doi: 10.1073/pnas.0809154105
20. Mao S, Sun W, Kissel T. Chitosan-based formulations for delivery of DNA and siRNA. *Adv Drug Deliv Rev* 2010;62(1):12-27. doi: 10.1016/j.addr.2009.08.004
21. Katas H, Alpar HO. Development and characterisation of chitosan nanoparticles for sirna delivery. *J Control Release* 2006;115(2):216-25. doi: 10.1016/j.jconrel.2006.07.021
22. Jadidi-Niaragh F, Atyabi F, Rastegari A, Mollarazi E, Kiani M, Razavi A, et al. Downregulation of CD73 in 4T1 breast cancer cells through siRNA-loaded chitosan-lactate nanoparticles. *Tumour Biol* 2016;37(6):8403-12. doi: 10.1007/s13277-015-4732-0

23. Raja MA, Katas H, Jing Wen T. Stability, intracellular delivery, and release of sirna from chitosan nanoparticles using different cross-linkers. *PLoS One* 2015;10(6):e0128963. doi: 10.1371/journal.pone.0128963

24. Ghasemi Z, Dinarvand R, Mottaghitalab F, Esfandyari-Manesh M, Sayari E, Atyabi F. Aptamer decorated hyaluronan/chitosan nanoparticles for targeted delivery of 5-fluorouracil to muc1 overexpressing adenocarcinomas. *Carbohydr Polym* 2015;121:190-8. doi: 10.1016/j.carbpol.2014.12.025

25. Saremi S, Atyabi F, Akhlaghi SP, Ostad SN, Dinarvand R. Thiolated chitosan nanoparticles for enhancing oral absorption of docetaxel: Preparation, in vitro and ex vivo evaluation. *Int J Nanomedicine* 2011;6:119-28. doi: 10.2147/ijn.s15500

26. Lengyel E, Prechtel D, Resau JH, Gauger K, Welk A, Lindemann K, et al. C-Met overexpression in node-positive breast cancer identifies patients with poor clinical outcome independent of Her2/neu. *Int J Cancer* 2005;113(4):678-82. doi: 10.1002/ijc.20598

19

Changes of Insulin Resistance and Adipokines Following Supplementation with *Glycyrrhiza Glabra L.* Extract in Combination with a Low C-alorie Diet in Overweight and Obese Subjects: a Randomized Double Blind Clinical Trial

Mohammad Alizadeh[1], Nazli Namazi[1,2*], Elham Mirtaheri[1*], Nafiseh Sargheini[3], Sorayya Kheirouri[4]

[1] *Nutrition Research Center, Faculty of Nutrition, Tabriz University of Medical Sciences, Tabriz, Iran.*
[2] *Diabetes Research Center, Endocrinology and Metabolism Clinical Sciences Institute, Tehran University of Medical Sciences, Tehran, Iran.*
[3] *Molecular Biomedicine, University of Bonn, Bonn, Germany.*
[4] *Department of Nutrition, Tabriz University of Medical Sciences, Tabriz, Iran.*

Keywords:
· Calorie restricted diet
· Licorice
· Adipokine
· Insulin Resistance
· Obesity

Abstract

Purpose: Adipose tissue is a highly active endocrine organ which plays a key role in energy homeostasis. The aim of this study was to determine the effects of dried licorice extract along with a calorie restricted diet on body composition, insulin resistance and adipokines in overweight and obese subjects.

Methods: Sixty-four overweight and obese volunteers (27 men, 37 women) were recruited into this double-blind, placebo-controlled, randomized, clinical trial. Participants were randomly allocated to the Licorice (n=32) or the placebo group (n=32), and each group received a low-calorie diet with either 1.5 g/day of Licorice extract or placebo for 8 weeks. Biochemical parameters, anthropometric indices, body composition and dietary intake were measured at baseline and at the end of the study.

Results: A total of 58 subjects completed the trial. No side effects were observed following licorice supplementation. At the end of the study, waist circumference, fat mass, serum levels of vaspin, zinc-α2 glycoprotein, insulin and HOMA-IR were significantly decreased in the intervention group, but only the reduction in serum vaspin levels in the licorice group was significant when compared to the placebo group (p<0.01).

Conclusion: Supplementation with dried licorice extract plus a low-calorie diet can increase vaspin levels in obese subjects. However, the anti-obesity effects of the intervention were not stronger than a low-calorie diet alone in the management of obesity.

Introduction

Adipose tissue is a highly active endocrine organ, which plays a key role in energy homeostasis, response to hormonal signals, metabolic regulation and adipokine secretion.[1] Current evidence suggests that adipose tissue secrets more than 50 signaling molecules and hormones, called adipokines.[1,2] Adipokines are involved in the regulation of thermogenesis, appetite, glucose metabolism, insulin sensitivity and other endocrine functions.[3] One adipokine is vaspin, a visceral adipose tissue-derived hormone which can be considered to be a new link between obesity and metabolic complications such as insulin resistance, type 2 diabetes and atherosclerosis.[4] Several studies have indicated an association between vaspin and body mass index (BMI); but the findings are contradictory. [5]

Zinc-alpha 2 glycoprotein (ZAG-2) is another adipokine which plays a main role in the mobilization and utilization of lipids.[5] It also can control fat mass (FM) and energy expenditure, induce lipolysis and act as a hormone-regulating lipid in glucose metabolism.[6] Some studies found an inverse relationship between ZAG, body mass index (BMI) and waist circumference (WC). It has also been suggested that ZAG may simulate adiponectin to protect against inflammation and the complications of obesity.[7]

Prior studies have indicated that some medicinal herbs, such as *Nigella sativa,*[8] green tea[9] and *Glycyrrhiza glabra*[10,11] are involved in the regulation of hormones and weight. *Glycyrrhiza glabra L.* (Fabaceae family), generally known as Mulaithi or Licorice, is a medicinal herb which is widely grown in the Mediterranean region and Southwest Asia. It contains various components with pharmacological properties, including glycyrrhizin, glabridin, flavonoids, beta-Glycyhrritinic acid, chalcones, isoflavones and triterpenoid saponins.[12,13] Licorice root is frequently used in traditional medicine, particularly for gastric and duodenal ulcers, dyspepsia and allergenic reactions. Human and animal models have not demonstrated any toxic or serious side effects of licorice consumption.[14]

It has been suggested that licorice root can alter body composition[10,11,15] and reduce insulin resistance.[16-18] However, there are limited clinical trials with contradictory results on the effects of licorice on obesity.[10,15,19] To the best of our knowledge, no clinical trials have evaluated the effects of licorice supplement with a low-calorie diet on the management of obesity and hormonal regulation. Accordingly, the primary aim of this study was to determine the effects of dried licorice extract together with a calorie restricted diet on anthropometric indices, body composition, insulin resistance and adipokines in overweight and obese subjects. The secondary aim was to evaluate the effects of licorice along with a low calorie diet on blood pressure and liver enzymes.

Material and Methods

Participants

In this double-blind randomized placebo-controlled clinical trial, 64 overweight and obese volunteers (27 men, 37 women) were recruited. Subjects were chosen by advertisement and dietitian referral from March to September 2012 at Tabriz University of Medical Sciences. A total of 64 subjects were enrolled based on FM variable in a previous study,[10] with α-value of 0.05, power of 90% and considering a 20% loss to follow up. Inclusion criteria were as follows: age 30-60 yrs old and BMI>25 kg/m.[2] The following were used as exclusion criteria cardiovascular disease, liver, thyroid and kidney disorders, diabetes, smoking, pregnancy or lactation of having taken any anti-obesity, vitamin and mineral supplements or herbal drugs in the 3 months prior to the study. Subjects who consumed any medications for hypertension or had Systolic Blood Pressure (SBP) $\geq$140 mmHg and Diastolic Blood Pressure (DBP) $\geq$ 90 mmHg were also excluded.

At the beginning of the trial, general characteristics including age, medication history and any family history of obesity were collected using a questionnaire.

Study Design and Intervention

Eligible participants were randomly allocated to the licorice (n=32) or placebo groups (n=32). Randomization was facilitated by random number table with a permuted block size of two. The participants were stratified for sex, age and BMI. All of the participants received a low-calorie diet; created by an expert dietitian who designed individualized diets with a 500 kcal deficit from the participates' energy requirements. The calories provided by the diets consisted of 55% carbohydrate, 15% protein and 30%. The intervention and placebo groups took 0.5 g/day (3 times a day 30 min before each meal) of dried licorice extract and placebo (corn starch), respectively for 8 consecutive weeks. To maintain blinding, a subject with no clinical involvement in the study performed the allocation. The patients and investigators remained blinded to the treatment assignment until data analysis.

Visits occurred every 20 days and supplements were distributed among the volunteers based on the allocation code after the randomization. Participants received a phone call every week to minimize withdrawal and ensure their adherence to the study protocol. The subjects were asked to maintain their usual physical activity level during the trial.

Licorice extract characteristics

The dried hydroalcoholic extract of licorice root (ethanol 70: water 30% v/v) was prepared by the Darook pharmacological company (Esfahan-Iran). It contained lowered Glycyrrhizin (<0.01%).

Measurements

Anthropometric indices, body composition, dietary intake, physical activity, blood pressure and biochemical parameters were measured at baseline and at the end of the study. Weight, height and WC were measured using standard methods. Assessment of dietary intake and physical activity levels were measured as explained in our previous study.[12]

Body composition measurements

BMI was calculated by dividing the weight in kilograms to the square of the height in meters. Body composition was measured using TANITA Bioelectrical Impedance Analysis (BC-418 MA, 50 kHz) after 12-14 hours fasting. We measured the amounts of FM and fat free mass (FFM) with an accuracy of $\pm$0.1 kg. Previous studies reported a significant correlation between TANITA and Dual Energy X-Ray absorptiometry (DEXA) test for the measurement of body composition.

Biochemical measurements

At the baseline and at the end of the trial, 10 mL of venous blood was collected after 12-14h fasting. The serum was separated from whole blood by centrifugation at 2500 rpm for 10 min. Serum levels of Fasting blood sugar (FBS) was measured on the day of sampling using Auto analyzer (Abbot Model Aclyon 300 USA) by commercially enzymatic kit (Pars Azmoon, Iran). The remaining serum samples were kept at -20 °C until measurement. Enzyme-linked immunosorbent assay (ELISA) method was used to determine insulin (Pars Azmoon, Iran), vaspin (Orgenium, Fenland) and ZAG-alpha 2 (Orgenium, Fenland) concentrations. Based on FBS and insulin levels, insulin resistance was evaluated using the homeostasis model assessment-insulin resistance (HOMA-IR) formula as follows:

HOMA-IR = fasting glucose (mg/dL) $\times$fasting insulin (μU/mL) /405[20]

Blood pressure measurement

Blood pressure was measured after 10 minutes rest in seated and relaxed position using a Microlife AG-30 mercury sphygmomanometer on the left arm. It was repeated after 5 min and the average of the two measurements was reported.

Statistical analysis

Data were analyzed using SPSS software version 13.0 (SPSS Inc., Chicago, IL, USA). The normality of the data distribution was evaluated by the one-sample Kolmogorov-Smirnov test. The results were expressed as mean±SD for variables with normal distribution, median (25th, 75th percentiles) for variables with non-normal distribution, and percentage (%) for qualitative variables. The Chi square test was used for the comparison of qualitative variables. Independent *t* tests (for baseline measurements) and analysis of covariance (ANCOVA) were used to compare quantitative variables between groups, controlling for confounding factors. The Mann-Whitney U test was used for comparison variables with non-normal distribution between two groups. Pair t-test was also used for within- group comparison. $p < 0.05$ was considered statistically significant.

Results

As presented in Figure 1, of the 64 participants, 58 subjects completed the study (intervention group, n=29; placebo group, n=29). The power of the study at the end of the study was 85%. Participants did not report any serious side effects for taking licorice supplement, except one who reported gastrointestinal problems and discontinued the study.

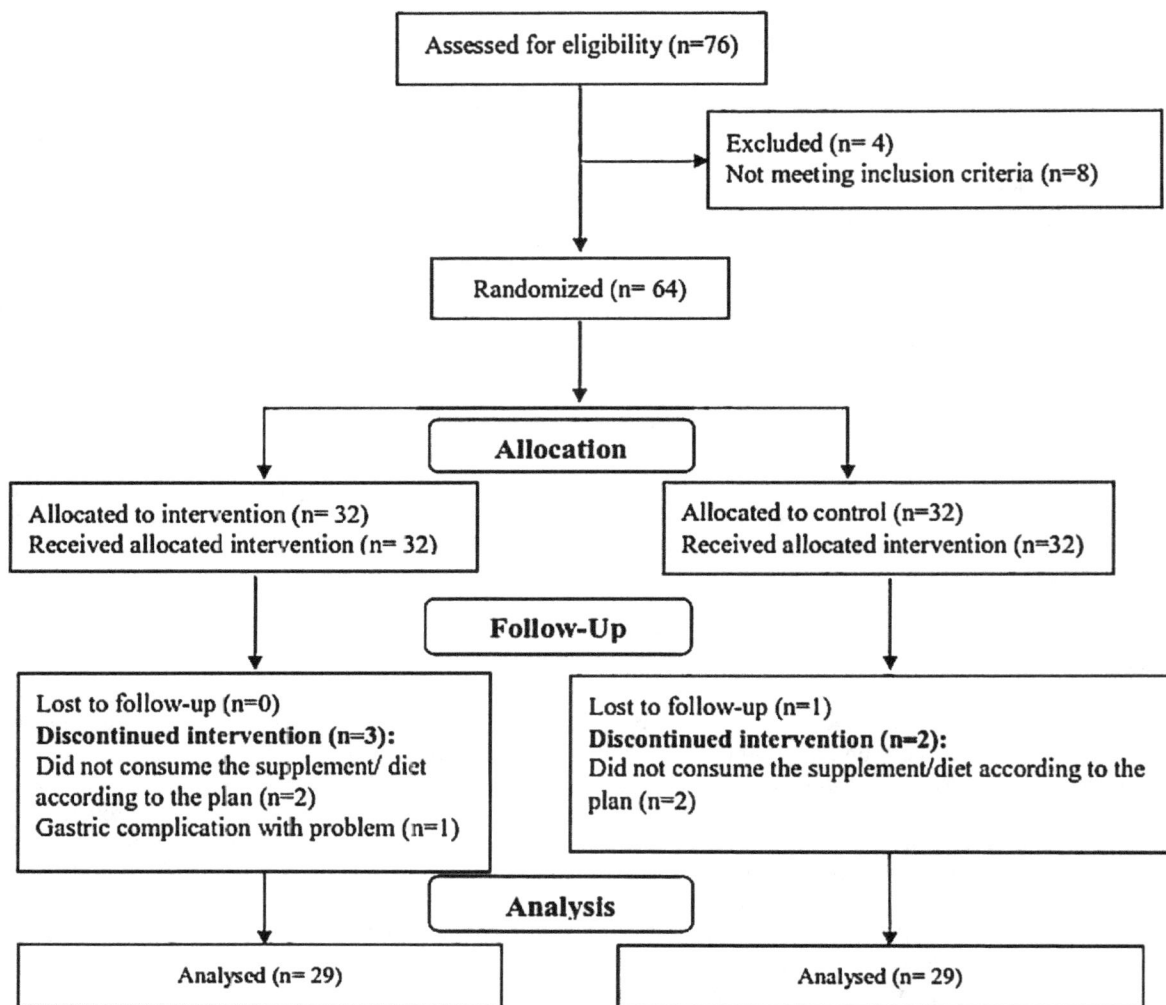

Figure 1. Flowchart of the study

There were no significant differences between the two study groups (except in height) at the baseline (Table 1). Table 3 shows anthropometric indices and body composition at baseline and at the end of the study. No significant differences were observed in the licorice and placebo groups at the start of the study. In the licorice group, a slight reduction (-2.3%) was observed in BMI at the end of the trial, but it was not significant within or between the groups (ANCOVA; adjusted for height and baseline value). FM decreased significantly at the end of the study in both groups when compared to the baseline (-7.2 vs. -6.5%; $p < 0.01$). However, a comparison of licorice and placebo groups did not indicate any significant reduction in FM after the intervention (p=0.6). In both the licorice and placebo groups, FFM slightly increased (0.3%; p=0.8) and significantly decreased (-1.3%; $p < 0.01$), respectively, but inter group comparisons did not show any significant differences in FFM at the end of the trial (p=0.7).

Table 1. Baseline characteristics of the study participants

-	Variables	Licorice group (n=29)	Placebo group (n=29)
-	Age (year)	36.0 ± 11.9*	33.6 ± 4.8
Sex (n(%))	Male	13 (44.8)	14 (48.2)
	Female	16 (55.2)	15 (51.8)
-	Weight(kg)	87.6 ± 15.5	81.9 ± 11.0
	Height(cm)	161.9 ± 8.3	158.4 ± 5.8
Physical activity (n(%))	Sedentary	18 (62.0)	16 (55.1)
	Moderate	11 (38.0)	13 (44.9)

* Mean± SD

No adverse effects were observed on blood pressure (Table 2) and biochemical tests (Table 3) (p>0.05 for all variables). In this present study, the licorice supplement contained less than 0.01% Glycyrrhizin, so no significant changes were observed in SBP and DBP after 8 weeks of the intervention.

Biochemical parameters are presented in Table 3. At baseline there were no significant differences between the two study groups in biochemical parameters, except in fasting blood sugar (FBS) levels. Serum levels of FBS was not affected by the intervention (p=0.8). However, comparison between the two groups indicated that, insulin concentrations and HOMA-IR decreased in both the groups after 8 weeks of the intervention, and that significant reductions in insulin and insulin resistance were only observed in the licorice group when compared to baseline (ANCOVA, adjusted for changes in weight, energy intake changes, and baseline values). Further, no significant reduction of the two factors were observed between the two groups (p<0.05 for both variables). Furthermore, levels of fat-derived hormones (vaspin and ZAG) also changed significantly following the licorice supplementation plus weight-loss diet when compared to baseline (-27.8 and 32.2%, respectively). Comparison of the licorice and placebo groups indicated that only the changes in serum levels of vaspin was significant at the end of the study (-27.8 vs. -4.2%, respectively).

Table 2. Comparison of anthropometric indices and body composition between Licorice and placebo groups at baseline and at the end of the trial

-	Variable	Licorice group (n=29)	Placebo group (n=29)	P-value** (Between groups)
BMI (Kg/m²)	Baseline	33.6±4.8*	32.7±3.7	0.4†
	End	32.8±4.8	32.3±3.5	0.2‡‡
	Pre to post P-value‡	0.3	0.6	
Waist circumference (cm)	Baseline	106.9±13.4	108.9±10.4	0.5†
	End	101.3±10.9	102.4±10.1	0.7
	Pre to post P-value‡	<0.01	<0.01	-
FM (Kg)	Baseline	31.7±8.3	30.6±6.7	0.5†
	End	29.4±10.6	28.6±6.3	0.6
	Pre to post P-value‡	<0.01	<0.01	-
FFM (Kg)	Baseline	55.9±10.7	51.3±8.0	0.04†
	End	56.1±12.0	50.6±5.1	0.7
	Pre to post P-value‡	0.8	<0.01	-
SBP (mmHg)	Baseline	110.2±10.1	110.5±10.5	0.4†
	End	109.0±10.0	110.0±10.4	0.8
	Pre to post P-value‡	0.2	0.2	-
DBP (mmHg)	Baseline	70.3±7.0	70.3±8.0	0.9†
	End	70.1±9.0	70.2±10.0	0.4
	Pre to post P-value‡	0.2	0.8	-

FM: Fat Mass; FFM: Fat Free Mass; SBP: Systolic Blood Pressure; DBP: Diastolic Blood Pressure
* Mean± SD
** ANCOVA (adjusted for energy intake changes and baseline values)
† Independent t-test
‡ Paired t-test
‡‡ ANCOVA (adjusted for height and baseline values)

Discussion

The present study highlights that licorice extract supplementation concurrently with a low-calorie diet, sufficiently attenuates serum levels of vaspin hormone in overweight and obese subjects with no significant side effects. The findings also revealed that a low-calorie while taking licorice supplementation was no more efficacious than a low-calorie diet alone on the management of obesity.

Table 3. Comparison of biochemical parameters between Licorice group and placebo group at baseline and at the end of trial

-	Variable	Licorice group (n=29)	Placebo group (n=29)	P-value (Between groups)**
FBS (mg/dL)	Baseline	98.5± 7.8*	93.2 ± 7.1	0.02†
	End	97.5 ± 7.3	93.5± 6.5	0.8
	Pre to post P-value‡	0.4	0.7	-
Vaspin (ng/mL)	Baseline	24.4±9.3	21.1±4.9	0.13†
	End	17.6±3.7	20.2±5.4	<0.01
	Pre to post P-value‡	0.01	0.1	-
ZAG (µg/mL)	Baseline	86.1±40.0	92.3±34.8	-
	End	113.9±57.5	101.3±40.2	0.5†
	Pre to post P-value‡	<0.01	0.4	0.4
Insulin (µU/mL)	Baseline	9.5 (5.3, 12.2)	9.5 (7.2, 13.5)	0.7†
	End	7.1 (5.0, 8.5)	9.2 (4.7, 11.0)	0.2
	Pre to post P-value‡	0.02	0.1	-
HOMA-IR	Baseline	2.3 (1.3, 3.0)	2.2 (1.3, 3.0)	0.8‡‡
	End	1.5 (1.2, 2.0)	2.0 (1.1, 2.5)	0.3
	Pre to post P-value‡	<0.01	0.4	-
AST (U/L)	Baseline	16.6±3.9	17.8±4.0	0.09†
	End	16.0±2.4	17.0±5.3	0.07
	Pre to post P-value‡	0.4	0.7	-
ALT (U/L)	Baseline	15.5±2.7	16.6±7.8	0.2†
	End	15.0±6.4	16.0±7.5	0.3
	Pre to post P-value‡	0.7	0.9	-

FBS: Fasting blood sugar; ZAG: Zinc alpha2 glyco protein; AST: Aspartate transaminase; ALT:Alanine aminotransferase
* Mean± SD
** ANCOVA (adjusted for weight changes, energy intake changes and baseline values)
† Independent t-test for variables with normal distribution and Mann-Whitney U test for variables with non-normal distribution
‡ Paired t-test
‡‡ ANCOVA (adjusted for FBS at baseline)

There are limited clinical trials with contradictory findings on the effects of licorice supplementation on anthropometric indices and body composition. Our findings were in accordance with two studies; Bell et al. reported that Glavonoid™ (Licorice Flavenoid Oil (LFO)) did not reduce body weight, FM and WC in overweight and grade I-II obese subjects after 8 weeks.[19] Moreover, Hajiaghamohammadi et al. reported that 2 g/day aqueous licorice extract did not reduce BMI in patients with non-alcoholic fatty liver disease after 8 weeks.[21] Our results were in opposition to Tominaga et al.'s study; who found that 300 and 1800 mg/day supplementation with Kaneka Glavonoid rich oil ™ (LFO) suppressed weight gain in overweight subjects with unhealthy lifestyle after 12 weeks. However, weight and BMI was increased at the end of the study in the placebo group. In addition, supplementation with 900 mg/day LFO decreased visceral fat in overweight subjects. They suggested that the reduction in FM was helpful in weight maintenance.[10] In another study in the U.S population, Tominaga et al. indicated that 300 mg/day LFO decreased WC and visceral fat after 12 weeks.[22]

Based on Armanina et al's., study, 3.5 g/day Licorice supplement decreased FM with no changes in BMI in normal weight subjects after 8 weeks.[15] Aoki et al. also indicated that adding 1 and 2% LFO to diet of obese mice for 8 weeks significantly slowed down weight gain and decreased abdominal white adipose tissue.[11] Differences in results of these studies may be due to differences in energy intake, physical activity level, dose and type of licorice (extract, oil), the duration of the intervention, BMI range and ethnic group. In our study, we compared the efficacy of licorice supplement concurrent with a calorie-restricted diet vs. a calorie-restricted diet alone. Based on evidence, differences between two groups were not significant at the end of the trial. It seems that licorice plus a weight loss diet prevents a reduction in FFM. However, they were not significant between the two intervention groups.

In this study, licorice extract with a calorie-restricted diet did not decrease serum levels of FBS, insulin concentrations, ZAG and HOMA-IR; but the intervention decreased serum levels of vaspin after 8 weeks. Limited clinical trials have evaluated the effects of licorice on glycemic status. In line with our study, Tominaga et al. found that 1800 mg/day LFO did not change FBS and insulin concentrations in overweight subjects after 12 weeks.[10] However, Luan et al. indicated that 10 µMg of glabridin, a main component of licorice, decreased insulin levels and insulin resistance in women with polycystic ovary syndrome after 12 months.[16] Zhao et al. demonstrated that 300 mg/day of licorice flavonoid decreased FBS and insulin levels in type 2 diabetic rats after 5 weeks,[17] and on Wu et al.'s study demonstrated that 40 mg/kg/day glabridin decreased FBS and insulin resistance in diabetic mice after 28 days.[18]

In our study, as no significant changes were observed in serum levels of FBS and insulin, insulin resistance did not change following the supplementation with Licorice extract. Reduction in body weight and fat mass are two main factors involve in improving insulin resistance in overweight and obese subjects. However, Licorice extract did not reduce these two anthropometric indices considerably. Therefore, no changes in insulin resistance might be due to this issue. In the current trial, we used the index of HOMA-IR to examine insulin resistance. There are several indices to assess this parameter.[23] Using different indices based on their different components can affect the results. Moreover, observing no changes in insulin resistance can be partially explained by the type of supplement. The aforementioned studies have examined licorice flavonoid, while our study assessed whole licorice extract. Different dosages, types of supplement, amounts of flavonoid, changes in weight, BMI at baseline, duration of the intervention, and methods for insulin resistant estimation are possible factors that can lead to different findings.

In our study, due to mineralcorticoid actions and vasopresser effects of Glycyrrhizin,[24,25] Glycyrrihizinhas been reduced to <0.01%. This could be attributed to the observation that the supplementation did not lead to any significant reduction in FBS and insulin concentrations. Furthermore, patient medical history, baseline BMI, dosages and form of licorice or its pure component and the duration of intervention can affect the final findings of each study.

To the best of our knowledge, our study was the first to evaluate the effects of supplementation with licorice extract on vaspin and ZAG hormone levels. Vaspin is an adipokine with insulin- sensitizing effects, and may be involved in obesity-associated diseases including type 2 diabetes, insulin resistance, atherosclerosis and cardiovascular disease. Therefore, it may be a possible target in the pharmaco-therapeutic treatment of obesity and its complications.[5,26] Handisurya et al. reported that

weight loss following gastric bypass decreased BMI and vaspin hormones in morbidly obese subjects after 12 months. They declared that visceral adipose tissue was the predominant localization for vaspin gene expression, and vaspin secretion decreased due to significant reductions in BMI after gastric bypass.[27] Based on Chung et al,. study lifestyle modification with orlistat decreased BMI and vaspin levels after 12 weeks. They hypothesized that weight loss (BMI reduction $\geq$ 2%) leads to a reduction in vaspin levels.[28] In this study, it seems that a larger reduction in BMI (-2.3%) in the licorice group compared to the placebo group might have resulted in a reduction in vaspin levels. However, due to the absence of adequate studies on the effects of licorice on vaspin levels, the underlying mechanisms are not clear. The results of our study contradict those of Koiuo et al. regarding changes in vaspin. They found that a calorie-restricted diet with orlistat or sibutramine decreased weight with no changes in vaspin concentrations after 6 months.[29] This discrepancy could be due to differences in the type of intervention, study duration and the rate of weight and BMI reduction.

Zinc-alpha 2 glycoprotein is an adipokine secreted from white and brown adipose tissues. Some studies have reported its possible effects on obesity and metabolic syndrome.[5,6] The expression of ZAG is regulated by TNF-alpha and PPAR-γ; thus, it may participate in lipid metabolism, enhance energy expenditure and skeletal muscle glucose transporters, inhibit of enzymes in lipogenesis pathways and stimulate adiponectin hormone expression.[30] In this study, there were no significant differences between the two groups. It seems that a greater reduction in weight or FM is needed to change levels of ZAG.

The main side effects of licorice are hypertension and hypokalemic-induced secondary disorders.[31] Glycyrrhizin plays a key role in occurring these side effects.[31] Therefore, in the present study we used a kind of licorice extract with reduced glycyrrhizin. Accordingly, except one who reported stomachache no side effects were reported.

This had some limitations. Firstly, the effects of licorice supplementation without calorie restricted diet were not evaluated. Secondly, the duration of the intervention was short and thirdly gene expressions of hormones were not measured. For future studies, we suggest that higher dosages and different forms (oil, pure components of licorice such as glabridin and flavonoids) of licorice extract are evaluated for their effect on the management of obesity.

Conclusion

We conclude that supplementation with dried licorice extract plus a low-calorie diet can increase vaspin levels in obese subjects, with no changes in insulin resistance and body composition. Overall, the effects of the intervention was not stronger than a low-calorie diet alone in the management of obesity.

Acknowledgments
We are grateful to the participants for their cooperation. The authors also would like to thank the Nutrition Research Center, Tabriz University of Medical Sciences for funding the project.

Ethical Issues
The trial was approved by the Ethics Committee of Tabriz University of Medical Sciences and written informed consent was obtained from each patient. The trial was registered on the Iranian registry of clinical trials (www.irct.ir/, IRCT2013062811288N3).

Conflicts of Interest
Authors declare no conflicts of interest

References
1. Galic S, Oakhill JS, Steinberg GR. Adipose tissue as an endocrine organ. *Mol Cell Endocrinol* 2010;316(2):129-39. doi: 10.1016/j.mce.2009.08.018
2. Bluher M. Adipose tissue dysfunction in obesity. *Exp Clin Endocrinol Diabetes* 2009;117(6):241-50. doi: 10.1055/s-0029-1192044
3. Poulos SP, Hausman DB, Hausman GJ. The development and endocrine functions of adipose tissue. *Mol Cell Endocrinol* 2010;323(1):20-34. doi: 10.1016/j.mce.2009.12.011
4. Auguet T, Quintero Y, Riesco D, Morancho B, Terra X, Crescenti A, et al. New adipokines vaspin and omentin. Circulating levels and gene expression in adipose tissue from morbidly obese women. *BMC Med Genet* 2011;12:60. doi: 10.1186/1471-2350-12-60
5. Bluher M. Vaspin in obesity and diabetes: Pathophysiological and clinical significance. *Endocrine* 2012;41(2):176-82. doi: 10.1007/s12020-011-9572-0
6. Gong FY, Zhang SJ, Deng JY, Zhu HJ, Pan H, Li NS, et al. Zinc-alpha2-glycoprotein is involved in regulation of body weight through inhibition of lipogenic enzymes in adipose tissue. *Int J Obes (Lond)* 2009;33(9):1023-30. doi: 10.1038/ijo.2009.141
7. Cabassi A, Tedeschi S. Zinc-alpha2-glycoprotein as a marker of fat catabolism in humans. *Curr Opin Clin Nutr Metab Care* 2013;16(3):267-71. doi: 10.1097/MCO.0b013e32835f816c
8. Mahdavi R, Alizadeh M, Namazi N, Farajnia S. Changes of body composition and circulating adipokines in response to nigella sativa oil with a calorie restricted diet in obese women. *J Herb Med* 2016; 6 (2):67-72.DOI: 10.1016/j.hermed.2016.03.003
9. Chan CC, Koo MW, Ng EH, Tang OS, Yeung WS, Ho PC. Effects of chinese green tea on weight, and hormonal and biochemical profiles in obese patients with polycystic ovary syndrome--a randomized placebo-controlled trial. *J Soc Gynecol Investig* 2006;13(1):63-8. doi: 10.1016/j.jsgi.2005.10.006
10. Tominaga Y, Mae T, Kitano M, Sakamoto Y, Ikematsu H, Nakagawa K. Licorice flavonoid oil effects body weight loss by reduction of body fat mass in overweight subjects. *J Health Sci* 2006;52(6):672-83. doi: 10.1248/jhs.52.672
11. Aoki F, Honda S, Kishida H, Kitano M, Arai N, Tanaka H, et al. Suppression by licorice flavonoids of abdominal fat accumulation and body weight gain in high-fat diet-induced obese c57bl/6j mice. *Biosci Biotechnol Biochem* 2007;71(1):206-14.
12. Mirtaheri E, Namazi N, Alizadeh M, Sargheini N, Karimi S. Effects of dried licorice extract with low-calorie diet on lipid profile and atherogenic indices in overweight and obese subjects: A randomized controlled clinical trial. *Eur J Integr Med* 2015;7(3):287-93. doi: 10.1016/j.eujim.2015.03.006
13. Ahn J, Lee H, Jang J, Kim S, Ha T. Anti-obesity effects of glabridin-rich supercritical carbon dioxide extract of licorice in high-fat-fed obese mice. *Food Chem Toxicol* 2013;51:439-45. doi: 10.1016/j.fct.2012.08.048
14. Parvaiz M, Hussain K, Khalid S, Hussnain N, Iram N, Hussain Z, et al. A review: Medicinal importance of glycyrrhiza glabra L.(fabaceae family). *Global J Pharmacol* 2014;8(1):8-13. doi: 10.5829/idosi.gjp.2014.8.1.81179
15. Armanini D, De Palo CB, Mattarello MJ, Spinella P, Zaccaria M, Ermolao A, et al. Effect of licorice on the reduction of body fat mass in healthy subjects. *J Endocrinol Invest* 2003;26(7):646-50. doi: 10.1007/bf03347023
16. Luan B-G, Sun C-X. Effect of glabridinon on insulin resistance, c-reactive protein and endothelial function in young women with polycystic ovary syndrome. *Bangladesh J Pharmacol* 2015;10(3):681-7. doi: 10.3329/bjp.v10i3.23648
17. Zhao H, Wang Y, Wu L, Yongping MA. Effect of licorice flavonoids on blood glucose, blood lipid and other biochemical indicators in type 2 diabetic rats. *China J Physiol* 2012;1:30-3.
18. Wu F, Jin Z, Jin J. Hypoglycemic effects of glabridin, a polyphenolic flavonoid from licorice, in an animal model of diabetes mellitus. *Mol Med Rep* 2013;7(4):1278-82. doi: 10.3892/mmr.2013.1330
19. Bell ZW, Canale RE, Bloomer RJ. A dual investigation of the effect of dietary supplementation with licorice flavonoid oil on anthropometric and biochemical markers of health and adiposity. *Lipids Health Dis* 2011;10:29. doi: 10.1186/1476-511x-10-29
20. Dai CY, Huang JF, Hsieh MY, Hou NJ, Lin ZY, Chen SC, et al. Insulin resistance predicts response to peginterferon-alpha/ribavirin combination therapy in chronic hepatitis c patients. *J Hepatol* 2009;50(4):712-8. doi: 10.1016/j.jhep.2008.12.017
21. Hajiaghamohammadi AA, Ziaee A, Samimi R. The efficacy of licorice root extract in decreasing transaminase activities in non-alcoholic fatty liver disease: A randomized controlled clinical trial.

Phytother Res 2012;26(9):1381-4. doi: 10.1002/ptr.3728

22. Tominaga Y, Kitano M, Mae T, Kakimoto S, Nakagawa K. Effect of licorice flavonoid oil on visceral fat in obese subjects in the united states. *Nutrafoods* 2014;13(1):35-43. doi: 10.1007/s13749-014-0002-9

23. Park SE, Park CY, Sweeney G. Biomarkers of insulin sensitivity and insulin resistance: Past, present and future. *Crit Rev Clin Lab Sci* 2015;52(4):180-90. doi: 10.3109/10408363.2015.1023429

24. Zadeh JB, Kor ZM, Goftar MK. Licorice (glycyrrhiza glabra linn) as a valuable medicinal plant. *Int J Adv Biol Biom Res* 2013;1(10):1281-8.

25. Shimoyama Y, Hirabayashi K, Matsumoto H, Sato T, Shibata S, Inoue H. Effects of glycyrrhetinic acid derivatives on hepatic and renal 11beta-hydroxysteroid dehydrogenase activities in rats. *J Pharm Pharmacol* 2003;55(6):811-7. doi: 10.1211/002235703765951429

26. Russell ST, Tisdale MJ. Antidiabetic properties of zinc-alpha2-glycoprotein in ob/ob mice. *Endocrinology* 2010;151(3):948-57. doi: 10.1210/en.2009-0827

27. Handisurya A, Riedl M, Vila G, Maier C, Clodi M, Prikoszovich T, et al. Serum vaspin concentrations in relation to insulin sensitivity following rygb-induced weight loss. *Obes Surg* 2010;20(2):198-203. doi: 10.1007/s11695-009-9882-y

28. Chung HK, Chae JS, Hyun YJ, Paik JK, Kim JY, Jang Y, et al. Influence of adiponectin gene polymorphisms on adiponectin level and insulin resistance index in response to dietary intervention in overweight-obese patients with impaired fasting glucose or newly diagnosed type 2 diabetes. *Diabetes care* 2009;32(4):552-8. doi: 10.2337/dc08-1605

29. Koiou E, Tziomalos K, Dinas K, Katsikis I, Kalaitzakis E, Delkos D, et al. The effect of weight loss and treatment with metformin on serum vaspin levels in women with polycystic ovary syndrome. *Endocr J* 2011;58(4):237-46.

30. Stejskal D, Karpisek M, Reutova H, Stejskal P, Kotolova H, Kollar P. Determination of serum zinc-alpha-2-glycoprotein in patients with metabolic syndrome by a new elisa. *Clin Biochem* 2008;41(4-5):313-6. doi: 10.1016/j.clinbiochem.2007.11.010

31. Nazari S, Rameshrad M, Hosseinzadeh H. Toxicological effects of glycyrrhiza glabra (licorice): A review. *Phytother Res* 2017;31(11):1635-50. doi: 10.1002/ptr.5893

20

Bioemulsifiers Derived from Microorganisms: Applications in the Drug and Food Industry

Mahmood Alizadeh-Sani[1,2], Hamed Hamishehkar[2], Arezou Khezerlou[1], Maryam Azizi-Lalabadi[1], Yaghob Azadi[2,3], Elyas Nattagh-Eshtivani[4], Mehdi Fasihi[4], Abed Ghavami[4], Aydin Aynehchi[4], Ali Ehsani[5]*

[1] Student Research Committee, Department of Food Sciences and Technology, Faculty of Nutrition and Food Sciences, Tabriz University of Medical Sciences, Tabriz, Iran.

[2] Drug Applied Research Center, Tabriz University of Medical Sciences, Tabriz, Iran.

[3] Student Research Committee, Tabriz University of Medical Sciences, Tabriz, Iran.

[4] Student Research Committee, Faculty of Nutrition and Food Sciences, Tabriz University of Medical Sciences, Tabriz, Iran.

[5] Department of Food Sciences and Technology, Faculty of Nutrition and Food Sciences, Tabriz University of Medical Sciences, Tabriz, Iran.

Keywords:
· Bioemulsifiers
· Emulsion stability
· Biosurfactants
· Microorganism

Abstract

Emulsifiers are a large category of compounds considered as surface active agents or surfactants. An emulsifier acts by reducing the speed of chemical reactions, and enhancing its stability. Bioemulsifiers are known as surface active biomolecule materials, due to their unique features over chemical surfactants, such as non-toxicity, biodegradability, foaming, biocompatibility, efficiency at low concentrations, high selectivity in different pH, temperatures and salinities. Emulsifiers are found in various natural resources and are synthesized by Bacteria, Fungi and Yeast. Bioemulsifier's molecular weight is higher than that of biosurfactants. Emulsion's function is closely related to their chemical structure. Therefore, the aim of this paper was to study the various bioemulsifiers derived from microorganisms used in the drug and food industry. In this manuscript, we studied organisms with biosurfactant producing abilities. These inexpensive substrates could be used in environmental remediation and in the petroleum industry.

Introduction

As it is clear, oil and water are incompatible. The mixture of oil and water lead to the production of an emulsion. When an emulsion stays still for a while, oil droplets begin to separate from water. In this regards, emulsifiers are used to stop this process. In fact, emulsifiers are used to prevent the emulsion from breaking. Examples of emulsions currently used in the food industry include milk, butter, margarine, mayonnaise and ice cream. Emulsifiers are a large category of compounds also known as surface active agents or surfactants. The word surfactant is used for molecules that migrate to the surface between phases.[1-6]

Bioemulsifiers are higher in molecular weight compared to biosurfactants since they are complex mixtures of heteropolysaccharides, lipopolysaccharides, lipoproteins and proteins.[7] Emulsifiers have double lipophilic and hydrophilic properties. On the other hand, emulsions are either oil-in-water (O/W) or water-in-oil (W/O). In oil emulsions, small droplets of oil form the dispersed phase and discrete in water, while in water emulsions, they are distributed as small droplets of water in oil.[8,9] Adding an emulsifier to an unmixable compound, reduces surface tension between the two phases and prevents it from separating. Therefore, the two liquids are able to form an emulsion. Since an emulsion consists of water-soluble and oil-soluble fragments, an emulsifier is placed on the surface of the area where the two liquids (water and oil) are connected. The water-soluble fragment ambulates towards the water fragment and the fat-soluble fragment places near the oil.[4,6,9-12]

Emulsifiers are substances that increase the uniformity of nutrients, such as fatty acids, fat-soluble vitamins, and amino acids. The function of emulsions is closely related to its chemical structure.[9] Physiologically, in animal's digestive system, the presence of bile salts, benefits fat absorption. Emulsifiers are surfactant materials widely used in food products.[9,13] Hydrophilic characteristics (water-friendliness) and lipophilic (lipid-friendliness) emulsifiers are sometimes referred as hydrophilic/lipophilic equilibrium (HLB), indicating the rate of emulsifier's inclination towards water or oil.[14-16] Emulsifiers are embedded in fat droplets and prevent the protein layer from collapsing. Other functions of emulsifiers in the food industry include:

1) Starch reaction: most emulsifiers have a lean fatty acid layer in their molecule which form an amylose mixture. This feature is very important in delaying bread and bakery products staling and reducing their adhesion to staple products such as potato puree and pasta.[10,11,17,18]

2) Generating interactions with proteins: emulsifiers have ionic structure which react with proteins in food products and produce a modifiable structure. For example, they

respond to the gluten present in wheat and increase protein elasticity, thereby increasing bakery products volume.[10,14,19]

3) Adhesion correction: some emulsifiers are added to food products containing sugar crystals that are scattered in fat and, by coating on glucose crystals, reduce adhesion. This feature affects the fluidity of molten chips and prevent fat appearance on the surface of chocolate.[11,20-22]

4) Creating foam: emulsifiers with saturated fatty acids stabilize the bottommost surface of aqueous solutions. Therefore, it is an important factor in creating foam in raw instant desserts.[4,11,21]

5) Tissue modification is a complex process that is performed on starch and reduces breakdown. For example, homogeneity usually occurs in pasta, bread and bakery products.[2,11]

6) Modifying the dispersion of liquids in another liquid in order to formulate clear solutions: many greed and colors require emulsifiers for solving.[11,14]

Today, due to emulsifier effect on human health and limited resources as well as expensivity, researchers have produced emulsifiers using natural resources, especially microorganisms.[19] According to findings, many microorganisms are able to produce compounds with emulsifying properties.[10] A number of these bioemulsifiers have been licensed by the International Organization for Animal Health, including WHO; but most of these compounds have been studied from a nutritional point of view. A large number of biomolecules are also used in the oil, food, drug and chemical industries.[11,17] The schematic and mechanism of action of important emulsifiers produced by microorganisms using biotechnological processes are presented in Figure 1.

Bioemulsifiers derived from yeast and fungi
Mannoprotein

Mannoprotein bioemulsifier is a glycoprotein with a molecular weight of about 14,000 to 15,800 Dalton. Within the cellular wall of *Saccharomyces spp.* and *Kluyveromyces marxianus* of yeast, mannoprotein molecules are present in glucan, networks, and released from the cell wall of yeast using pressurized heat treatments. This bioemulsifier is able to stabilize oil-in-water emulsions (O/W). According to researchers, bioemulsifiers can be used for producing mayonnaise along with carboxymethyl cellulose (CMC), instead of using expensive ingredients such as ginseng for mayonnaise formulation. Bakery's yeast (*Saccharomyces cerevisiae*) is an affordable, inexpensive and non-toxic source used for producing this bioemulsifier. Mannoprotein is stable in pH = 3-11. Removing mannoprotein molecules from bakery yeast cell is possible using thermal and enzymatic processes (β-1 and 3 glucanases). Mannoprotein molecules are formed from a polypeptide chain with short and long mannose links. When the protein portion of the mannoprotein molecule is detached by the protease enzyme, the mannoprotein emulsifier disappears. In an industrial scale, this

bioemulsifier is active at concentrations equal to or greater than 5% sodium chloride.[10-12,19,23,24]

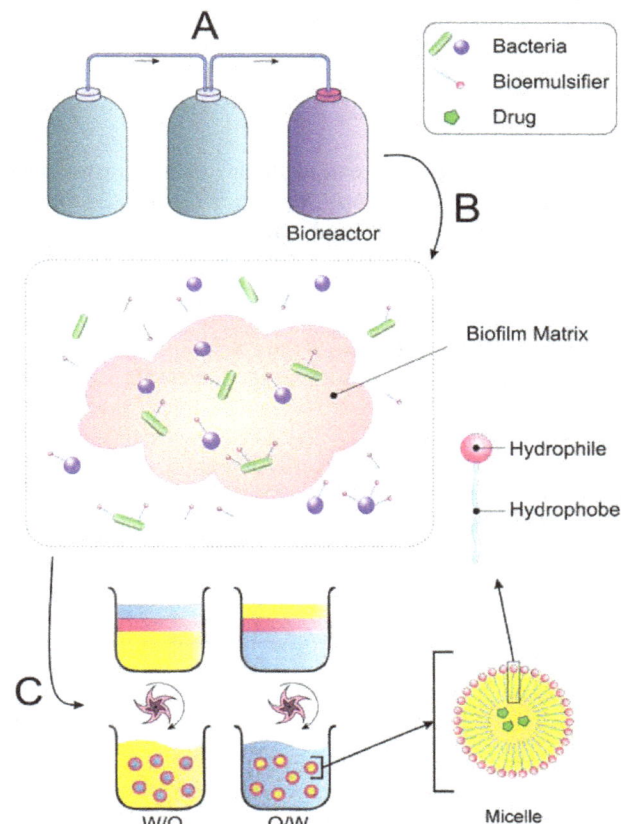

Figure 1. The schematic and mechanism of action of bioemulsifiers in emulsion systems. A: The cultivation, preparation, purification and isolation of microorganisms producing bioemulsifiers. B: Bioemulsifiers produced by microorganisms. C: Emulsion production, adding bioemulsifiers to emulsion systems and assessing their stability.

Liposan

Liposan bioemulsifier is a water-soluble emulsifier obtained from extracting organic solvents fermented by *Candida lipolytica* yeast. Liposan is produced in the extracellular layer and consists of 83% carbohydrate and 17% protein. The presence of protein fractions in the bioemulsifier polymer molecule is essential for its emulsifying properties. The carbohydrate part is a heteropolysaccharide, composed of glucose, galactose, galactose-amine and galacturonic acid molecules. The maximum liposomal properties of liposan are observed at pH = 2-5. Liposan is resistant to temperatures less than 70 °C, but after heating at 100 °C for one hour, 60% of its emulsifiable strength reduces. Liposan causes the stability of various types of emulsions in oil, such as hydrocarbons, vegetable oils including cottonseed, soybean, sunflower, corn, ground, safflower and olive oil.[10,25-30]

Candida tropicalis yeast

During the fed-batch process, *Candida* yeast species produce an extracellular bioemulsifier. This bioemulsifier is very effective in fixing emulsions of many types of hydrocarbons, especially aromatic compounds. The amount of emulsifier produced and its activity increases during fermentation by limiting nitrogen (N) source. Extracting this bioemulsifier from *Candida tropicalis* cells using hot water shows better results in terms of increasing emulsion strength.[11,14,17,31-34]

Rhodotorula yeast
This bioemulsifier is an extracellular emulsifier produced by the *Rhodotorula glutinis* yeast. It is formulated during fed-batch fermentation and glucose utilization under limited nitrogen conditions at 30 °C and pH = 4.[32,33,35-37]

Phaffia yeast
Phaffia rhodozyma is a *basidiomycetous* pink yeast. It has been known as a natural source of astaxanthin and many other nutrients. Also, it is currently being used as an ingredient in feeds. It grows on carbohydrate, hydrocarbon and a mixture of carbohydrate and lipid polymers. Fermentation is accomplished in a culture medium chain with sucrose as the carbon source for 3 days

at 22 °C and centrifuged at 150 rpm. Experiments have shown that adding sodium citrate, stimulates bioemulsifiers production.[10,11,38,39] Table 1 and 2 show bioemulsifiers produced by yeast and fungi.

Table 1. List of bioemulsifiers producing yeast

Microorganism's	Bioemulsifiers	Ref.
Torulopsis petrophilum	Sophorolipids	40
Torulopsis apicola	Sophorolipids	41
Pseudozyma rugulosa	Mannosylerythritol lipids	42
Pseudozyma aphidis	Mannosylerythritol lipids	43
Kurtzmanomyces sp.	Mannosylerythritol lipids	44
Kurtzmanomyces sp. I-11	Mannosylerythritol lipids	45
Debaryomyces polymorphus	Carbohydrate protein-lipid complex	32
Saccharomyces cerevisiae	Mannoprotein	23
Kluyveromyces marxianus	Mannoprotein	12
Rhodotorula glutinis	Polymeric bioemulsifier	46

Table 2. List of bioemulsifiers producing fungi

Microorganism's	Bioemulsifiers	Ref.
Candida tropicalis	Mannan-fatty acid	47
Candida lipolytica Y-917	Sophorous lipid	39
Candida utilis	NDA	39
Candida ingens	Fatty acids	48
Candida lipolytica UCP0988	Carbohydrate-protein-lipid complex	49
Candida tropicalis	Liposan	28
Candida bombicola	Sophorolipids	50
Candida (torulopsis) apicola	Sophorolipids	51
Candida lipolytica ATCC 8662	Carbohydrate-protein complex	52
Penicillium chrysogenum	Polyketide derivative	53
Yarrowia lipolytica IMUFRJ 50682	Carbohydrate-protein complex	27,54
Yarrowia lipolytica NCIM 3589	Bioemulsifier	54
Yarrowia lipolytica IMUFRJ 50682	Yansan	55
Ustilago maydis	Cellobiose lipids	56
Candida sphaerica UCP0995	Sophorolipids	57
Candida. glabrata UCP0995	Sophorolipids	58
Pseudomonas. aeruginosa	Rhamnolipids	59

Bioemulsifiers derived from bacteria
Lauryl fructose
This bioemulsifier is produced by the lipase enzyme obtained from *Pseudomonas spp.*[60] in a culture media containing dry pyridine. This bioemulsifier has emulsification properties for a variety of hydrocarbons, edible oils, and oil based oils such as margarine and shortening. In a water-containing environment, Laura fructose reduces surface tension from 72 to 29 (MN / m). Also, it reduces the intermolecular reaction of water and hydrocarbons from 50 to 6 when combined with water-insoluble oil compounds.[10,11,61-63] In Table 3, bio-emulsifiers produced by bacteria are presented.

Alasan or E-KA53
Alasan is a biomolecular bacterium produced by the *Acinetobacter radioresistant* bacteria. The molecular composition of this complex bioemulsifier consists of polysaccharides and proteins with high molecular weight (100,000 - 230,000 Daltons). If the protein portion is damaged and digested using proteolytic enzymes, the bioemulsifier polymer turns into a thick polysaccharide and loses its emulsifying properties. Heating with alcohol at 50 °C may lead to 2.5 times increase in polysaccharide concentration, while the protein portion and the emulsifying properties of the molecule remain unchanged. Heating at 60-90 °C reduces viscosity and increases emulsifying activity as much as 5.8 times than the initial

value. The emulsifying properties of alasan are affected by pH and magnesium ion concentrations. This bioemulsifier is an extracellular product and is used extensively in the food industry. Alasan is produced during *Acinetobacter* bacterium fermentation in a fed-batch fermentation system. The ultimate product consists of 2.2 g of emulsifier per liter of culture fluid. Alcohols stabilize a wide range of oil-in-water (O/W) emulsions, such as n-alkanes, alkaline compounds, liquid paraffin, soybean oil, coconut oil and raw oils. The emulsifying activity of alasan increase approximately 2-3 times, when

heated at 100 °C under neutral or alkaline conditions. This bioemulsifier is completely active in pH = 3.3-9.2 and its maximum emulsifier activity is at pH = 5. Magnesium ions increase the activity of emulsifiers both at lower (3.3-4.5) and higher pH (5.5-9.3) than that of the optimal pH. Alasan activity is higher in an environment containing 20 mL citrate than that of same concentrations of acetate or Tris-HCl. According to studies, we can indicate that this bioemulsifier is a high molecular weight anion heteropolysaccharide combined with a protein component such as alanine.[10,11,21,64-70]

Table 3. List of bioemulsifiers producing bacteria

Microorganism's	Bioemulsifiers	Ref.
Pseudomonas fluorescens	Viscosin	[71]
Pseudomonas aeruginosa	Rhamnolipids	[72]
Pseudomonas fluorescens	Carbohydrate-lipid complex	[39]
Bacillus amyloliquefaciens,	Surfactin/Iturin	[73]
Bacillus subtilis	Subtilisin	[74]
Bacillus subtilis	Lichenysin	[75]
Bacillus licheniformis K51, Bacillus subtilis	Peptide lipids	[76]
Bacillus pumilus A1	Rhamnolipids	[77]
Bacillus sp. AB-2	Hydrocarbon-lipid-protein	[78]
Acinetobacter calcoaceticus	Emulsan	[79]
Acinetobacter radioresistens	Alasan	[39]
Acinetobacter calcoaceticus RAG1	Emulsan	[80]
Rhodococcus erythropolis	Glycoprotein	[81]
Rhodococcus sp. 33	Uronic acids	[82]
Cyanobacteria	Trehalose dicorynomycolate	[83]
Clostridium pasteurianum	Polysaccharide	[84]
Debaryomyces polmorphus	Whole cell	[85]
Halomonas eurihalina	Carbohydrate-lipid complex	[86]
Halomonas	Emulsifier HE39 & HE67	[87]
Lactobacillus paracasei	Glycoprotein	[88]
Leuconostoc mesenteriods	Dextran	[89]
Serratia marcescens, Serrated rubidea	Serrawettin	[90]
Bacillus pseudomycoides BS6	Lipopeptide	[91]
Pseudomonas. cepacia CCT6659	Rhamnolipids	[92]
Bacillus. licheniformis R2	Lipopeptide	[93]

Emulsan

Emulsan is an extracellular poly-anionic bioemulsifier produced by *Acinetobacter calcoaceticus RAG 1* bacteria. In fact, emulsan is a lipoheteropolysaccharide polymer containing D-galactose-amine produced during the stationary phase. This bioemulsifier is a poly-anionic and amphiphilic compound which is able to stabilize the hydrocarbon emulsion in water by creating a very thin layer between the hydrocarbon droplets and water. Maximum concentration is obtained when culture media containing 12 carbon-based fatty acids are used as the carbon source. Emulsan production is possible with fermentation methods such as batch, chemo-stat, immobilized cell system and self-cycling fermentation (SCF). Based on SCF methods, bioemulsifier production could increase about 50 times compared to the batch

method. Another type of emulsan considered as bio-emulsion is produced by *Acinetobacter calcoaceticus*, which is used in the formulation and production of soft cheese and ice creams as well as creams and skin-protecting materials. Different types of emulsions produced from these bacteria include alpha-amyloemulsan, Apo-alpha-oleo-emulsan, and beta-emulsan, which are used for treating skin infections are widely used in the food industry. These compounds are mostly poly-anionic lipoheteropolysaccharides that are produced by different species of *Acinetobacter venetianus rag-1t* ATCC 31012- and *Streptomyces* NRRL.B- 15615, NRRL.B-15847 or ATCC 31926 and few other species.[7,70,94-98]

Cyanobacteria

A variety of *cyanobacteria* (Genus phormidium, ATCC 39161) (Oscillatoriales) bacterium produce bioemulsifiers that can be used for producing hydrocarbon and oil emulsions in a fluid environment such as water. This bacterium is obtained from using precise separation methods from riverside water, which subsequently grow on a suitable culture medium under favorable conditions and produce an extracellular bioemulsifier sphincter. The molecular weight of this polymeric bioemulsifier is more than 200,000 Dalton. According to chemical tests, it contains sugars, fatty acids, and a protein fractions. Also, more accurate tests using IR spectrophotometry have shown that it is contains amide, carboxylic and amino groups. This bioemulsifier is used for producing various types of oil-in-water emulsions (O/W).[99-101]

Pseudomonas cepacia bacteria

This bioemulsifier which in terms of molecular characteristics, is considered as a mixture of glycolic acid, is produced after *Pseudomonas cepacia* bacteria growth and propagation on sunflower oil (as the carbon source) medium. The production of this bioemulsifier is carried out by *Pseudomonas cepacia* bacteria by adding 1.7 % of sunflower oil per liter of culture medium when oxygen and nitrogen levels are controlled. This bioemulsifier is used as a natural source of disintegrating agents used for decomposing and neutralizing polychlorinated biphenyls, especially polychlorinated biphenyls. Polychlorinated biphenyls are toxic and with carcinogenic compounds produced by pesticides during various chemical processes which are able to contaminate industrial wastewater and cultivated soils.[102-105]

Bacillus stearothermophilus

During growth, *Bacillus stearothermophilus VR-8* produces an extracellular bioemulsifier on a medium containing 4% crude oil. The optimum temperature for producing this bioemulsifier is 50 °C, which at this temperature, 0.6 gr/L bioemulsifier is produced. This emulsifier is purified by acetone and dialysis and contains 46% protein, 16% carbohydrate and 10% fat. Its emulsifier activity is stable over a wide range of temperatures, i.e. 50-80 °C, and pH = 2-8, and salt concentrations (5% chlorine, 5% calcium chloride or 1% chlorine magnesium). The emulsifying properties of this bioemulsifier are related to its stability in a wide range of pH (liposomal at pH = 2-5 and a maximum of 70 °C) and temperatures. This emulsifier is used for removing crude oil from reservoirs and eliminating the remaining oil of crude oil tanks. Hereby, recovery of crude oil, increases by complete scouring of oil remained on storage chamber.[9,106-110]

Sphingomonas bacteria

Presence of polycyclic aromatic hydrocarbons (PAH) in water resources due to their low solubility, is somewhat problematic. When the molecular weight of these compounds (PAH) are reduced, available microorganisms metabolize them. A number of degrading bacteria have been isolated from multi-ring aromatic hydrocarbons of contaminated soils, which produce bioemulsifiers and active compounds, most notably strain No. 107 of *Sphingomonas* bacteria. This bacterium grows on culture media containing a variety of aromatic hydrocarbon compounds and create clear spots on the medium. Also in liquid culture media, this bacterium uses aromatic hydrocarbons as the main source of energy and carbon. Notably, this bioemulsifier has emulsifying properties similar to high molecular weighting polycyclic hydrocarbons.[111-114]

Discussion

Biosurfactants have received great attention due to their safety and biodegradable properties. Although biosurfactants have various functions,their practical application is limited. Biosurfactants worldwide production was approximately 17 million tons in 2000 and is expected to have a growth rates of 3-4% per year globally. Biosurfactants have many advantages in comparison to synthesized components, such as, biodegradability (easily decomposed by microorganism), low toxicity (Effective Concentration =50), availability of raw materials (produced from cheap materials), physical factors (components which are not affected by temperature, pH and ionic strength tolerances), surface and interface activity (lower surface tension) ,biocompatibility and digestibility, commercial laundry detergents, bio pesticide, medical function (antimicrobial activity, anti-cancer activity, anti-adhesive agents, immunological adjuvants, antiviral activity, gene delivery), food processing industry, cosmetic industry and increasing oil recovery. Considering, biosurfactants applications and their affect on nutrient, micronutrient and environmental factors, their production still remains a challeng. It is expected that in the near future, a new strain of microorganisms will be developed for using as biosurfactants in industries.

Conclusion

Nowadays, emulsifiers are widely used in the food and drug industry. Therefore, using emulsifiers derived from natural resources are preferred to synthetic emulsifiers because of their nutritional benefits. As a result, using bioemulsifiers derived from microbial sources are beneficial and may be a significant alternative for synthesized emulsifiers. Thus, they can be used efficiently in the food and drug industry in acceptable and recommended quantities.

Acknowledgments

This review was conducted at Tabriz University of Medical Sciences, Tabriz, Iran.
Compliance with Ethical standards.

Ethical Issues

This article does not contain any studies with human participants or animals performed by any of the authors.

Conflict of Interest
The authors declare no conflict of interests.

References
1. Hasenhuettl GL, Hartel RW. Food emulsifiers and their applications. USA: Springer; 2008.
2. Whitehurst RJ. Emulsifiers in food technology. United Kingdom: John Wiley & Sons; 2008.
3. Krog N. Functions of emulsifiers in food systems. *J Am Oil Chem Soc* 1977;54(3):124-31.
4. Krog NJ, Sparso FV. Food emulsifiers and their chemical and physical properties. New York: Marcel Dekker Inc; 1997.
5. Hasenhuettl GL. Synthesis and commercial preparation of food emulsifiers. Food emulsifiers and their applications: *Springer*; 2008. 11-37.
6. Lauridsen JB. Food emulsifiers: Surface activity, edibility, manufacture, composition, and application. *J Am Oil Chem Soc* 1976;53(6):400-7.
7. Uzoigwe C, Burgess JG, Ennis CJ, Rahman PK. Bioemulsifiers are not biosurfactants and require different screening approaches. *Front Microbiol* 2015;6: 245.
8. Calvo C, Manzanera M, Silva-Castro GA, Uad I, Gonzalez-Lopez J. Application of bioemulsifiers in soil oil bioremediation processes. Future prospects. *Sci Total Environ* 2009;407(12):3634-40. doi: 10.1016/j.scitotenv.2008.07.008
9. Calvo C, Toledo FL, Pozo C, Martínez-Toledo MV, González-López J. Biotechnology of bioemulsifiers produced by micro-organisms. *J Food Agric Environ* 2004;2(3):238-43.
10. Shepherd R, Rockey J, Sutherland IW, Roller S. Novel bioemulsifiers from microorganisms for use in foods. *J Biotechnol* 1995;40(3):207-17.
11. Nitschke M, Costa S. Biosurfactants in food industry. *Trends Food Sci Tech* 2007;18(5):252-9.
12. Lukondeh T, Ashbolt NJ, Rogers PL. Evaluation of kluyveromyces marxianus fii 510700 grown on a lactose-based medium as a source of a natural bioemulsifier. *J Ind Microbiol Biotechnol* 2003;30(12):715-20.
13. Bach H, Gutnick D. Potential applications of bioemulsifiers in the oil industry. *Stud Surf Sci Catal* 2004;151:233-81.
14. Zajic J, Panchal C, Westlake D. Bio-emulsifiers. *CRC Crit Rev Microbiol* 1976;5(1):39-66.
15. Sineriz F, Hommel R, Kleber H. Production of biosurfactants. Argentina: Encyclopedia of life support systems, semanticscholar; 2001.
16. Satpute SK, Banpurkar AG, Dhakephalkar PK, Banat IM, Chopade BA. Methods for investigating biosurfactants and bioemulsifiers: A review. *Crit Rev Biotechnol* 2010;30(2):127-44. doi: 10.3109/07388550903427280
17. Campos JM, Stamford TL, Sarubbo LA. Production of a bioemulsifier with potential application in the food industry. *Appl Biochem Biotechnol* 2014;172(6):3234-52. doi: 10.1007/s12010-014-0761-1
18. Mnif I, Besbes S, Ellouze R, Ellouze-Chaabouni S, Ghribi D. Improvement of bread quality and bread shelf-life by bacillus subtilis biosurfactant addition. *Food Sci Biotechnol* 2012;21(4):1105-12.
19. Torabizadeh H, Shojaosadati S, Tehrani H. Preparation and characterisation of bioemulsifier fromsaccharomyces cerevisiaeand its application in food products. *LWT-Food Sci Technol* 1996;29(8):734-7.
20. Mnif I, Ghribi D. Glycolipid biosurfactants: Main properties and potential applications in agriculture and food industry. *J Sci Food Agric* 2016;96(13):4310-20. doi: 10.1002/jsfa.7759
21. Kosaric N, Sukan FV. Biosurfactants: Production: Properties: Applications. Canada: CRC Press; 2010.
22. Gutierrez T, Rhodes G, Mishamandani S, Berry D, Whitman WB, Nichols PD, et al. Polycyclic aromatic hydrocarbon degradation of phytoplankton-associated arenibacter spp. And description of arenibacter algicola sp. Nov., an aromatic hydrocarbon-degrading bacterium. *Appl Environ Microbiol* 2014;80(2):618-28. doi: 10.1128/AEM.03104-13
23. Cameron DR, Cooper DG, Neufeld R. The mannoprotein of saccharomyces cerevisiae is an effective bioemulsifier. *Appl Environ Microbiol* 1988;54(6):1420-5.
24. Barriga JA, Cooper DG, Idziak ES, Cameron DR. Components of the bioemulsifier from s. Cerevisiae. *Enzyme Microb Tech* 1999;25(1):96-102.
25. Cirigliano MC, Carman GM. Purification and characterization of liposan, a bioemulsifier from candida lipolytica. *Appl Environ Microbiol* 1985;50(4):846-50.
26. Cirigliano MC, Carman GM. Isolation of a bioemulsifier from candida lipolytica. *Appl Environ Microbiol* 1984;48(4):747-50.
27. Amaral P, Da Silva J, Lehocky M, Barros-Timmons A, Coelho M, Marrucho I, et al. Production and characterization of a bioemulsifier from yarrowia lipolytica. *Process Biochem* 2006;41(8):1894-8.
28. Sarubbo L, Porto A, Campos-Takaki G. The use of babassu oil as substrate to produce bioemulsifiers by candida lipolytica. *Can J Microbiol* 1999;45(5):423-6.
29. Souza F, Salgueiro A, Albuquerque C. Production of bioemulsifiers by yarrowia lipolytica in sea water using diesel oil as the carbon source. *Braz J Chem* 2012;29(1):61-7.
30. Fracchia L, Cavallo M, Martinotti MG, Banat IM. Biosurfactants and bioemulsifiers biomedical and related applications–present status and future potentials. *Bio Sci Eng Technol* 2012.
31. Batista RM, Rufino RD, Luna JM, de Souza JE, Sarubbo LA. Effect of medium components on the production of a biosurfactant from candida tropicalis applied to the removal of hydrophobic contaminants in soil. *Water Environ Res* 2010;82(5):418-25.
32. Amaral PF, Coelho MAZ, Marrucho IM, Coutinho JA. Biosurfactants from yeasts: Characteristics, production and application. *Adv Exp Med Biol* 2010;672:236-49.

33. Campos-Takaki GM, Sarubbo LA, Albuquerque CDC. Environmentally friendly biosurfactants produced by yeasts. *Adv Exp Med Biol* 2010;672:250-60.

34. Accorsini FR, Mutton MJR, Lemos EGM, Benincasa M. Biosurfactants production by yeasts using soybean oil and glycerol as low cost substrate. *Braz J Microbiol* 2012;43(1):116-25.

35. Satpute SK, Banat IM, Dhakephalkar PK, Banpurkar AG, Chopade BA. Biosurfactants, bioemulsifiers and exopolysaccharides from marine microorganisms. *Biotechnol Adv* 2010;28(4):436-50. doi: 10.1016/j.biotechadv.2010.02.006

36. Mnif I, Ghribi D. High molecular weight bioemulsifiers, main properties and potential environmental and biomedical applications. *World J Microbiol Biotechnol* 2015;31(5):691-706. doi: 10.1007/s11274-015-1830-5

37. Eliwa E-S, El-Hofi M. B-galactosidase (β-gal) from the yeast rhodotorula ingeniosa and its utilization in ice milk production. *Biotechnol* 2010;13(1):02.

38. Feng H-f, DU Q-j, LUAN J, SUN Y-m. Biosurfactant production by ochrobactrum sp. With alkane as carbon source. *J Ind Microbiol* 2015;3:011.

39. Shekhar S, Sundaramanickam A, Balasubramanian T. Biosurfactant producing microbes and their potential applications: A review. *Crit Rev Environ Sci Technol* 2015;45(14):1522-54.

40. Cooper DG, Paddock DA. Torulopsis petrophilum and surface activity. *Appl Environ Microbiol* 1983;46(6):1426-9.

41. Rau U, Hammen S, Heckmann R, Wray V, Lang S. Sophorolipids: A source for novel compounds. *Ind Crop Prod* 2001;13(2):85-92.

42. Morita T, Konishi M, Fukuoka T, Imura T, Kitamoto D. Discovery of pseudozyma rugulosa nbrc 10877 as a novel producer of the glycolipid biosurfactants, mannosylerythritol lipids, based on rdna sequence. *Appl Microbiol Biotechnol* 2006;73(2):305.

43. Rau U, Nguyen LA, Schulz S, Wray V, Nimtz M, Roeper H, et al. Formation and analysis of mannosylerythritol lipids secreted by pseudozyma aphidis. *Appl Microbiol Biotechnol* 2005;66(5):551-9. doi: 10.1007/s00253-004-1672-9

44. Konishi M, Morita T, Fukuoka T, Imura T, Kakugawa K, Kitamoto D. Production of different types of mannosylerythritol lipids as biosurfactants by the newly isolated yeast strains belonging to the genus pseudozyma. *Appl Microbiol Biotechnol* 2007;75(3):521.

45. Kakugawa K, Tamai M, Imamura K, Miyamoto K, Miyoshi S, Morinaga Y, et al. Isolation of yeast kurtzmanomyces sp. I-11, novel producer of mannosylerythritol lipid. *Biosci Biotechnol Biochem* 2002;66(1):188-91. doi: 10.1271/bbb.66.188

46. Johnson V, Singh M, Saini VS, Adhikari DK, Sista V, Yadav NK. Bioemulsifier production by an oleaginous yeastrhodotorulaglutinis iip-30. *Biotechnol lett* 1992;14(6):487-90.

47. Miura Y. Mechanism of liquid hydrocarbon uptake by microorganisms and growth kinetics. *Adv Biochem Eng* 2017;9:31-56. doi: 10.1007/BFb0048090

48. Amezcua-Vega C, Poggi-Varaldo HM, Esparza-Garcia F, Rios-Leal E, Rodriguez-Vazquez R. Effect of culture conditions on fatty acids composition of a biosurfactant produced by candida ingens and changes of surface tension of culture media. *Bioresour Technol* 2007;98(1):237-40. doi: 10.1016/j.biortech.2005.11.025

49. Rufino R, Sarubbo L, Campos-Takaki G. Enhancement of stability of biosurfactant produced by candida lipolytica using industrial residue as substrate. *World J Microb Biot* 2007;23(5):729-34. doi: 10.1007/s11274-006-9278-2

50. Cavalero DA, Cooper DG. The effect of medium composition on the structure and physical state of sophorolipids produced by candida bombicola atcc 22214. *J Biotechnol* 2003;103(1):31-41.

51. Hommel R, Weber L, Weiss A, Himmelreich U, Rilke O, Kleber H-P. Production of sophorose lipid by candida (torulopsis) apicola grown on glucose. *J Biotechnol* 1994;33(2):147-55. doi: 10.1016/0168-1656(94)90107-4

52. Huang L, Zhang B, Gao B, Sun G. Application of fishmeal wastewater as a potential low-cost medium for lipid production by lipomyces starkeyi hl. *Environ Technol* 2011;33(15-16):1975-81.

53. Gao SS, Li XM, Du FY, Li CS, Proksch P, Wang BG. Secondary metabolites from a marine-derived endophytic fungus penicillium chrysogenum qen-24s. *Mar Drugs* 2010;9(1):59-70. doi: 10.3390/md9010059

54. Zinjarde SS, Pant A. Emulsifier from a tropical marine yeast, yarrowia lipolytica ncim 3589. *J Basic Microbiol* 2002;42(1):67-73. doi: 10.1002/1521-4028(200203)42:1<67::AID-JOBM67>3.0.CO;2-M

55. Coelho M, Amaral P, Belo I. Yarrowia lipolytica: An industrial workhorse. *Appl Microbiol Microb Biotechnol* 2010;2:930-40.

56. Teichmann B, Linne U, Hewald S, Marahiel MA, Bolker M. A biosynthetic gene cluster for a secreted cellobiose lipid with antifungal activity from ustilago maydis. *Mol Microbiol* 2007;66(2):525-33. doi: 10.1111/j.1365-2958.2007.05941.x

57. Ben Belgacem Z, Bijttebier S, Verreth C, Voorspoels S, Van de Voorde I, Aerts G, et al. Biosurfactant production by pseudomonas strains isolated from floral nectar. *J Appl Microbiol* 2015;118(6):1370-84. doi: 10.1111/jam.12799

58. Luna JM, Rufino RD, Sarubbo LA, Rodrigues LR, Teixeira JA, de Campos-Takaki GM. Evaluation antimicrobial and antiadhesive properties of the biosurfactant lunasan produced by candida sphaerica UCP 0995. *Curr Microbiol* 2011;62(5):1527-34. doi: 10.1007/s00284-011-9889-1

59. Gusmão CAB, Rufino RD, Sarubbo LA. Laboratory production and characterization of a new biosurfactant from Candida glabrata UCP1002 cultivated in vegetable fat waste applied to the removal of

hydrophobic contaminant. *World J Microb Biot* 2010;26(9):1683-92. doi: 10.1007/s11274-010-0346-2

60. Santos CA, Bezerra MS, Pereira HS, Santos ES, Macedo GR. Production and recovery of rhamnolipids using sugar cane molasses as carbon source. *J Chem Eng Chem Eng* 2010;4(11): 27.

61. Mohammadi S, Abbasi S, Scanlon M. Development of emulsifying property in persian gum using octenyl succinic anhydride (osa). *Int J Biol Macromol* 2016;89:396-405. doi: 10.1016/j.ijbiomac.2016.04.006

62. Kiran GS, Selvin J, Manilal A, Sujith S. Biosurfactants as green stabilizers for the biological synthesis of nanoparticles. *Crit Rev Biotechnol* 2011;31(4):354-64. doi: 10.3109/07388551.2010.539971

63. dos Santos SC, Fernandez LG, Rossi-Alva JC, de Abreu Roque MR. Evaluation of substrates from renewable-resources in biosurfactants production by pseudomonas strains. *Afr J Biotechnol* 2010;9(35).

64. Hames EE, Vardar-Sukan F, Kosaric N. 11 patents on biosurfactants and future trends. Biosurfactants: Production and Utilization Processes, Technologies, and Economics. USA: CRC press, Taylor & Francis group; 2014.

65. Perfumo A, Smyth T, Marchant R, Banat I. Production and roles of biosurfactants and bioemulsifiers in accessing hydrophobic substrates. Handbook of hydrocarbon and lipid microbiology. Germany: Springer; 2010.

66. Jagtap S, Yavankar S, Pardesi K, Chopade B. Production of bioemulsifier by acinetobacter species isolated from healthy human skin. *Indian J Exp Biol* 2010;48(1):70-6.

67. Cameotra SS, Makkar RS, Kaur J, Mehta SK. Synthesis of biosurfactants and their advantages to microorganisms and mankind. *Adv Exp Med Biol* 2010;672:261-80.

68. Ron E, Rosenberg E. Role of biosurfactants. Handbook of hydrocarbon and lipid microbiology: Germany: Springer; 2010.

69. Vijayakumar S, Saravanan V. Biosurfactants-types, sources and applications. *Res J Microbiol* 2015;10(5):181-92.

70. Foght JM, Gutnick DL, Westlake DW. Effect of emulsan on biodegradation of crude oil by pure and mixed bacterial cultures. *Appl Environ Microbiol* 1989;55(1):36-42.

71. Banat IM, Franzetti A, Gandolfi I, Bestetti G, Martinotti MG, Fracchia L, et al. Microbial biosurfactants production, applications and future potential. *Appl Microbiol Biotechnol* 2010;87(2):427-44. doi: 10.1007/s00253-010-2589-0

72. Jadhav M, Kalme S, Tamboli D, Govindwar S. Rhamnolipid from pseudomonas desmolyticum ncim-2112 and its role in the degradation of brown 3rel. *J Basic Microbiol* 2011;51(4):385-96. doi: 10.1002/jobm.201000364

73. Arguelles-Arias A, Ongena M, Halimi B, Lara Y, Brans A, Joris B, et al. Bacillus amyloliquefaciens ga1 as a source of potent antibiotics and other secondary metabolites for biocontrol of plant pathogens. *Microb Cell Fact* 2009;8(1):63. doi: 10.1186/1475-2859-8-63

74. Abriouel H, Franz CM, Omar NB, Gálvez A. Diversity and applications of bacillus bacteriocins. *FEMS Microbiol Rev* 2010;35(1):201-32. doi: 10.1111/j.1574-6976.2010.00244.x

75. Yakimov MM, Golyshin PN. Coma-dependent transcriptional activation of lichenysin a synthetase promoter in bacillus subtilis cells. *Biotechnol Prog* 1997;13(6):757-61. doi: 10.1021/bp9700622

76. Begley M, Cotter PD, Hill C, Ross RP. Identification of a novel two-peptide lantibiotic, lichenicidin, following rational genome mining for lanm proteins. *Appl Environ Microbiol* 2009;75(17):5451-60. doi: 10.1128/AEM.00730-09

77. Banat IM, Makkar RS, Cameotra SS. Potential commercial applications of microbial surfactants. *Appl Microbiol Biotechnol* 2000;53(5):495-508.

78. Banat IM. Biosurfactants production and possible uses in microbial enhanced oil recovery and oil pollution remediation: A review. *Bioresour Technol* 1995;51(1):1-12. doi: 10.1016/0960-8524(94)00101-6

79. Rosenberg E, Barkay T, Navon-Venezia S, Ron E. Role of acinetobacter bioemulsans in petroleum degradation. Novel approaches for bioremediation of organic pollution. USA: Springer; 1999.

80. Kim S-Y, Oh D-K, Kim J-H. Biological modification of hydrophobic group in acinetobacter calcoaceticus RAG-1 emulsan. *J Biosci Bioeng* 1997;84(2):162-4. doi: 10.1016/S0922-338X(97)82548-2

81. Hirrlinger B, Stolz A, Knackmuss H-J. Purification and properties of an amidase from rhodococcus erythropolis mp50 which enantioselectively hydrolyzes 2-arylpropionamides. *J Bacteriol* 1996;178(12):3501-7. doi: 10.1128/jb.178.12.3501-3507.1996

82. Aizawa T, Neilan BA, Couperwhite I, Urai M, Anzai H, Iwabuchi N, et al. Relationship between extracellular polysaccharide and benzene tolerance of rhodococcus sp. 33. *Actinomycetologica* 2005;19(1):1-6. doi: 10.3209/saj.19.1

83. Nerurkar AS, Hingurao KS, Suthar HG. Bioemulsifiers from marine microorganisms. *J Sci Ind Res* 2009;68(4):273-7

84. Mortenson LE. Ferredoxin and atp, requirements for nitrogen fixation in cell-free extracts of clostridium pasteurianum. *Proc Natl Acad Sci U S A* 1964;52:272-9.

85. Yang Q, Yediler A, Yang M, Kettrup A. Decolorization of an azo dye, reactive black 5 and mnp production by yeast isolate: Debaryomyces polymorphus. *Biochem Engine J* 2005;24(3):249-53. doi: 10.1016/j.bej.2004.12.004

86. Ates O, Oner ET, Arga KY. Genome-scale reconstruction of metabolic network for a halophilic extremophile, chromohalobacter salexigens dsm 3043. *BMC Syst Biol* 2011;5(1):12. doi: 10.1186/1752-0509-5-12

87. Gutierrez T, Mulloy B, Black K, Green DH. Glycoprotein emulsifiers from two marine halomonas species: Chemical and physical characterization. *J Appl Microbiol* 2007;103(5):1716-27. doi: 10.1111/j.1365-2672.2007.03407.x

88. Gudina EJ, Teixeira JA, Rodrigues LR. Isolation and functional characterization of a biosurfactant produced by lactobacillus paracasei. *Colloids Surf B Biointerfaces* 2010;76(1):298-304. doi: 10.1016/j.colsurfb.2009.11.008

89. Sarwat F, Ul Qader SA, Aman A, Ahmed N. Production & characterization of a unique dextran from an indigenous leuconostoc mesenteroides cmg713. *Int J Biol Sci* 2008;4(6):379-86.

90. Wei YH, Lai HC, Chen SY, Yeh MS, Chang JS. Biosurfactant production by serratia marcescens ss-1 and its isogenic strain smðr defective in spnr, a quorum-sensing luxr family protein. *Biotechnol lett* 2004;26(10):799-802.

91. Li J, Deng M, Wang Y, Chen W. Production and characteristics of biosurfactant produced by Bacillus pseudomycoides BS6 utilizing soybean oil waste. *Int Biodeter Biodegr* 2016; 112:72–9. doi: 10.1016/j.ibiod.2016.05.002

92. Silva RCFS, Rufino RD, Luna JM, Farias CBB, Filho HJB, Santos VA, et al. Enhancement of biosurfactant production from Pseudomonas cepacia CCT6659 through optimisation of nutritional parameters using response surface methodology. *Tenside Surfact Det* 2013;50(2):137-42. doi: 10.3139/113.110241

93. Joshi SJ, Desai AJ. Bench-scale production of biosurfactants and their potential in ex-situ MEOR application. *Soil Sediment Contam* 2013;22(6):701–15. doi: 10.1080/15320383.2013.756450

94. Fondi M, Orlandini V, Emiliani G, Papaleo MC, Maida I, Perrin E, et al. Draft genome sequence of the hydrocarbon-degrading and emulsan-producing strain acinetobacter venetianus rag-1t. *J Bacteriol* 2012;194(17):4771-2. doi: 10.1128/JB.01019-12

95. Mousavian S, Rahimi K. Emulsan production by acinetobacter calcoaceticus rag-1 ATCC-31012. 2010;7(26): 117-25.

96. Goldman S, Shabtai Y, Rubinovitz C, Rosenberg E, Gutnick DL. Emulsan in acinetobacter calcoaceticus rag-1: Distribution of cell-free and cell-associated cross-reacting material. *Appl Environ Microbiol* 1982;44(1):165-70.

97. Rubinovitz C, Gutnick DL, Rosenberg E. Emulsan production by acinetobacter calcoaceticus in the presence of chloramphenicol. *J Bacteriol* 1982;152(1):126-32.

98. Pines O, Gutnick D. Role for emulsan in growth of acinetobacter calcoaceticus rag-1 on crude oil. *Appl Environ Microbiol* 1986;51(3):661-3.

99. Shilo M, Fattom A. Cyanobacterium-produced bioemulsifier composition and solution thereof. Google Patents; 1987. No. 4,693,842.

100. Susilaningsih D. Biosurfactant properties of extracellular pink pigment produced by a freshwater cyanobacterium, oscillatoria sp. *Microbiol Indones* 2010;1(3).

101. Shete A, Wadhawa G, Banat I, Chopade B. Mapping of patents on bioemulsifier and biosurfactant: A review. *J Sci Ind Res* 2006;65:91-115.

102. Kanaly RA, Harayama S. Biodegradation of high-molecular-weight polycyclic aromatic hydrocarbons by bacteria. *J Bacteriol* 2000;182(8):2059-67.

103. Fiebig R, Schulze D, Chung J-C, Lee S-T. Biodegradation of polychlorinated biphenyls (pcbs) in the presence of a bioemulsifier produced on sunflower oil. *Biodegradation* 1997;8(2):67-75.

104. Aislabie J, Lloyd-Jones G. A review of bacterial-degradation of pesticides. *Aust J Soil Res* 1995;33(6):925-42. doi: 10.1071/SR9950925

105. Van Dyke MI, Lee H, Trevors JT. Applications of microbial surfactants. *Biotechnol Adv* 1991;9(2):241-52. doi: 10.1016/0734-9750(91)90006-H

106. Gurjar M, Khire J, Khan M. Bioemulsifier production by bacillus stearothermophilus vr-8 isolate. *Lett Appl Microbiol* 1995;21(2):83-6. doi: 10.1111/j.1472-765X.1995.tb01012.x

107. Rosenberg E, Ron EZ. High- and low-molecular-mass microbial surfactants. *Appl Microbiol Biotechnol* 1999;52(2):154-62.

108. Rosenberg E, Ron EZ. Bioemulsans: Microbial polymeric emulsifiers. *Curr Opin Biotechnol* 1997;8(3):313-6.

109. Ilori MO, Amobi CJ, Odocha AC. Factors affecting biosurfactant production by oil degrading aeromonas spp. Isolated from a tropical environment. *Chemosphere* 2005;61(7):985-92. doi: 10.1016/j.chemosphere.2005.03.066

110. de Acevedo GT, McInerney MJ. Emulsifying activity in thermophilic and extremely thermophilic microorganisms. *J Ind Microbiol* 1996;16(1):1-7. doi: 10.1007/BF01569914

111. Willumsen PA, Karlson U. Screening of bacteria, isolated from pah-contaminated soils, for production of biosurfactants and bioemulsifiers. *Biodegradation* 1996;7(5):415-23. doi: 10.1007/BF00056425

112. Ron EZ, Rosenberg E. Biosurfactants and oil bioremediation. *Curr Opin Biotechnol* 2002;13(3):249-52. doi: 10.1016/S0958-1669(02)00316-6

113. Dagher F, Deziel E, Lirette P, Paquette G, Bisaillon JG, Villemur R. Comparative study of five polycyclic aromatic hydrocarbon degrading bacterial strains isolated from contaminated soils. *Can J Microbiol* 1997;43(4):368-77.

114. Leys NM, Ryngaert A, Bastiaens L, Top EM, Verstraete W, Springael D. Culture independent detection of sphingomonas sp. Epa 505 related strains in soils contaminated with polycyclic aromatic hydrocarbons (pahs). *Microb Ecol* 2005;49(3):443-50. doi: 10.1007/s00248-004-0011-0

21

A Review about Regulatory Status and Recent Patents of Pharmaceutical Co-Crystals

Arun Kumar (iD), **Sandeep Kumar** (iD), **Arun Nanda*** (iD)

Department of Pharmaceutical Sciences, Maharshi Dayanand University, Rohtak-124001, India.

Abstract

Pharmaceutical Co-crystals are not new, they have gained much attention since the last decade among scientists and pharmaceutical industry. Pharmaceutical co-crystals are multicomponent systems composed of two or more molecules and held together by non-covalent interactions. The development of pharmaceutical co-crystals, a new solid crystalline form, offer superior physico-chemical properties (such as melting point, stability, solubility, permeability, bioavailability, taste masking, etc.) without altering the pharmacological properties. Recently, with the upsurge in the growth of Pharmaceutical co-crystals, the major concern is over the regulatory status of co-crystals. With the new guidelines from United States Food and Drug Administration (USFDA) and European Medicines Agency (EMA), the status has become even more complicated due to significantly different opinions. This review highlights whether co-crystals fulfil the requirements for the grant of a patent or not and how cocrystals are going to affect the present scenario of pharmaceuticals.

Keywords:
· Pharmaceutical Co-crystals
· Crystal Engineering
· Regulatory guidelines
· Patents

Introduction

Pharmaceutical co-crystals have established a new paradigm in the solid-state modification. The formation of API co-crystal offers a wide range of physical and chemical enhancements to the properties of drugs without altering their chemical nature, thereby maintaining its pharmaceutical importance as such.[1] This is evident from the fact that regulatory bodies like United States Food and Drug Administration (USFDA) and European Medicines Agency (EMA) have published regulatory guidelines to clarify the status of co-crystals in their respective regions. Pharmaceutical and Biotechnology companies rely upon intellectual protection for safeguarding their products. In order to maintain revenues generated through these products as a means to recover the resources and money spent on research and development, the presence of proper regulatory guidelines is expected to significantly affect the development and quality control as well as intellectual properties aspects of pharmaceutical cocrystals and their formulations.[2]

However, the concern that remains unanswered is whether the standard development and manufacturing processes that were initially designed for salt-based formulations can also be used for co-crystal based formulations in order to achieve the desired product quality that is required to ensure the safety and efficacy.[3] Moreover, from regulatory perspective the addition of another component to the drug formulation could mandate additional bioequivalence, clinical and toxicity studies.

This article focuses on listing recent developments regarding regulatory status of co-crystals in different regulatory regions, the effect of these regulatory guidelines and intellectual protection in the field of crystal engineering. Another point to be probed is whether co-crystals are eligible for patent protection or not as per the literature and guidelines available on pharmaceutically acceptable co-crystals.

Pharmaceutical Co-Crystals

Poor solubility has been a crucial issue in the development of a pharmaceutical dosage form. Amorphous solids may be considered as a good choice but these solids have their own limitations related to stability.[4] The composition and the arrangement of molecules/ions in a crystal lattice directly affects the crystal properties, it means that exerting control over the composition by selecting a co-former from a wide range can lead to co-crystals of desired physicochemical properties. This was the reason crystal engineering gained impetus in pharmaceuticals for the enhancement of stability/solubility of pharmaceutical formulations.[5] Co-crystals can be made for both complex drugs containing sensitive functional groups as well as for drugs containing non-ionizable moieties and that is the unique advantage of co-crystals over salts. The other key advantages of co-crystals are that co-former modifies only the physicochemical properties of drug without altering the molecular structure and pharmacological properties of the drug.[6]

---

*Corresponding author: Arun Nanda, Email: an.pharmsciences@mdurohtak.ac.in

Cocrystals are a long known but understudied class of crystalline solids. In 1844, Wöhler was the first to obtain a co-crystal of the 1:1 ratio between Benzoquinone and Hydroquinone (Quinhydrone).[7] Desiraju in 1989 defined crystal engineering as "the understanding of intermolecular interactions in the context of crystal packing and in the utilization of such understanding in the design of new solids with desired physical and chemical properties".[8] However, pharmaceutical co-crystals have attracted interest from scientists in the past decade and now much of work has been done in this field, mainly because co-crystallization utilizes non-covalent interactions and supramolecular synthons to control the organisation of molecules inside the crystal lattice, co-crystals possess better thermodynamic stability, purity and processing characteristics over amorphous solids.[9]

In 2004, Almarsson and Zaworotko proposed the least controversial definition of co-crystals as "co-crystals are those that are formed between an active pharmaceutical ingredient (API) and a co-former also called as crystal former (CF), which under ambient conditions are solids. This definition is not limited to two components, that the co-crystal can be multi-component". The components in the co-crystal interact by hydrogen bonding or other non-ionic and non-covalent interactions such as halogen or π-π interactions.[10] In 2011, a bilateral meeting jointly sponsored by the Indo–U.S. Science and Technology Forum (IUSSTF) was held on Pharmaceutical Cocrystals and Polymorphs where meeting a generally accepted definition of co-crystals was evolved which reads as follows "Cocrystals are solids that are crystalline single-phase materials composed of two or more different molecular and/or ionic compounds generally in a stoichiometric ratio which are neither solvates nor simple salts".[11] USFDA defined that cocrystals are crystalline materials which are composed of two or more molecules in the same crystalline lattice and associated by non-ionic and non-covalent bonds.[12,13] Pharmaceutical co-crystals belong to a subclass of co-crystals wherein one of the components is a biologically active substance (an API) while the other one the co-former is drug or food grade substance (generally regarded as safe). Inside the crystal lattice the two components interact through non-covalent interactions such as hydrogen bonding in fixed stoichiometric ratio.[14]

The foundation of crystal engineering lies in the concept of supramolecular chemistry. The basic tenet of supramolecular chemistry is the molecular recognition between complementary molecular fragments giving rise to self-organization of molecules to give a supramolecular function.[15] Co-crystallization has been shown to significantly modify the physicochemical properties of drug substances such as the, permeability, bioavailability, solubility and dissolution rate, compaction and tableting, physical form, biochemical and hydration stability, melting point, etc.[6,14,16-18] Selection of suitable co-formers and screening of co-crystals for a drug are the main challenges to overcome during the process of cocrystal development. Selection of co-formers is mainly done by researchers using theoretical

or experimental approaches. Different approaches i.e. hydrogen bonding propensity, Cambridge Structure Database, supramolecular synthons,[18] ΔpKa values,[19] Fabine's method,[20] COSMO-RS screening,[21] Hansen solubility parameters,[22] virtual cocrystal screening,[23] thermal methods (including DSC screening,[24] hot stage microscopy[25] and saturation method[26,27]) and others methods are reported in the literature by the scientists for the selection of the appropriate co-former for a drug and screening of cocrystals.

Academicians and scientists reported various methods (such as solution based, grinding, and other advanced methods freeze drying, spray drying, hot melt extrusion, supercritical carbon dioxide processing, ultrasound crystallization and microfluidic jet dispersion) for the synthesis of cocrystals with their pros and cons.[14,28-31] Bavishi and Borkhataria described the "Spring and Parachute" concept for better understanding in the improvement of solubility and dissolution rate of drug.[32] Different characterization techniques such as structural analysis (crystallographic studies, Hirshfeld surface analysis and spectroscopic characterization), thermal analysis (Differential scanning calorimetry, thermogravimetric analysis and hot stage microscopy) and pharmaceutical characterizations (solubility and dissolution profile, stability, bioavailability and pharmacokinetic studies) have been used for determining the successful synthesis and pharmaceutical utility of cocrystals.[14,18,33]

A co-crystal is also possible between two biologically active molecules that is drug: drug co-crystal. The motive behind multidrug cocrystals is towards developing combination therapies, prevention of multi-drug resistance, synergistically increasing the action of drugs, reducing side effects, etc.[34] Bhatt et al., reported a co-crystal between Lamivudine and Zidovudine (both anti-viral drugs active against HIV).[35]

Regulatory prospects and patentability issues of Co-Crystals

Once a pharmaceutical cocrystal with promising results is developed, the next step would be gaining regulatory approval so that it can be brought to market. However, the lack of clear regulatory guidelines is a major issue to tackle with. Over the last decade, cocrystal development has seen enormous growth, there are even few patents granted for cocrystals. For an invention, in order to be patentable, the invention must fulfil the three conditions such as novelty, non-obviousness and utility or usefulness.[36,37]

Novelty

Desiraju in his book "Pharmaceutical salts and co-crystals: retrospect and prospects" mentioned that pharmaceutical co-crystals are new composition of matter and hence should satisfy the requirement of novelty for the grant of patent.[38] Andrew Trask in his article titled "An Overview of Pharmaceutical Cocrystals as Intellectual Property" also stated that pharmaceutical co-crystals should satisfy the novelty condition as equally as salts. Both Desiraju and Andrew emphasised that since co-former screening is a daunting work and co-formers are selected from a huge official list of GRAS compounds and the result of co-crystallization is not easily predictable, co-crystals may or may not be formed. Apart from this, the properties of the synthesized co-crystals cannot be anticipated. But the situation is completely different, FDA didn't even consider co-crystals in the same class as that of salts or polymorphs.[39]

Non-obviousness

Non-obviousness means that if someone skilled in the relevant field of technology and familiar with its subject matter invented it with comparative ease; such an "invention" would be novel but obvious to that person. Desiraju described that unlike salt formation wherein an acid is necessary to form a salt with a base, the identification of a co-former is hardly an ever routine.[38] According to Trask, in spite of a number of co-crystals screening methods available, there is no confirmed way to predict whether two molecules will form a hydrogen bond and a co-crystal will be formed. There are a lot of factors that govern the co-crystallization process and still there is a need to better understanding of this process. Moreover, co-crystal structure cannot be predicted from the available sources. Hence co-crystals well satisfy the Non-obviousness criteria too.[39]

Utility

In case of Pharmaceutical co-crystals, the only criteria that needs to be demonstrated in order to obtain a patent is utility or application of the invention. Co-crystals offer opportunities similar to that of polymorphs. They are clearly new substances, problems of inherent anticipation are not likely to arise so often and more of them can be made for any given API, expanding the pharmaceutical space around it and consequently the types of advantageous properties that may be accessed.[38] As per Trask, co-crystal of an API shares the same patentable therapeutic utility as its parent API. The enormous research on co-crystals in the past decade indicates that co-crystals offer vast opportunities for enhancement of the properties of an API, which in turn increases its utility and hence also the chances of patentability.[39]

Regulatory Perspectives

USFDA was the first regulatory body to publish guidelines for pharmaceutical co-crystals in 2013; the guidance classified Pharmaceutical co-crystals as drug product intermediate and treated them similar to API-excipient molecular complexes. Further the document stated that:

- The API and the co-former should exist in neutral states and interaction among them should be non-covalent/non-ionic.
- The value of ΔpKa should be less than 1 that is ΔpKa [pKa (base) - pKa (acid)] < 1.

- The API and the co-former should completely dissociate before reaching the site of pharmacological activity.[12]

The revised guidelines of FDA published in 2016, classify the pharmaceutical co-crystals as a special case of solvates and hydrates and placed pharmaceutical co-crystals in the regulatory classification similar to that of a polymorph of the API. Additionally, FDA required an *in-vitro* evaluation based on dissolution and/or solubility is generally considered sufficient to demonstrate that the active drug dissociates completely from the co-former.[13]

EMA's opinion on Pharmaceutical co-crystals differs considerably from that of FDA. EMA published a paper in 2014 about cocrystals and placed co-crystals in the same class as that of salts. The regulations also classify that co-crystals are eligible for generic application in the same way as salts. For a co-crystal to be considered as New Active Substance status (NAS), the co-crystals should demonstrate the difference in efficacy and/or safety with respect to that of API. NAS status for other routes of administration will be dependent on the therapeutic moiety that is present at the site of pharmacological action when compared to that of the authorised product.[40] The USFDA and EMA classification of Pharmaceutical co-crystals is summarised in Table 1.

Patents on Co-Crystals: Case Studies

Over the past decade, Pharmaceutical co-crystals have seen enormous growth and a large number of research papers and patents have been filed all over the world and till date, a number of patents related to co-crystals and multi-drug co-crystals have been approved. Some of the recently approved pharmaceutical co-crystal formulations and list of approved patents on pharmaceutical co-crystals in USA, Europe, International (worldwide) and multi-drug co-crystals patents have been enlisted in the Table 2, Table 3, Table 4 and Table 5 respectively.

Entresto

The US Food and Drug Administration (FDA) on July 7, 2015, approved a multidrug co-crystal formulation of sacubitril and valsartan (brand name Entresto, Novartis) to reduce the risk for cardiovascular and chronic heart failure. Entresto was a new oral combination approved through fast-track review.[41]

Lexapro

Lexapro is a co-crystal formulation composed of escitalopram and was approved in 2009 under the brand name Lexapro, for the treatment of major depressive and anxiety disorders.[42]

Steglatro

The Food and Drug Administration (USFDA) has approved Ertugliflozin co-crystal formulation (Ertugliflozin cocrystal with 5-oxo-proline) under the brand name Steglatro™.[43,44]

Suglat® (Ipragliflozin: L-proline)

An Ipragliflozin: L-Proline co-crystal of the molecular ratio 1:1 was developed by Astellas Pharma and Kotobuki Pharmaceuticals, Ipragliflozin is a sodium-glucose co-transporter-2 (SGLT2) inhibitor. The co-crystal formulation was approved and is available under the trade name Suglat® in Japan.[45,46]

TAK-020—Gentisic acid Co-crystals

Takeda pharmaceuticals developed a new co-crystal-based formulation named TAK-020 developed for the treatment of rheumatoid arthritis (Bruton's tyrosine kinase inhibitor). The co-crystal has completed phase-I clinical trials.[46]

Table 1. Comparison between United States Food & Drug Administration and European Medicines Agency guidelines[3]

Regulatory considerations	Food & Drug Administration guidance (2013 & 2016)	European Medicines Agency reflection paper (2015)
Regulatory category	Polymorph of the Active Pharmaceutical Ingredient	Active Pharmaceutical Ingredient
Composition	Active Pharmaceutical Ingredient & a food or drug grade co-former	Active Pharmaceutical Ingredient and co-former in fixed stoichiometric ratio
Interaction in crystal	Non-ionic/non-covalent interactions	Non-ionic/non-covalent interactions
Co-former role	Excipient	Reagent
New Chemical Entity /New Active Substance Registration	No	Possible if shown difference in efficacy/safety
Similarity with Active Pharmaceutical Ingredient	Similar	Similar unless demonstrated different efficacy/safety
Classification	Polymorph of Active Pharmaceutical Ingredient	Salts of Active Pharmaceutical Ingredient
Cocrystal and salt	Differences in interaction and regulatory pathways	Regulation dependent on efficacy/safety
Drug Master File/Active Substance Master File requirement	No	Required for New Active Substance registration

Aripiprazole

Aripiprazole is a co-crystal formulation available in the market under the brand name Abilify®, Abilify consists of co-crystals comprising aripiprazole and fumaric acid. Aripiprazole is a psychotropic drug useful for the treatment of schizophrenia.[47]

Tramadol-Celecoxib (1:1) Cocrystal

E-58425 comprising celecoxib and tramadol (1:1) was developed by Enantia and Esteve, R&D, Spain, and patented by Laboratorios Del. This is an example of multidrug cocrystal, which is under clinical development. Synergistic action between its components will help to achieve the therapeutic benefits at lower and tolerable doses of each component. A phase II proof-of-concept study in acute postoperative pain has shown that the cocrystals demonstrated superior efficacy and safety over both placebo and a standard. The co-crystal based formulation is currently in phase-III of clinical trials.[48-50] Some other patents about the novel cocrystals of tiotropium bromide and ticagrelor drugs have also been granted to Boehringer Ingelheim Pharma Gmbh Co and Astrazeneca respectively.[51]

Table 2. Composition patents issued in the USA for pharmaceutical cocrystals[2]

US Patent No.	Date of issue	Assignee	Compound(s)	Ref.
US6001996	14 Dec, 1999	Eli Lilly & Co., Inc.	Complexes of (carba)cephalosporins with parabens	52
US7446107	4 Nov, 2008	TransForm Pharmaceuticals, Inc.	Itraconazole; cocrystals with acarboxylic acid	53
US7625910	1 Dec, 2009	Astra Zeneca AB	AZD1152; a phosphate prodrug and maleic acid cocrystal	54
US8097592	17 Jan, 2012	Astellas Pharma Inc., Kotobuki Pharmaceutical Co. Ltd.	SGLT-2 Inhibitor, l-proline cocrystal	55
US8124603	28 Feb, 2012	Thar Pharmaceutical	Meloxicam with various carboxylic acids, aliphatic and aromatic, and maltol and ethyl maltol	56
US8163790	24 Apr, 2012	New Form Pharmaceuticals, Inc.	Metronidazole cocrystals with gentisic acid and gallic acid (specific x-ray reflections in each case) and a cocrystal of imipramine HCl and (+)-camphoric acid	57
US20170044176 A1	16 Feb, 2017	Euticals Spa	Cocrystal of tiotropium bromide and lactose monohydrate	58
US20170224724 A1	10 Aug, 2017	University Of South Florida	Co-crystal (ICC) of lithium with salicylic acid and 1-proline	59
US20170101433 A1	13 Apr, 2017	Amri Sci. Llc.	Co-crystal of progesterone and a co-former selected from the group consisting of vanillic acid, benzoic acid, salicylic acid, cinnamic acid, and vanillin	60

Table 3. European patents on Co-Crystals[2]

Patent no.	Date of issue	Assignee	Componds	Ref.
EP1755388B1	6 Oct, 2010	TransForm Pharmaceuticals, Inc.	Mixed cocrystals of modafinil	61
EP2185546B1	26 Oct, 2011	Vertex Pharmaceuticals, Inc.	Cocrystals and pharmaceutical compositions, telaprevir (VX-950)	62
EP2334687B1	4 Jan, 2012	Pfizer Inc.	SGLT-2 inhibitors, l-proline and pyroglutamic acid cocrystals	63
EP2300472B1	18 Jan, 2012	Boehringer Ingelheim Intl. GmBH	Glucocorticoid analogs, phosphoric acid and acetic acid cocrystals	64
EP2114924B1	25 Jan, 2012	Vertex Pharmaceuticals Inc.	Cocrystals of telaprevir with 4-hydroxybenzoic acid; solvates	65
EP2288606B1	15 Feb, 2012	Bayer Pharma Ag	Rivaroxaban cocrystal with malonic acid	66
EP1608339B1	21 Mar, 2012	McNeil PPC	Celecoxib cocrystal with nicotinamide	67
EP3210975 A1	30 Aug, 2017	Enantia, S.L.	Cocrystals of Lorcaserin hydrochloride and an organic diacid	68
EP3240575 A1	8 Nov, 2017	Dr. Reddy's Laboratories Ltd.	co-crystal of carfilzomib with maleic acid	69

Table 4. International patents on Co-Crystals

Patent no.	Date of issue	Assignee	Compounds	Ref.
WO2017191539 A1	9 Nov, 2017	Aurobindo Pharma Limited	dl-proline co-crystal of dapagliflozin	70
WO2017172811 A1	5 Oct, 2017	Intra-Cellular Therapies, Inc.	Co-crystal forms of 1-(4-fluoro-phenyl)-4-((6bR,10aS)-3-methyl-2,3,6b,9,10,10a-hexahydro-1H,7H-pyrido[3' 4':4,5]pyrrolo[1,2,3-de]quinoxalin-8-yl)-butan-1-one and isonicotinamide and nicotinamide.	71
WO2017144598 A1	31 Aug, 2017	Enantia, S.L.	Cocrystals of Lorcaserin hydrochloride and an organic diacid	72
WO2017115284 A1	6 Jul 2017	Leiutis Pharmaceuticals Pvt, Ltd.	Adipic acid co-crystal of Agomelatine	73
WO2016156127 A1	6 Oct 2016	Ratiopharm Gmbh	Co-crystal of ibrutinib and carboxylic acid	74

Table 5. Patents on multi-drug Co-Crystals[34]

Drug combination	Therapeutic category	Refs.
ASA–theanine	NSAID and psychoactive	75
Cyprodinil–dithianon	Fungicides	76
Ciprofloxacin and norfloxacin with various co-crystal formers	Antibacterial	77
Mesalamine with alpha amino acids, flavones, and nutraceuticals	Anti-inflammatory	78
Metformin–oleoylethanolamide	Antidiabetic and anti-obesity	79
Quercetin–metformin	Antioxidant and antidiabetic	80

Co-crystals and Evergreening of Patents

Ever-Greening and follow on patent are used to refer the patents that are filled to protect the additional aspects of further improvements to an invention. This provision of follow on patents to an existing invention was included in law so as to encourage further research as a means to obtain pharmaceutical products that are much safer and effective. While the terms "ever-greening patent" and "follow-on patent" are both used to refer to patents that protect pharmaceutical formulations, new forms of active agents, processes for manufacturing active agents, new uses for pharmaceutical products, new combinations of active agents, new dosing regimens, most of the pharmaceutical companies have ill practiced in this provision and have created picket fences of minor improvements filled over the parent patent and hence successfully thwarting any generic entry in the market and maintaining their monopoly for extended periods of time. While, Co-crystallisation is an approach that results in drug products that seem to satisfy the conditions of novelty, non-obviousness and utility but it may definitely stimulate investigation of older APIs for new benefits and this may in turn lead to ever greening of existing drug patents.[81]

Conclusion

Co-crystallization is a flourishing approach with direct application to the pharmaceutical industry. It is quite evident from the amount of interest shown by both academia and pharmaceutical industry that in near future pharmaceutical cocrystals will be one of the viable and important solid forms of pharmaceuticals that should be available in the market. The value of co-crystals to the pharmaceutical industry should become clearer, particularly with respect to several relevant legal and regulatory issues, as products containing cocrystal technology emerge from pharmaceutical development pipelines into the market. It will also lead to screening of older API's to see new benefits and improvements of existing drugs. Co-crystal formation offers tremendous scope for controlled modification of the key pharmaceutical properties such as dissolution rate, solubility, compressibility, melting point, stability, bioavailability and permeability. There is a need to explore into an understanding of cocrystallization mechanism, *in-vivo* behaviour of cocrystal for better therapeutics and other unanswered questions like polymorphic transformation, the concepts of supramolecular synthesis, and crystal engineering remain largely underexploited. Pharmaceutical cocrystals generally appear patentable when measured against the criteria of novelty, utility, and non-obviousness as evident from the fact that number of patents filed throughout the world by various pharmaceutical industries and research groups are also increasing at a fast pace. The challenges that lie ahead include scaling up the production of the pharmaceutical cocrystals, preceded by discovery of new scale up methods, and high throughput screening of the possible co-crystal with various co-formers and their polymorphs.

Acknowledgments

Authors thank Maharshi Dayanand University, Rohtak and University Grant Commission, New Delhi for providing University Research Fellowship and Basic Scientific Research Fellowship respectively, for working in the project.

Ethical Issues

Not applicable.

Conflict of Interest

The authors declare no conflict of interests.

References

1. Vishweshwar P, McMahon JA, Bis JA, Zaworotko MJ. Pharmaceutical co-crystals. *J Pharm Sci* 2006;95(3):499-516. doi: 10.1002/jps.20578

2. Almarsson O, Peterson ML, Zaworotko M. The A to Z of pharmaceutical cocrystals: a decade of fast-moving new science and patents. *Pharm Pat Anal* 2012;1(3):313-27. doi: 10.4155/ppa.12.29

3. Izutsu KI, Koide T, Takata N, Ikeda Y, Ono M, Inoue M, et al. Characterization and Quality Control of Pharmaceutical Cocrystals. *Chem Pharm Bull (Tokyo)* 2016;64(10):1421-30. doi: 10.1248/cpb.c16-00233

4. Leuner C, Dressman J. Improving drug solubility for oral delivery using solid dispersions. *Eur J Pharm Biopharm* 2000;50(1):47-60. doi: 10.1016/S0939-6411(00)00076-X

5. Perlovich GL, Manin AN. Design of Pharmaceutical Cocrystals for Drug Solubility Improvement. *Russ J Gen Chem* 2014;84(2):407-14. doi: 10.1134/S107036321402042X

6. Bolla G, Nangia A. Pharmaceutical cocrystals: walking the talk. *Chem Commun (Camb)* 2016;52(54):8342-60. doi: 10.1039/C6CC02943D

7. Wohler F. Untersuchungen über des chinons. *Annalen Chem Pharm* 1844;51:145-63.

8. Desiraju GR. Crystal Engineering: The Design of Organic Solids. Amsterdam: Elsevier; 1989.

9. Desiraju GR. Supramolecular synthons in crystal engineering—A new organic synthesis. *Angew Chem Int Ed Engl* 1995;34(21):2311-27. doi: 10.1002/anie.199523111

10. Almarsson Ö, Zaworotko MJ. Crystal engineering of the composition of pharmaceutical phases. Do pharmaceutical co-crystals represent a new path to improved medicines? *Chem Commun (Camb)* 2004;0(17):1889-96. doi: 10.1039/B402150A

11. Aitipamula S, Banerjee R, Bansal AK, Biradha K, Cheney ML, Choudhury AR, et al. Polymorphs, salts, and cocrystals: What's in a name? *Cryst Growth Des* 2012;12(5):2147-52. doi: 10.1021/cg3002948

12. Guidance for Industry: Regulatory Classification of Pharmaceutical Co-Crystals. Center for Drug Evaluation and Research, United States Food and Drug Administration. https://www.fda.gov/downloads/Drugs/Guidances/UCM281764.pdf. Accessed on: 5 Jan 2018.

13. Guidance for Industry: Regulatory Classification of Pharmaceutical Co-Crystals. Revision-1. Center for Drug Evaluation and Research, United States Food and Drug Administration. http://www.fda.gov/Drugs/GuidanceCompliance/Regulatoryinformation/Guidances/UCM516813.pdf. Accessed on: 5 Jan 2018.

14. Qiao N, Li M, Schlindwein W, Malek N, Davies A, Trappitt G. Pharmaceutical cocrystals: An overview. *Int J Pharm* 2011;419(1-2):1-11. doi: 10.1016/j.ijpharm.2011.07.037

15. Desiraju GR. Chemistry beyond the molecule. *Nature* 2001;412(6845):397-400. doi: 10.1038/35086640

16. Schultheiss N, Newman A. Pharmaceutical cocrystals and their physicochemical properties. *Cryst Growth Des* 2009;9(6):2950-67. doi: 10.1021/cg900129f

17. Duggirala NK, Perry ML, Almarsson O, Zaworotko MJ. Pharmaceutical cocrystals: along the path to

improved medicines. *Chem Commun (Camb)* 2016;52(4):640-55. doi: 10.1039/C5CC08216A

18. Kumar S, Nanda A. Pharmaceutical Cocrystals: An Overview. *Indian J Pharm Sci* 2017;79(6):858-71. doi: 10.4172/pharmaceutical-sciences.1000302

19. Cruz-Cabeza AJ. Acid-base crystalline complexes and the pK_a rule. *CrystEngComm* 2012;14(20):6362-5. doi: 10.1039/C2CE26055G

20. Laszlo F. Cambridge structural database analysis of molecular complementarity in cocrystals. *Cryst Growth Des* 2009;9(3):1436-43. doi: 10.1021/cg800861m

21. Abramov YA, Loschen C, Klamt A. Rational coformer or solvent selection for pharmaceutical cocrystallization or desolvation. *J Pharm Sci* 2012;101(10):3687-97. doi: 10.1002/jps.23227

22. Mohammad MA, Alhalaweh A, Velaga SP. Hansen solubility parameter as a tool to predict cocrystal formation. *Int J Pharm* 2011;407(1-2):63-71. doi: 10.1016/j.ijpharm.2011.01.030

23. Musumeci D, Hunter CA, Prohens R, Scuderi S, McCabe JF. Virtual cocrystal screening. *Chem Sci* 2011;2(5):883-90. doi: 10.1039/C0SC00555J

24. Lu E, Rodriguez-Hornedo N, Suryanarayanan R. A rapid thermal method for cocrystal screening. *CrystEngComm* 2008;10(6):665-8. doi: 10.1039/B801713C

25. Berry DJ, Seaton CC, Clegg W, Harrington RW, Coles SJ, Horton PN, et al. Applying hot-stage microscopy to co-crystal screening: a study of nicotinamide with seven active pharmaceutical ingredients. *Cryst Growth Des* 2008;8(5):1697-712. doi: 10.1021/cg800035w

26. Ross SA, Lamprou DA, Douroumis D. Engineering and manufacturing of pharmaceutical co-crystals: a review of solvent-free manufacturing technologies. *Chem Commun (Camb)* 2016;52(57):8772-86. doi: 10.1039/C6CC01289B

27. Malamatari M, Ross SA, Douroumis D, Velaga SP. Experimental cocrystal screening and solution based scale-up cocrystallization methods. *Adv Drug Deliv Rev* 2017;117:162-77. doi: 10.1016/j.addr.2017.08.006

28. Douroumis D, Ross SA, Nokhodchi A. Advanced methodologies for cocrystal synthesis. *Adv Drug Deliv Rev* 2017;117:178-95. doi: 10.1016/j.addr.2017.07.008

29. Karki S, Friscic T, Jones W, Motherwell WD. Screening for pharmaceutical cocrystal hydrates via neat and liquid-assisted grinding. *Mol Pharm* 2007;4(3):347-54. doi: 10.1021/mp0700054

30. Aher S, Dhumal R, Mahadik K, Paradkar A, York P. Ultrasound assisted cocrystallization from solution (USSC) containing a non-congruently soluble cocrystal component pair: Caffeine/maleic acid. *Eur J Pharm Sci* 2010;41(5):597-602. doi: 10.1016/j.ejps.2010.08.012

31. Alhalaweh A, Velaga P. Formation of cocrystals from stoichiometric solutions of incongruently saturating

systems by spray drying. *Cryst Growth Des* 2010;10(8):3302-5. doi: 10.1021/cg100451q

32. Bavishi DD, Borkhataria CH. Spring and parachute: How cocrystals enhance solubility. *Prog Cryst Growth Charact Mater* 2016;62(3):1-8. doi: 10.1016/j.pcrysgrow.2016.07.001

33. Pindelska E, Sokal A, Kolodziejski W. Pharmaceutical cocrystals, salts and polymorphs: Advanced characterization techniques. *Adv Drug Deliv Rev* 2017;117:111-46. doi: 10.1016/j.addr.2017.09.014

34. Thipparaboina R, Kumar D, Chavan RB, Shastri NR. Multidrug co-crystals: towards the development of effective therapeutic hybrids. *Drug Discov Today* 2016;21(3):481-90. doi: 10.1016/j.drudis.2016.02.001

35. Bhatt PM, Azim Y, Thakur TS, Desiraju GR. Co-crystals of the anti-HIV drugs lamivudine and zidovudine. *Cryst Growth Des* 2009;9(2):951-7. doi: 10.1021/cg8007359

36. USPTO. United States Patent and Trademark Office. [10 Jan 2018]; Available from: http://www.uspto.gov.

37. EPO. European Patent Office. [10 Jan 2018]; Available from: http://www.epo.org.

38. Desiraju GR. Pharmaceutical salts and co-crystals: retrospect and prospects. In: Wouters J, Quéré L, editors. Pharmaceutical Salts and Co-crystals. Cambridge: RSC Publishing; 2011. PP. 1-8.

39. Trask AV. An overview of pharmaceutical cocrystals as intellectual property. *Mol Pharm* 2007;4(3):301-9. doi: 10.1021/mp070001z

40. Reflection paper on the use of cocrystals of active substances in medicinal products. Committee for Medicinal Products for Human Use. European Medicines Agency. http://www.ema.europa.eu/docs/en_GB/document_library/Scientific_guideline/2015/07/WC500189927.pdf . Accessed on: 5 Jan 2018.

41. Fala L. Entresto (Sacubitril/Valsartan): First-in-Class Angiotensin Receptor Neprilysin Inhibitor FDA Approved for Patients with Heart Failure. *Am Health Drug Benefits* 2015;8(6):330-4.

42. Harrison WT, Yathirajan HS, Bindya S, Anilkumar HG, Devaraju. Escitalopram oxalate: co-existence of oxalate dianions and oxalic acid molecules in the same crystal. *Acta Crystallogr C* 2007;63(Pt 2):o129-31. doi: 10.1107/S010827010605520X

43. Mascitti V, Thuma BA, Smith AC, Robinson RP, Brandt T, Kalgutkar AS, et al. On the importance of synthetic organic chemistry in drug discovery: reflections on the discovery of antidiabetic agent ertugliflozin. *MedChemComm* 2013;4(1):101-11. doi: 10.1039/C2MD20163A

44. Pfizer.com. Press Release Pfizer. [10 Jan 2018]; Available from: https://www.pfizer.com/news/press-release/press-release-detail/fda_approves_sglt2_inhibitor_steglatro_ertugliflozin_and_fixed_dose_combination_steglujan_ertugliflozin_and_sitagliptin_for_adults_with_type_2_diabetes.

45. Poole RM, Dungo RT. Ipragliflozin: first global approval. *Drugs* 2014;74(5):611-7. doi: 10.1007/s40265-014-0204-x

46. Chavan RB, Thipparaboina R, Yadav B, Shastri NR. Continuous manufacturing of co-crystals: challenges and prospects. *Drug Deliv Transl Res* 2018;19:1-4. doi: 10.1007/s13346-018-0479-7

47. Devarakonda SN, Vyas K, Bommareddy SR, Padi PR, Raghupathy B. Inventors; Reddy's Laboratories Ltd, Reddy's Laboratories Inc, assignee. Aripiprazole co-crystals. United States patent application US 2009; 12/278,022.

48. esteve.es. [8 Jan 2018]; Available from: http://www.esteve.es/EsteveFront/es/en/jsp/idi_rd_po rtfolio_E-58425.jsp.

49. clinicaltrials.gov. United States National Library of Medicine. [15 Feb 2018]; Available from: https://clinicaltrials.gov/ct2/show/NCT03108482?con d=co-crystals&rank=1.

50. clinicaltrialsregister.eu. EU Clinical Trials Register. [15 Feb 2018]; Available from: https://www.clinicaltrialsregister.eu/ctr-search/search?query=E-58425.

51. freshpatents.com. Fresh Patents. [15 Feb 2018]; Available from: http://www.freshpatents.com/-dt20111020ptan20110257215.php.

52. Amos JG, Indelicato JM, Pasini CE, Reutzel SM. Complexes of cephalosporins and carbacephalosporins with parabens. US Patent 6001996A. Eli Lilly and Co Ltd (GB); 1995.

53. Remenar J, MacPhee M, Peterson M, Morissette S, Almarsson O. Crystalline forms of conazoles and methods of making and using the same. US Patent 7446107. TransForm Pharmaceuticals Inc; 2002.

54. Sependa GJ, Storey R. AZD1152; a phosphate prodrug and maleic acid cocrystal. US Patent 7625910. Astra Zeneca AB.

55. Imamura M, Nakanishi K, Shiraki R, Onda K, Sasuga D, Yuda M. Cocrystal of C-glycoside derivative and L-proline. US Patent 8097592. Astellas Pharma Inc./Kotobuki Pharmaceutical Co. Ltd; 2006.

56. Hanna M, Shan N, Cheney ML, Weyna DR. In vivo studies of crystalline forms of meloxicam. US Patent 8124603. Grunenthal GmbH/Thar Pharmaceuticals; 2008.

57. Childs SL. Metronidazole cocrystals and imipramine cocrystals. US Patent 8163790. New Form Pharmaceuticals, Inc; 2006.

58. Grisenti P, Argese M, Scrocchi R, Livieri A, Guazzi G. Crystalline form of tiotropium bromide with lactose. US Patent 20170044176 A1. Euticals Spa; 2014.

59. Tan J, Shytle RD. Ionic cocrystal of lithium, lispro, for the treatment of fragile x syndrome. US Patent 20170224724 A1. University Of South Florida; 2016.

60. Albert E, Andres P, Bevill MJ, Smit J, Nelson J. Cocrystals of progesterone. US Patent 20170101433 A1. AMRI SSCI LLC; 2012.

61. Oliveira M, Peterson M. Mixed co-crystals and pharmaceutical compositions comprising the same. EU Patent 1755388B1. TransForm Pharmaceuticals, Inc.

62. Zhang Y, Connelly PR, Johnston S. Co-crystals and pharmaceutical compositions comprising the same. EU Patent 2185546B1. Vertex Pharmaceuticals, Inc; 2011.

63. Mascitti V, Collman BM. Dioxa-bicyclo[3.2.1.]octane-2,3,4-triol derivatives. EU Patent 2334687B1. Pfizer Inc.

64. Ingelheim Pharma Gmbh & Co. Kg Boehringer, Betageri R, Bosanac T, Burke MJ, Harcken C, Kim S, et al. Glucocorticoid mimetics, methods of making them, pharmaceutical compositions, and uses thereof. EU Patent 2300472B1. Boehringer Ingelheim Intl. GmBH.

65. Connelly PR, Kadiyala I, Stavropolus K, Zhang Y, Johnston S, Bhisetti GR, et al. Co-crystals and pharmaceutical compositions comprising the same. EU Patent 2114924B1. Vertex Pharmaceuticals Inc; 2007.

66. Grunenberg A, Queckenberg KF, Reute C, Keil B, Gushurst KS, Still EJ. New co-crystal compound of rivaroxaban and malonic acid. EU Patent 2288606B1. Bayer Pharma Ag.

67. Almarsson Ö, BourgholHM, Peterson M, Zaworotko MJ, Moulton B, Hornedo NR. Pharmaceutical co-crystal of celecoxib-nicotinamide. EU Patent 1608339B1. University of South Florida Johnson and Johnson Consumer Inc University of Michigan; 2003.

68. Tesson N, Esther C. Cocrystals of lorcaserin. EU Patent 3210975 A1. ENANTIA SL; 2016.

69. Kumar R, Vasam NS, Makireddy SR, Murki V, Ganorkar R, Jose J, et al. Co-crystal of carfilzomib with maleic acid and process for the preparation of pure carfilzomib. EU Patent 3240575 A1. Dr. Reddy's Laboratories Ltd; 2014.

70. Kumar S, Kishore N, Vittal, Sivakumaran MS. Process for the preparation dl-proline co-crystal of dapagliflozin. WO Patent 2017191539A1. Aurobindo Pharma Limited; 2016.

71. Wennogle LP, Li P, Aret E. Novel co-crystals. WO Patent 2017172811 A1. Intra-Cellular Therapies, Inc; 2016.

72. Tesson N, Gordo CE. Cocrystals of lorcaserin. WO Patent 2017144598 A1. Enantia, S.L; 2016.

73. Kocherlakota C, Banda N. Novel co-crystal forms of agomelatine. WO Patent 2017115284 A1. Leiutis Pharmaceuticals Pvt, Ltd; 2015.

74. Albrecht W, Geier J, Sebastian, Perez D. Co-crystals of ibrutinib with carboxylic acids. WO Patent2016156127 A1. Ratiopharm Gmbh; 2015.

75. Smith AJ, Kim SH, Duggirala NK, Jin J, Wojtas L, Ehrhart J, et al. Improving lithium therapeutics by crystal engineering of novel ionic cocrystals. *Mol Pharm* 2013;10(12):4728-38. doi: 10.1021/mp400571a

76. Ong TT, Kavuru P, Nguyen T, Cantwell R, Wojtas L, Zaworotko MJ. 2:1 Cocrystals of homochiral and achiral amino acid zwitterions with Li⁺ salts: Water-stable zeolitic and diamondoid metal-organic materials. *J Am Chem Soc* 2011;133(24):9224-7. doi: 10.1021/ja203002w

77. Kruthiventi A, Roy S, Goud R, Javed I, Nangia A, Reddy JS. Synergistic pharmaceutical cocrystals. WO Patent 2009136408A4. Institute Of Life Sciences, S.O.C., University Of Hyderabad.

78. Dandela R, Reddy JS, Viswanadha GS, Nagalapalli R, Solomon AK, Gaddamanugu G, et al. Novel cocrystals/molecular salts of mesalamine to be used as improved anti-inflammatory drug. WO Patent 2012090224A1. Nutracryst Therapeutics Private Limited; 2010.

79. Reddy JS, Dandela R, Viswanadha GS, Nagalapalli R, Solomon AK, Javed I, et al. Novel cocrystals / molecular salts of metformin with oleoylethanolamide as an effective anti-diabetic + anti- obesity agent. WO Patent 2012090225A2. Nutracryst Therapeutics Private Limited; 2010.

80. Kruthiventi AK, Javed I, Jaggavarapu SR, Nagalapalli R, Viswanadha GS, Anand SK. Pharmaceutical co-crystals of quercetin. WO Patent 2010134085A1. Nutracryst Therapeutics Private Limited; 2009.

81. Kumar A, Nanda A. Ever-greening in Pharmaceuticals: Strategies, Consequences and Provisions for Prevention in USA, EU, India and Other Countries. *Pharm Regul Aff* 2017;6:1-6. doi: 10.4172/2167-7689.1000185

22

Effect of *Onopordon acanthium* L. as Add on Antihypertensive Therapy in Patients with Primary Hypertension Taking Losartan: a Pilot Study

Roshanak Ghods[1,2]*, Manouchehr Gharouni[3], Massoud Amanlou[4], Niusha Sharifi[4], Ali Ghobadi[1,2], Gholamreza Amin[5]

[1] *Research Institute for Islamic and Complementary Medicine, Iran University of Medical Sciences, Tehran, Iran.*

[2] *School of Persian Medicine, Iran University of Medical Sciences, Tehran, Iran.*

[3] *Faculty of Medicine, Tehran University of Medical Sciences, Tehran, Iran.*

[4] *Department of Medicinal Chemistry, Faculty of Pharmacy, Tehran University of Medical Sciences, Tehran, Iran.*

[5] *Department of Pharmacognosy, Faculty of Pharmacy, Tehran University of Medical Sciences, Tehran, Iran.*

Keywords:
· *Onopordon acanthium* L
· Hypertension
· Blood pressure
· Angiotensin converting enzyme
· Persian medicine

Abstract

Purpose: *Onopordon acanthium* L. is known for its medicinal properties. Our recent study showed that its seed extract is a novel natura angiotensin-converting-enzyme inhibitor (ACEI). This study was carried out to investigate its possible antihypertensive effects in patients receiving losartan.

Methods: This uncontrolled clinical trial was carried out among 20 patients (30-60y) with uncontrolled hypertension despite receiving 50 mg losartan (stage I & II) in two hospitals in Iran. After completing informed consent, patients were treated by 2 capsules [each 1g of *Onopordon acanthium seed extract* (OSE)] as add-on therapy, two times per day.

Results: 18 patients completed the study (50.94 ±8.37y). Mean systolic blood pressure (SBP) at the baseline was 151.9 ± 13.74mmHg and at the end of the study, it was 134.6 ± 18.25 mmHg and mean diastolic blood pressure (DBP) was 97.41 ± 10.36 at the baseline and was 85.71 ± 7.481 after 8 weeks. OSE significantly reduced SBP and DBP at the end of 8 weeks (P=0.003, 95% CI: -19.7, -15.1; P=0.0006, 95% CI: -10.23, -13.15; respectively). No evidence of hepatic or renal toxicity was detected.

Conclusion: Based on the results of this study OSE has antihypertensive property with no significant adverse effects. However, because of the low number of samples, this medication may be not safely administered. The results of this study could be the basis for further studies with larger sample size.

IRCT registration number: IRCT2013020712391N.

Introduction

Hypertension (HTN) is a global concern and affects approximately 75 million adults in the United States and if left untreated increases risk of stroke, myocardial infarction, vascular disease, and chronic kidney disease.[1,2] Diagnosis and treatment of high blood pressure are essential to prevent mortality and morbidity.[2,3] Hypertension may be treated by using routine drugs such as angiotensin-converting-enzyme (ACE) inhibitors, beta-blockers, diuretics, calcium channel blockers, alpha-blockers, and peripheral vasodilators,[3,4] improving lifestyle factors including weight loss, quitting smoking, reducing sodium intake, regular exercise and limiting alcohol consumption.[5] These recommendations may be used alone or in combination with others[4]. Losartan is an oral medication that belongs to a class of drugs called angiotensin receptor blocker (ARBs) which was approved by the U.S. Food and Drug Administration (FDA) in April 1995. Losartan blocks the angiotensin receptor, relaxes muscle cells and dilates blood vessels and reduces blood pressure.[6,7]

Our recent study showed that the OSE is a novel natural inhibitor agent and inhibit angiotensin-converting-enzyme by 80.2 ± 2 % at concentration of 330 μg/ml, and exerted antioxidant activity (IC$_{50}$ value of 2.6 ± 0.04 mg/ml).[8] This plant has been well known under the name "Khaje Bashi"[9] and has long been used in folk medicine as a hypotensive, cardiotonic and diuretic agent.[10] Also it has been noted in Persian Medicine (PM) literatures as diuretic, diaphoretic, antipyretic, analgesic. Cotton thistle or Scotch thistle are its common names. It is a flowering plant belonging to the Compositae (Asteraceae) family and is widely naturalized almost globally, particularly in Europe and Western Asia and is a vigorous biennial plant with coarse, spiny leaves and conspicuous spiny-winged stems.[11] In modern medicine, *O. acanthium* has been reported to be a bactericide, cardiotonic, hypotensive and hemostatic agent and is used against hypotonicity.[12-14] This species has several bioactive components among which sesquiterpene lactones have been found to have numerous biological properties including antibacterial,

*Corresponding author: Roshanak Ghods, Email: Ghods.r@iums.ac.ir

anti-inflammatory, anti-malarial, and hypotensive effects.[15] Since the antihypertensive effect of *O. acanthium* seed extract has not been studied on patients in follow up of our previous in vitro study, we conducted this trial to investigate the possible antihypertensive effects of OSE on patients with stage I-II hypertension who were under treatment with losartan, a chemical ACE inhibitor, as add-on therapy.

Materials and Methods
Plant material
O. acanthium L. dried seeds were purchased from the local market in Tehran (Grand Bazaar), Iran. The seeds were identified by Prof. Gholamreza Amin and were kept under the voucher number PMP–714 at the herbarium of Faculty of Pharmacy, Tehran University of Medical Sciences.

Preparation of the extract and drug formulation
The extract was prepared in the laboratory of traditional pharmacy at faculty of Traditional Medicine, Tehran university of medical sciences via maceration method using ethanol as the solvent (1:8) at three time points (24, 48 and 72 h). The three extracts were mixed, filtered and evaporated. The total evaporated extract was freeze-dried and grinderies to obtain a powder for preparing the capsule. Each capsule contained 1g of the freeze-dried powder equal to 11 gram of dried seeds, and all the physiochemical quality control (QC) tests were performed on the capsules.

Toxicology evaluation
To measure the toxic dose of total extract of OSE (*Khaje Bashi* plant), rats were used and kept at the Animal house of the Faculty of Pharmacy, Tehran University of Medical Sciences. Animals were kept in standard light (12 hours of light and 12 hours of darkness), room temperature (25-35 °C) with adequate water and food. 12 male albino NMRI mice were divided into three groups (4 animals per group). The whole extract of the plant was taken in dried form and stored in a dark bottle in the refrigerator until it was tested. Due to its low solubility, the extract was dissolved in dimethyl sulfoxide (DMSO) at a desired concentration and diluted with normal saline at a rate of 1:3 and made as a monotonous suspension.

The solution was injected intraperitoneally (i.p.). Animals received the same amount of DMSO in different dose groups. Animals' condition (lethargy and movement) and animal death were investigated for 24-48 hours. In each group, mortality rate was reported and plotted against the dose used. The dose that causes 50 percent of deaths in animals or "Lethal Dose, 50%" (LD_{50}) was calculated based on the curve.

Considering that no studies have been done on the toxicity of this plant, in the first step, 0.5, 1, 2, 3.5 and 5 g/kg of body weight were used to find the dose range, but no mortality or change was observed in animals. In the next step, doses of 6-20 g/kg were used, and in dose 20, all animals died. In the next stage, the range of 6-13.5 g/kg

was tested in 6 groups of animals. The results were calculated as a percentage of death for each group. LD_{50} was calculated using non-linear sigmoid regression and Probit method. Meanwhile, the relationship between effective dose and effect was analyzed using Pearson's relationship and according to the results of these experiments, the lethal dose (LD_{50} value of 8.44 ± 0.04 g/kg) was determined. According to these results, the extract of this plant was classified in "practically non-poisonous ".

Clinical trial design
This open-labeled, non-randomized, uncontrolled clinical trial, a pilot study, was performed on 20 patients, who were under losartan treatment (50mg/d) for at least 6 weeks before starting the study and their blood pressure constantly remained higher than 140/90 (stage I&II) hypertension according to the seventh report of the joint national committee (JNC VII) report.[16] Sample size was calculated as follow: based on predicted 14 mmHg reduction of systolic blood pressure (d=14) at the end point (after 8 weeks), standard deviation 20 (σ=20, power 80%, confidence interval (CI) of 95% ($Z_{1-\alpha/2}$=1.96) and taking into account a correlation of 0.5 between frequent measurements and considering 20 % loss to follow, 20 patients were enrolled to determine the effective dose of therapy. Each individual took 2 capsules, two times a day (2 g/BD) and blood pressure was checked every other week. If blood pressure has increased more than 15 mmHg, the patients would have dropped out the study.

The primary outcome measure was systolic and diastolic blood pressure that was measured using aneroid sphygmomanometer (F. Bosch, Model: 0123, Germany). Metabolic parameters (lipid profile, liver function tests, BUN, Cr, FBS) were measured two times during the study (at the beginning and at the end of study) at Noor laboratory to evaluate the general health status of the patients.

Participants
The patients (30-60 y) were selected from Imam Khomeini & Amir-alam hospitals of Tehran University of medical sciences. Patients with history of malignant hypertension, blood pressure higher than 200/140 mmHg and whom needed multi-drug treatment or emergency IV drug infusion, history of secondary hypertension, end organ damages (EOD), sudden increase of blood pressure to greater than 15 mmHg at any time during the study, cardiac arrhythmias, symptomatic valvular heart diseases (except mitral valve prolapse) were excluded from the study. Other exclusion criteria were: diabetes type 1& 2, liver disorders, pregnancy breast feeding, cured or uncured malignancies during the last 5 years, serum potassium >5.2 or <3.5 mEq/L in the first visit, drug or alcohol abuse. The procedure was explained to all patients and written informed consents were obtained. Patients were examined at the beginning of the study and then every two weeks, and their arterial blood pressure was measured. The researcher's contact number was also

provided to patients in order to report any problems between every two visits. In addition, patients were asked at each session about possible complications such as coughing, severe headache, visual impairment, any types of arrhythmias, and orthostatic hypotension, and were recorded. Demographic and baseline data, medical history and any concomitant medications of enrolled patients were recorded. The study protocol was approved by the ethics committee of Research Institute for Islamic and Complementary Medicine of Iran University of Medical Sciences at 09/10/2012 with reference number 732/P26/M/T.

Statistical methods
The changes in blood pressure were analyzed using repeated measures ANOVA analysis. P value <0.05 was considered significant. The LD_{50} was calculated using nonlinear sigmoid regression and Probit technique. Moreover, the correlation between effect and administered dose was analyzed using Pearson correlation test.

Results and Discussion
Cytotoxicity of the extract was performed in mice by injecting different doses of OSE (0.5-13.5 g/kg) to measure the minimum toxic dose of OSE and LD_{50} was 8.44 ± 0.04 g/kg. Sampling began on May 21, 2013 and continued for five months, till October 23, 2013. 54 patients were assessed. Only 24 patients met the inclusion criteria whom four were not willing to participate in the study. At the end, 18 patients (of 20) completed the study and two patients were left the study due to increased blood pressure more than 160/100 mmHg in one patient after 2 days and another, after 3 days from starting point. Based on the ethical issues and respect to the patients' right, they were excluded and researcher referred both of them to the cardiologist to be treated with two or more drugs (Figure 1).

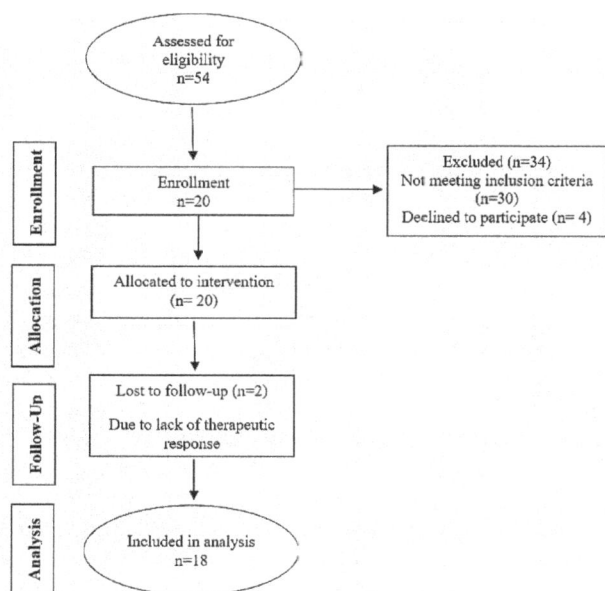

Figure 1. The trial flowchart

Patients took 2 capsules two times a day (2 g/BD) and were visited every other week and systolic and diastolic blood pressure and any possible side effects were recorded (Table 1).

Table 1. Blood pressure changes (before and after the study)

Blood pressure(mmHg)	Time	Mean ± SD
Systolic blood pressure (SBP)	at baseline	151.9 ± 13.74
	after 8 weeks	134.6 ± 18.25
Diastolic blood pressure (DBP)	at baseline	97.41 ± 10.36
	after 8 weeks	85.71 ± 7.48

After treatment for at least 8 weeks, systolic and diastolic blood pressure decreased significantly (P=0.003, 95% CI: -19.7, -15.1; P=0.0006, 95% CI: -10.23, -13.15; respectively) (Table 2). Moreover systolic and diastolic blood pressure decreased after 45 days treatment (P=0.025, 95% CI: -15.4, -10.6; P=0.034, 95% CI: -7.71, -7.85; respectively). At the end of the study, OSE decreased systolic and diastolic blood pressure 17.3 and 11.7 mmHg, respectively. (Figure 2, A & B).

Table 2. Baseline characteristics of participants and changes in systolic and diastolic BP.

Demographic characteristics		
Age	y (mean ± SD)	50.94 ± 8.73
BMI	kg/m² (mean ± SD)	30.4 ± 4.84
Male	n (%)	7 (35)
Sample size	n	20
Blood pressure(mmHg)		
Systolic blood pressure (SBP)	After 2 weeks	~ -11
	After 4 weeks	~ -9.9
	After 6 weeks	~ -13
	After 8 weeks	~ -17.3
Diastolic blood pressure (DBP)	After 2 weeks	~ -4.3
	After 4 weeks	~ -4.59
	After 6 weeks	~ -7.79
	After 8weeks	~ -11.7

We did not observe hepatic or renal toxicity as the result of *O. acanthium* extract consumption in patients during the study.

The results of these tests showed no significant changes (CBC, FBS, TG, Chol, LDL, HDL, SGOT, SGPT, BUN, Cr). As shown in the following diagrams, although these changes were not significant, in some cases, such as glucose, cholesterol, triglyceride, LDL, VLDL, and BUN, there was a tendency to reduction. Based on these results, HDL levels show a modest increase. The levels of sodium and creatinine were almost constant. The amount of potassium and liver enzymes were in the normal range (Figures 3 & 4). In general the changes of liver enzymes levels before and after treatment was not significant (P=0.1481; P=0.1400, respectively) (Figure 5).

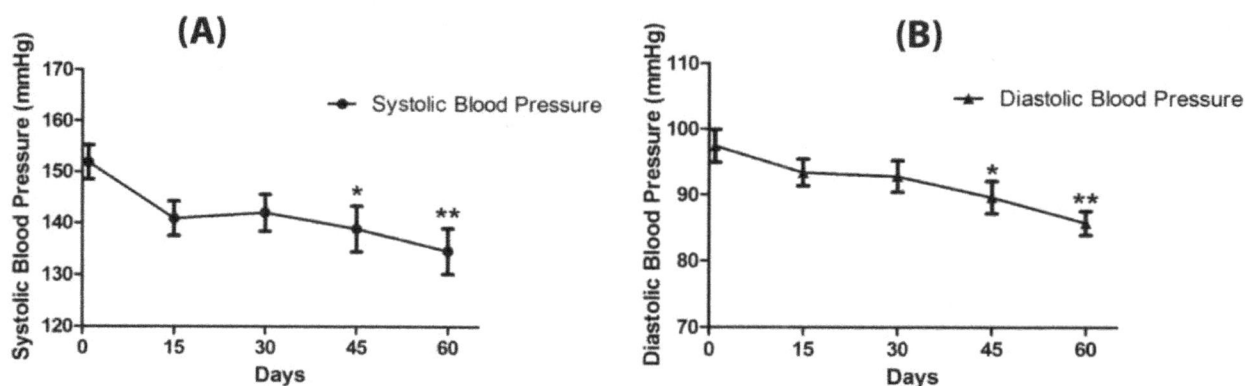

Figure 2. Blood pressure changes during treatment. Systolic (A) and diastolic blood pressures (B) have been measured at multiple time points: on the first day of investigation, 15, 30, 45, and 60 days after treatment (mean ± SEM). Decline of blood pressure at different time points have been compared with the blood pressure at the beginning of the investigation. There was a significant decline of blood pressure beyond 45 days of treatment when compared with the blood pressure before treatment (the asterisks indicate $P < 0.05$, repeated measures ANOVA analysis).

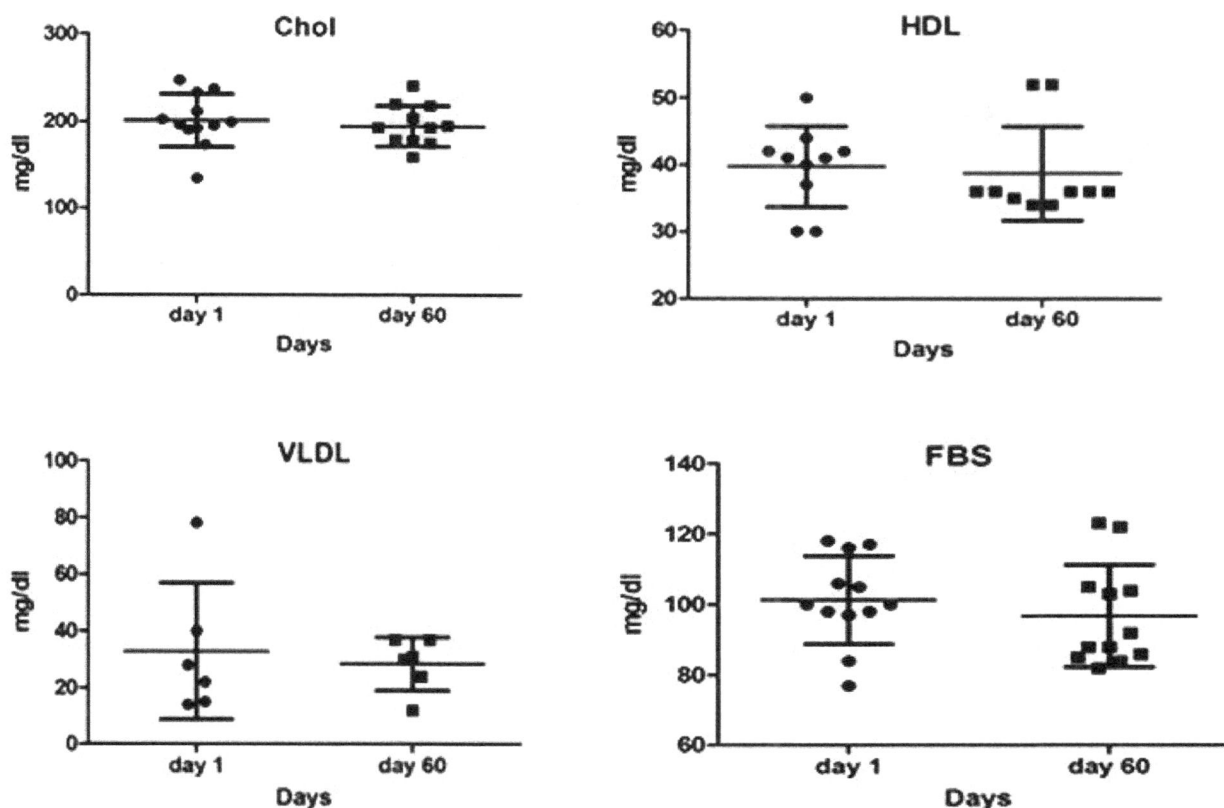

Figure 3. Changes in metabolic factors compared with the beginning of the intervention. After analysis, student t-test did not change significantly. $P < 0.05$ was considered as a significant level.

Regarding the side effects, we detected mild dyspnea in two patients after 2 weeks. Also two patients showed dizziness and feeling of heaviness in the head in the first month of treatment that resolved later.

These data indicated that 4 g/day of *O. acanthium* seed extract for 8 weeks significantly decreases systolic and diastolic blood pressure in patients with stage I and II primary essential hypertension under losartan treatment. In line with our recent findings in which a novel compound was extracted and identified from *O. acanthium* named Onopordia, OSE showed antioxidant and angiotensin converting enzyme inhibitor (ACEI) activity (80.2 ± 2 %). Its potential of blood pressure decreasing can be due to its different components such as sesquiterpenes and flavoncid.[8] There is no study on evaluating the effects of *O. acanthium* on blood pressure; however, some studies around the world have evaluated the hypotensive effect of some popular and well-known hypotensive herbal medicines.

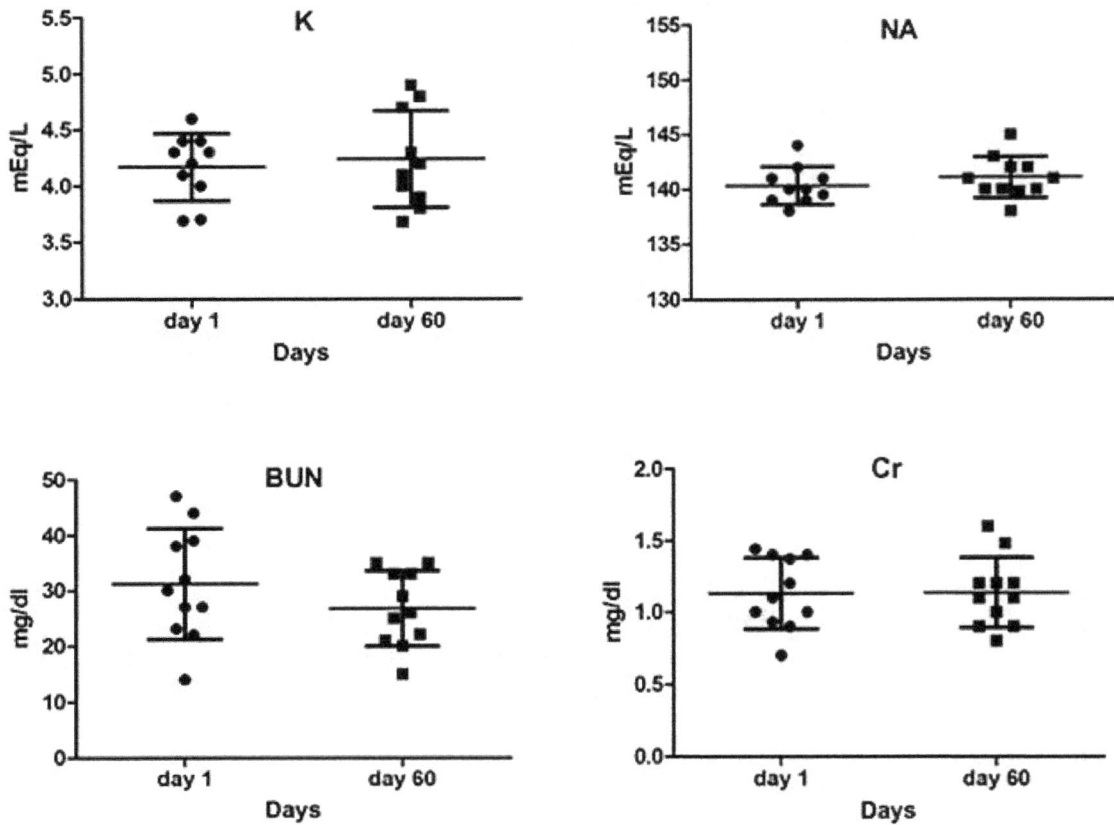

Figure 4. Changes in electrolytes and renal tests compared with the beginning of the intervention. After analysis, student t-test did not change significantly. P <0.05 was considered as a significant level.

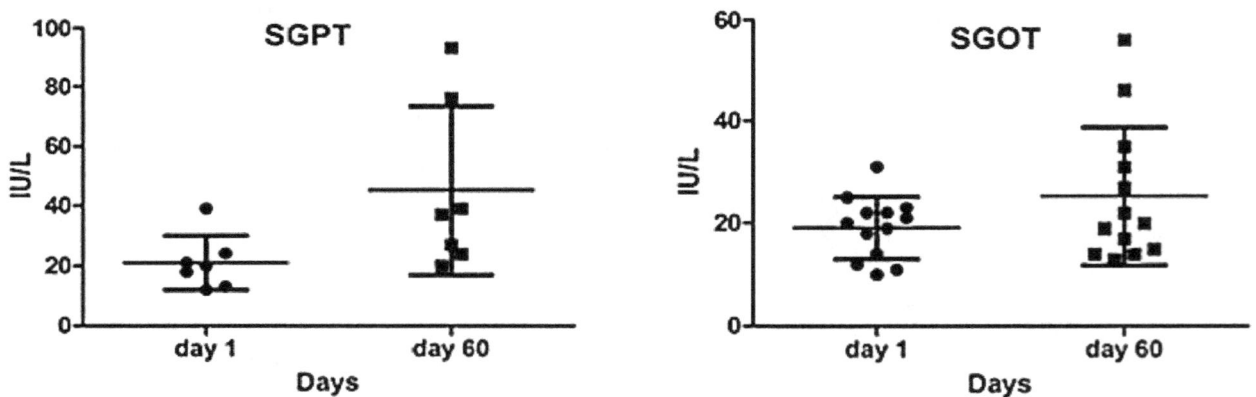

Figure 5. Changes in the liver function tests compared to the beginning of the intervention. After analysis, student t-test did not change significantly. P <0.05 was considered as a significant level.

Asgary et al., in a study in Iran, administered *Achillea wilhelmsii* to 120 patients for 8 weeks and showed significant decline of systolic and diastolic blood pressure (P=0.005 and P=0.003, respectively).[17] Walker et al., administered 500 mg/day of dried, full-spectrum aqueous-alcoholic extract of hawthorn (*Crataegus laevigata*) leaves and flowers to 36 patients with essential HTN for 10 weeks and found that diastolic blood pressure decreased in 19 patients. However the difference was not significant (P=0.08).[18] In a follow up study Walker et al., evaluated the hypotensive effect of *Crataegus laevigata*, 1200mg/day for 16 weeks on 76 patients and indicated significant decrease in diastolic (P=0.03) but no significant decrease in systolic blood pressure (P=0.32).[19] Consistent with these findings Ried, et al. indicated that treatment with aged garlic extract for 12 weeks lowered systolic blood pressure 10.2 mmHg.[20] Furthermore Susalit, et al., investigated the hypotensive effect of olive (*Olea europaea*) leaf extract, 500 mg/daily for 8 weeks on 232 patients and indicated the extract lowered 10 mmHg systolic blood pressure.[21] Moreover, several other herbal agents were studied independently and showed hypotensive effect. Examples are Sour Cherry (*Prunus cerasus* L.), *Nigella sativa* seed extract, pomegranate juice, *Hibiscus sabdariffa* and canola oil with sunflower oil.[22-29] In this study, OSE lowered systolic blood pressure by 17.3 mmHg that is more potent than all studied hypotensive agents. Similar effects have been reported about aged garlic extract and olive leaf extract that showed a reduction of about 10 mmHg of systolic blood pressure. The reasons for such discripency is not clear but it may be due to the presence of both ACEI and diuretic activity in OSE. This finding was in line with previous report by Sharifi, et al., that revealed OSE has more hypotensive effect than other 50 herbal agents which has been assessed.[8]

Several limitations are inherent to the present study. Recruiting hypertensive patients categorized in the first and second stage of hypertension who were also treated with losartan was very difficult. The majority of hypertensive patients had to use two or more drugs to control their blood pressure, due to lack of good response to one-drug therapy. The limitation of recruiting hypertensive patients in this study was consistent with the one in the other studies. The withdrawal of the patients was also an obstacle to obtain the desired results with higher power of analysis.

Conclusion
OSE synergistically with diuretic and plasma ACE inhibitor activity reduced blood pressure (both systolic and diastolic) in the patients under treatment with losartan, and did not show remarkable side effects in patients with primary hypertension. Because of the low number of samples, this medication may be not safely recommended. Further clinical trials is needed for increasing certainty with larger sample size and placebo.

Acknowledgments
This study was part of a postgraduate thesis entitled: "Investigating the Effect of Onopordon Acanthium Seed on Primary Hypertension Reduction in Patients under Treatment by Losartan"; and was supported by a grant from Tehran University of Medical Sciences. The funding source had no involvement in any part of the study. We would like to thank the participants for their contribution to the maintenance of our patient record without which this project would have been impossible. Special thanks to Mr. Hadi Salehi, for his kindly efforts for extraction and drug preparation. We would like to thank Dr. Mohsen Amin assistant Prof. at Faculty of Pharmacy, Tehran University of Medical Sciences for his help in data analysis and manuscript editing.

Ethical Issues
The study protocol was approved by the ethics committee of Research Institute for Islamic and Complementary Medicine of Iran University of Medical Sciences at 09/10/2012 with reference number 732/P26/M/T.

Conflict of Interest
The authors have declared no conflicts of interest.

References
1. Chockalingam A. Impact of world hypertension day. *Can J Cardiol* 2007;23(7):517-9. doi: 10.1016/S0828-282X(07)70795-X
2. Chockalingam A. World hypertension day and global awareness. *Can J Cardiol* 2008;24(6):441-4. doi: 10.1016/S0828-282X(08)70617-2
3. Sever PS, Messerli FH. Hypertension management 2011: Optimal combination therapy. *Eur Heart J* 2011;32(20):2499-506. doi: 10.1093/eurheartj/ehr177
4. Kalra S, Kalra B, Agrawal N. Combination therapy in hypertension: An update. *Diabetol Metab Syndr* 2010;2:44. doi: 10.1186/1758-5996-2-44
5. Williams B, Poulter NR, Brown MJ, Davis M, McInnes GT, Potter JF, et al. Guidelines for management of hypertension: Report of the fourth working party of the british hypertension society, 2004-bhs iv. *J Hum Hypertens* 2004;18(3):139-85. doi: 10.1038/sj.jhh.1001683
6. Habashi JP, Judge DP, Holm TM, Cohn RD, Loeys BL, Cooper TK, et al. Losartan, an at1 antagonist, prevents aortic aneurysm in a mouse model of marfan syndrome. *Science* 2006;312(5770):117-21. doi: 10.1126/science.1124287
7. Abadir PM, Foster DB, Crow M, Cooke CA, Rucker JJ, Jain A, et al. Identification and characterization of a functional mitochondrial angiotensin system. *Proc Natl Acad Sci U S A* 2011;108(36):14849-54. doi: 10.1073/pnas.1101507108
8. Sharifi N, Souri E, Ziai SA, Amin G, Amini M, Amanlou M. Isolation, identification and molecular docking studies of a new isolated compound, from onopordon acanthium: A novel angiotensin converting enzyme (ace) inhibitor. *J Ethnopharmacol* 2013;148(3):934-9. doi: 10.1016/j.jep.2013.05.046
9. Amin G. The most common iranian traditional medicinal plants. 2nd ed. Tehran: Tehran University of Medical Sciences and Research Center for Medical Ethics and History; 2008.
10. Ugur A, Sarac N, Duru ME. Chemical composition and antimicrobial activity of endemic *onopordum caricum*. *Middle-East J Sci Res* 2011;8(3):594-8.
11. Stace C. New flora of the british isles. 3rd ed. UK: Cambridge University Press; 2010.

12. Khalilov L, Khalilova A, Shakurova E, Nuriev I, Kachala V, Shashkov A, et al. Pmr and 13c nmr spectra of biologically active compounds. Xii. Taraxasterol and its acetate from the aerial part of onopordum acanthium. *Chem Nat Compd* 2003;39(3):285-8. doi: 10.1023/A:1025478720459

13. Reichard S, Seebacher L. Addendum to a report, Analysis and Assessment of the Invasive risk of Onopordum Illyricum. University of Washington, College of Forest Resources, Center for Urban Horticulture; 2001.

14. Tyumkina T, Nuriev I, Khalilov L, Akhmetova V, Dzhemilev U. Pmr and 13 c nmr spectra of biologically active compounds. Xiii.* structure and stereochemistry of a new phenylpropanoid glycoside isolated from "onopordum acanthium" seeds. *Chem Nat Compd* 2009;45(1):61-5. doi: 10.1007/s10600-009-9254-9

15. Esmaeili A, Saremnia B. Preparation of extract-loaded nanocapsules from "onopordon leptolepis" Dc. *Ind Crop Prod* 2012;37(1):259-63. doi:10.1016/j.indcrop.2011.12.010

16. National High Blood Pressure Education P. The seventh report of the joint national committee on prevention, detection, evaluation, and treatment of high blood pressure. Bethesda (MD): National Heart, Lung, and Blood Institute (US); 2004.

17. Asgary S, Naderi GH, Sarrafzadegan N, Mohammadifard N, Mostafavi S, Vakili R. Antihypertensive and antihyperlipidemic effects of achillea wilhelmsii. *Drugs Exp Clin Res* 2000;26(3):89-93.

18. Walker AF, Marakis G, Morris AP, Robinson PA. Promising hypotensive effect of hawthorn extract: A randomized double-blind pilot study of mild, essential hypertension. *Phytother Res* 2002;16(1):48-54.

19. Walker AF, Marakis G, Simpson E, Hope JL, Robinson PA, Hassanein M, et al. Hypotensive effects of hawthorn for patients with diabetes taking prescription drugs: A randomised controlled trial. *Br J Gen Pract* 2006;56(527):437-43.

20. Ried K, Frank OR, Stocks NP. Aged garlic extract lowers blood pressure in patients with treated but uncontrolled hypertension: A randomised controlled trial. *Maturitas* 2010;67(2):144-50. doi: 10.1016/j.maturitas.2010.06.001

21. Susalit E, Agus N, Effendi I, Tjandrawinata RR, Nofiarny D, Perrinjaquet-Moccetti T, et al. Olive (olea europaea) leaf extract effective in patients with stage-1 hypertension: Comparison with captopril. *Phytomedicine* 2011;18(4):251-8. doi: 10.1016/j.phymed.2010.08.016

22. Ataee-jafari A, Hosseini S, Heshmat R, Parviz M, Raeeszade S, Yoosefi M, et al. Effect of sour cherry (*prunus cerasus* l.) on cardiovascular risk factors in patients with diabet type ii. *Iran J Diabetes Lipid Disord* 2006;5(4):365-70.

23. Ashraf R, Khan RA, Ashraf I, Qureshi AA. Effects of allium sativum (garlic) on systolic and diastolic blood pressure in patients with essential hypertension. *Pak J Pharm Sci* 2013;26(5):859-63.

24. Saberi M, Kazemi-saleh D, Booloorian V. Effect of olive leaf on mild to moderate and common drug resistant hypertension. *J Med Plants* 2009;3(27):52-9.

25. Dehkordi FR, Kamkhah AF. Antihypertensive effect of nigella sativa seed extract in patients with mild hypertension. *Fundam Clin Pharmacol* 2008;22(4):447-52. doi: 10.1111/j.1472-8206.2008.00607.x

26. Sohrab G, Sotoode G, Siasi F, Neyestani T, Rahimi A. Effect of pomegranate juice consupmtion on blood pressure in type 2 diabetic patients. *Iran J Endocrinol Metab* 2009;9(4):399-405.

27. Wahabi HA, Alansary LA, Al-Sabban AH, Glasziuo P. The effectiveness of hibiscus sabdariffa in the treatment of hypertension: A systematic review. *Phytomedicine* 2010;17(2):83-6. doi: 10.1016/j.phymed.2009.09.002

28. McKay DL, Chen CY, Saltzman E, Blumberg JB. Hibiscus sabdariffa l. Tea (tisane) lowers blood pressure in prehypertensive and mildly hypertensive adults. *J Nutr* 2010;140(2):298-303. doi: 10.3945/jn.109.115097

29. Seied-ebrahimi S, Shidfar F, heydari I, Haghighi L, Gohari M-r, Hoseini S. Comparison of the effect of canola oil with sunflower oil on blood pressure,lipid profile, apoproteins, lipoprotein (a), total antioxidant capacity and crp in hyperlipidemic postmenopausal women. *Iran J Nutr Sci Food Technol* 2011(2):21-9.

23

Effect of Ghrelin on Caspase 3 and Bcl2 Gene Expression in H2O2 Treated Rat's Bone Marrow Stromal Cells

Alireza Abdanipour[1] iD, Masoud Dadkhah[2], Mohsen Alipour[2] iD, Hadi Feizi[2]* iD

1 Department of Anatomical Sciences, Faculty of Medicine, Zanjan University of Medical Sciences, Zanjan, Iran.
2 Department of Physiology and Pharmacology, Faculty of Medicine, Zanjan University of Medical Sciences, Zanjan, Iran.

Keywords:
· Ghrelin
· Caspase 3
· Bcl2
· H2O2
· Rat
· BMSCs

Abstract

Purpose: The antiapoptotic effect of ghrelin in various cell lines including bone marrow stromal cells (BMSCs) has been proved. However, the real mechanism of this effect is not clear. Caspase3 and Bcl2 are well-known pro- and antiapoptotic regulatory genes in eukaryotes. The aim of the study was to find out the effect of ghrelin on Caspase 3 and Bcl2 change in BMSCs.

Methods: Rat BMSCs were cultivated in DMEM. Passage 3 BMSCs were treated with ghrelin 100 µM for 48 h. Real-time PCR for Caspase 3 and Bcl2 was carried out from B (untreated BMSCs), BH (BMSCs treated with 125 µM H2O2), BGH (BMSCs treated with 100 µM ghrelin then 125 µM H2O2) and BG (BMSCs treated with 100 µM ghrelin) groups. For immunofluorescence, cells were incubated with anti Caspase 3 and Bcl2monoclonal antibodies. Primary antibodies were visualized using the FITC method. All data are presented as means ± SEM. Values of $P<0.05$ were considered statistically significant.

Results: Ghrelin decreased mRNA expressions of *Caspase-3* significantly as compared to the BH group ($P<0.05$). Also, Bcl-2 gene expression showed an increment in BG group as compare with BH and BGH groups ($P<0.05$). A high present of *Bcl-2* positive cells were observed in the BGH group while *Caspase-3* positive cells were significantly decreased in the BGH group compared with the BH group ($P<0.05$).

Conclusion: Ghrelin probably enhances BMSCs viability through regulation of pro- and antiapoptotic genes Caspase 3 and Bcl2. However the signaling pathway of this effect should be elucidated in the future.

Introduction

Ghrelin is an endogenous peptide that has some well known physiological functions especially in controlling the metabolism and food intake.[1] It acts through a receptor belong to G protein-coupled receptors named GSR1α.[2] This receptor has been found in different tissues including kidneys, adrenal glands, thyroid, breast, ovary, placenta, testis, prostate, liver, gallbladder, lung, skeletal muscles, myocardium, skin, and bone.[3] Since its discovery, ghrelin has been shown to be involved in many physiological and pathophysiological roles such as regulation of glucose and lipid metabolism, modulation of immunity, stimulation of gastric motility, cardiovascular function, modulation of appetite, stress, anxiety, taste sensation and behavior in nervous system, as well as metabolic complications, chronic inflammation, gastroparesis or cancer-associated anorexia and cachexia.[4,5] One of the recently introduced roles of ghrelin is the antiapoptotic and cell injury protection.[6]

Bone marrow stromal cells (BMSCs) are a population of progenitor cells for skeletal tissue constituents.[7] These cells are capable to differentiate into bone, cartilage, and adipocytes.[8] BMSCs also support hematopoietic stem cells structurally and physiologically.[9] BMSCs have been applied in several cell therapy strategies in order to tissue repair and functional recovery.[10,11] Therefore, autologous BMSCs can be isolated from bone marrow and used as a credible source of stem cells for restoring injured tissue function. However, previous studies have shown that transplanted BMSCs do not accommodate well within diseased tissues.[12] There is evidence that these cells are suffered due to host immune responses and die because of apoptosis.[13]

Apoptosis is a programmed cell-suicide in which some gene products are responsible as apoptotic effectors proteins and some of them act as antiapoptosis regulators.[14] Caspases are a gene family that acts in a cascade manner and caspase3 is one of the final effectors leading to apoptosis.[15] Among the anti-apoptotic genes, Bcl2 is considered to be one of the most important and well-known genes.[16] Due to the apoptosis inducers, oxidative stress is a common cause and H2O2 is a mediator of this phenomenon.[17]

Recently we have shown that ghrelin increases the BMSCs viability and protect them against the H2O2 induced damage.[18] Consequently, using ghrelin, as an endogenous peptide, that enhances BMSC's resistance to apoptosis would improve the therapeutic potential of these cells. However, to find out the mechanism of this phenomenon, in the present study we are going to examine the probable effects of this peptide on the Caspase 3 and Bcl2 gene expression in H2O2 treated rat's BMSCs.

Materials and Methods
BMSCs culture and drug treatments
Male Wistar rat of 4-6 weeks were sacrificed under deep anesthesia using ketamine–xylazine (K, 100 mg/kg; X, 10 mg/kg). The lower limbs were removed with a pair of scissors separating it from the hip joint and put on a sterile gauze. The accompanied soft tissue (muscles, fasciae, and tendons) was removed, and femurs and tibiae were separated and put in a dish containing phosphate buffered saline (PBS, Gibco, Life Technologies, USA) and penicillin/streptomycin (Gibco, Life Technologies, USA). The dish was transferred under a laminar hood. The bones were subsequently washed again with PBS and put on a sterile gauze to dry. Both ends of the bones were cut, then with an insulin syringe containing high glucose Dulbecco's Modified Eagle Medium (DMEM, Gibco, Life Technologies, USA) and 1% penicillin/streptomycin, all the contents of the bone's lumen were flushed directly to 25 cm2 culture flask (SPL, life sciences, Korea) without any additional manipulation. The flushing was done several times, so that the lumen became pale. Rat BMSCs were initially cultivated in DMEM (Dulbecco's Modified Eagle Medium), supplemented with 20% FBS (Gibco), 100 U/ml penicillin, and 100 mg/ml streptomycin in 4 experimental groups as B (untreated BMSCs), BH (BMSCs treated with 125 µM H2O2), BG (BMSCs treated with 100 µM ghrelin) and BGH (BMSCs treated with 100 µM ghrelin then 125 µM H2O2). The cells were incubated at 37°C (5% CO2) in 25 cm2 plastic flask. The medium refreshed every 2-3 days until cells became confluent. The cells were harvested with trypsin–EDTA and passaged up to three times. To induce BMSC, ghrelin was freshly prepared. Passage 3 BMSCs were cultured in 96-well plates (5000 cells/well) in DMEM medium supplemented with different concentration of ghrelin (0.1, 1, 10 and 100 µM) for 24 and 48 h.

Real-time PCR
Real-time PCR was carried out with RNA from B (untreated BMSCs), BH (BMSCs treated with 125 µM H2O2), BGH (BMSCs treated with 100 µM ghrelin then 125 µM H2O2) and BG (BMSCs treated with 100 µM ghrelin) groups. In all groups, 1,000 ng purified RNA from cultured cells was used to synthesize 20 µlcDNA, using Revert aid™ first strand cDNA synthesis kit (Fermentas, Germany) according to the manufacturer's instructions. cDNA (25ng) was used to quantify Caspase3 and Bcl2 mRNA levels. As an internal control, primers for GAPDH were used. All primers have been listed in Table 1. The PCR reaction was synthesized in a 12.5µl volume (sense and anti-sense primers, cDNA, Sybr green,) and carried out for 40 cycles (Applied Biosystems cycler). For analyzing relative changes in mRNA levels, we used the delta CT method (Pfaffl method).

Table 1. Sequences of Oligonucleotide Primers

Name	Sequence (5' → 3')
Caspase3(Forward)	GGTATTGAGACAGACAGTGG
Caspase3(Reverse)	CATGGGATCTGTTTCTTTGC
Bcl2 (Reverse)	ATCGCTCTGTGGATGACTGAGTAC
Bcl2 (Reverse)	AGAGACAGCCAGGAGAAATCAAAC
GAPDH (Forward)	CAAGGTCATCCATGACAACTTTG
GAPDH (Reverse)	GTCCACCACCCTGTTGCTGTAG

Immunostaining
BMSCs were cultured on cover slides and fixed in 3% paraformaldehyde for 20 min at RT, followed by a permeabilization step in 100% methanol for 30 min at RT (room temperature). For immunofluorescence, cells were incubated with anti-CD90 (for BMSCs) and Anti-Caspase3 and Bcl2 (for produced erythroid Progenitor Cells) monoclonal antibodies, followed by incubation with a fluorescein isothiocyanate (FITC)–conjugated Rabbit anti-Mouse antibody (millipore). Nuclei were counterstained with DAPI. For indirect immunoperoxidase labeling, 100 µM treated BMSCs (for 48 h) were permeabilized with 0.4% Triton X-100, followed by FCS 10% for 60 minutes to block endogenous peroxidase. Then were incubated with anti-CD90 and Caspase3 and Bcl2 antibodies overnight at 4°C. Primary antibodies were visualized using the FITC method.

Statistics
Statistical analysis was performed using the SPSS15 software. All data are presented as means ± SEM. To compare multiple means in groups, one-way ANOVA followed by Tukey's post hoc comparison was used. Values of $P < 0.05$ were considered statistically significant.

Results
BMSCs expansion and identification
The Ethics Committee for animal studies at the University of Zanjan University (ZUMS) confirmed the

experiment conducted in this study. The primary culture of the isolated BMSCs is presented in Figure 1-A-D. The results showed, after 12 hours, the cells were attached to the flask and most of them were rounded (Figure 1-A). Adherent cells were cultured and became heterogeneous after 12 or 16 days (passage 4) (Figure 1-D). Following,

the cells were immunostained with anti-CD90 (mesenchymal stem cells markers) antibody and incubated with FITC conjugated secondary antibody. The result showed, 100% of the cells were immunoreactive to CD90 (Figure 1-E, F).

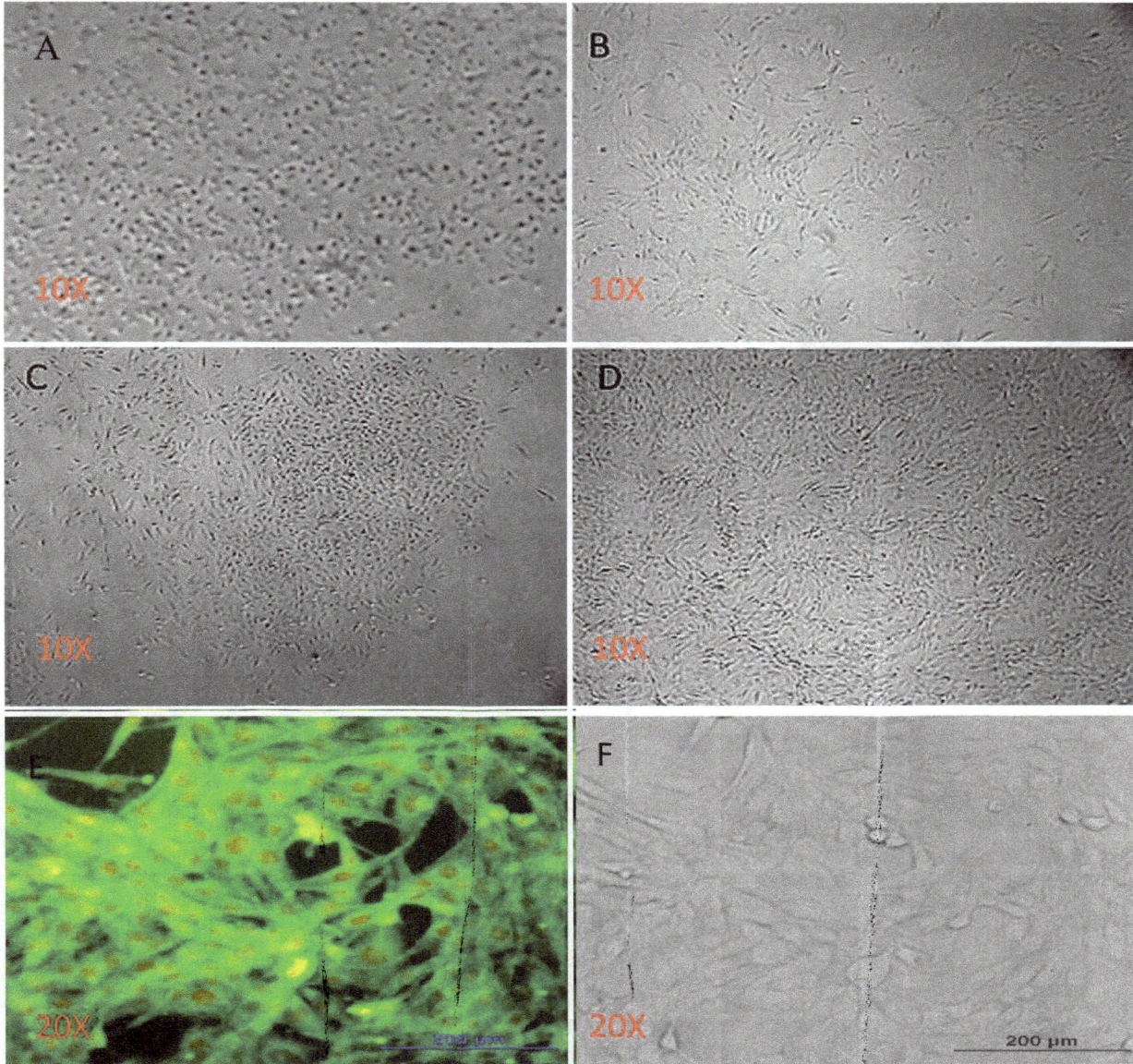

Figure 1. Micrographs of bone marrow stromal cells (BMSCs). A in primary culture the BMSCs had round shapes (after 12 hrs). **B;** The cells are fibroblast-like cells after 48 hours. **C;** Cells at the stage of the first passage and formation of colonies. **D;** BMSCs have a more uniform spindle shape after 4 passages. **E, D;** represents Phase contrast micrographs of BMSCs and immunostaining of CD90 at same field respectively. The cells were immunostained with relevant primary antibodies and labeled with FITC-conjugated secondary antibody (green color shows positive cells) and the red colors are ethidium bromide counterstaining of the nuclei

Bcl-2 and Caspase-3 genes expression rates

Decreasing of both genes expressions in BGH and other groups (BH and BG) at 48 hrs were confirmed by quantitative real-time RT-PCR. The results of the mRNA expression pattern have been shown in the (Figure 2). Our data showed that mRNA expressions of **Caspase-3** gene significantly decreasing when Ghrelin was used (BGH;0.83 ± 0.09, BG; 1.04 ± 0.07) as compare to the BH group (1.97 ± 0.14). Also, the result showed,

increasing of the Bcl-2 gene in BG group (1.89 ± 0.12) as compare with BH (0.57 ± 0.05) and BGH (0.47 ± 0.06).

Immunostaining of Bcl-2 and Caspase-3

To determine the protective effect of Ghrelin, *Bcl-2* and *Caspase-3* protein expression were detected using immunocytochemistry technique. The results were shown in the Figures 3 and 4. The percentage of *Bcl-2* (Figure 3 left panel) and *Caspase-3* (Figure 3 right panel)

Positive cells were calculated in 5 samples. A high present of *Bcl-2* (9.52 ± 1.31) and *Caspase-3* (37.01 ± 2.15) positive cells were observed in the BGH and BH groups respectively. But the low percentage of *Bcl-2* (1.46 ± 0.68) positive cells were visible in the B group. The percentage of *Caspase-3* positive cells was significantly decreased in the BGH group (26.09 ± 2.8) compared with the BH group (37.02 ± 2.15).

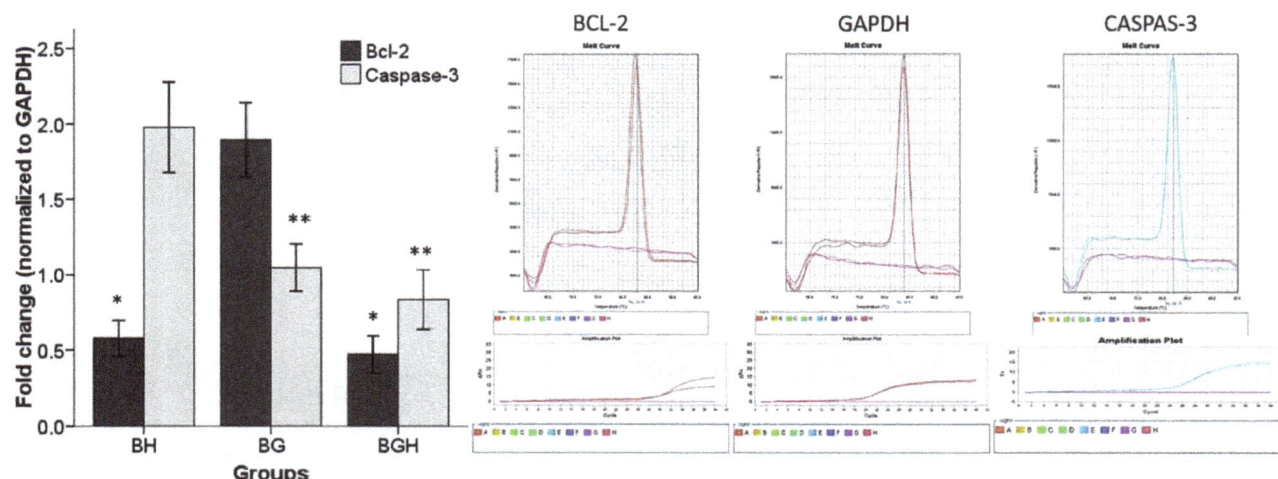

Figure 2. Bcl-2 and Caspase-3 genes expression. Fold change ratio of *Bcl-2* and *Caspase-3* mRNA of BMSCs treated with 100 μM concentrations of Ghrelin for 48 hrs and various experimental groups. Real-time PCR results have been presented as relative expression normalized to GAPDH mRNA amplification. Amplification of the Bcl-2 and Caspase-3 mRNA derived from BH, BG and BGH groups showing increases level of Bcl-2 mRNA and decreasing *Caspase-3* mRNAin the BG and (BG, BGH) groups respectively. The bars indicate the mean ± SEM. P<0.05 *(compared to BG group), **(compared to BH group). B (untreated BMSCs), BH (BMSCs treated with 125 μM H2O2), BG (BMSCs treated with 100 μM ghrelin) and BGH (BMSCs treated with 100 μM ghrelin then 125 μM H2O2)

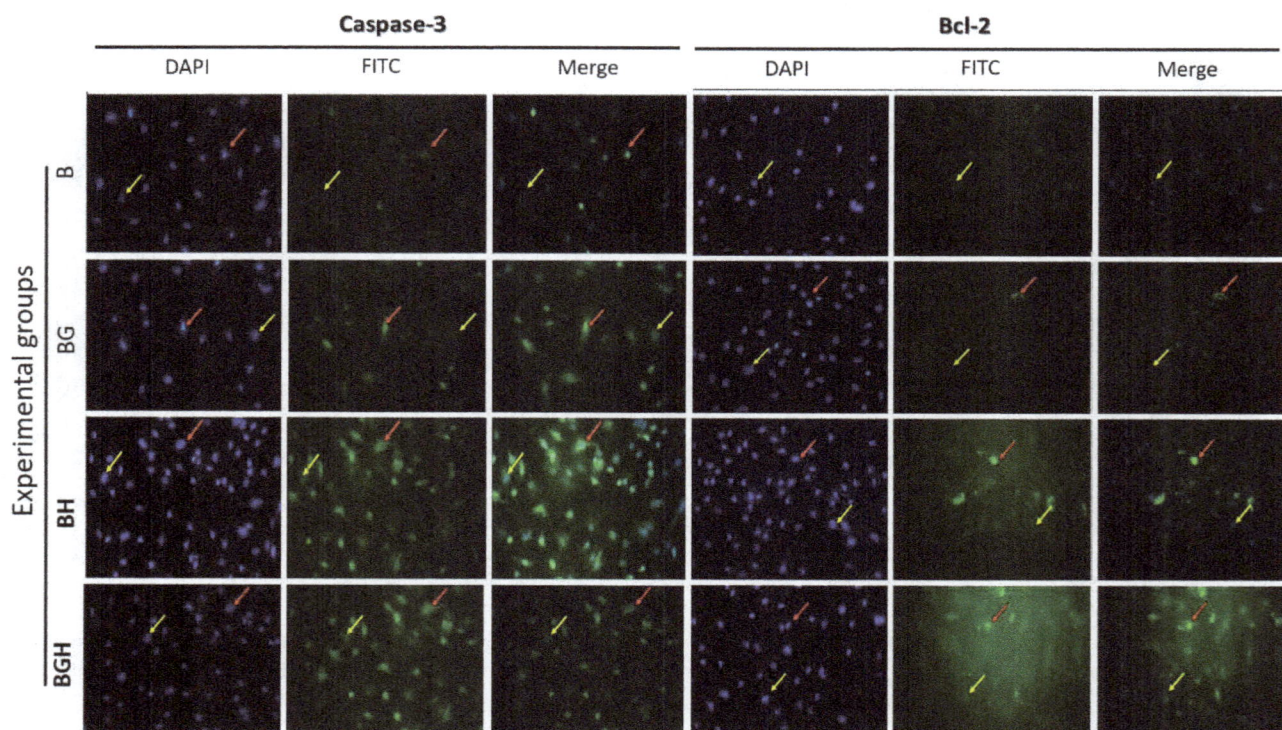

Figure 3. *Bcl-2* and *Caspase-3* protein expression. Representative immunostaning-photomicrographs showing Bcl-2 (left panel) and Caspase-3 (right panel) immuncreactivity in the B, BG, BH and BGH experimental groups after 48 hrs of treatments. Red arrows indicate to immunopositive cells and yellow arrows indicate to negative cells. Magnification, 200×. B (untreated BMSCs), BH (BMSCs treated with 125 μM H2O2), BG (BMSCs treated with 100 μM ghrelin) and BGH (BMSCs treated with 100 μM ghrelin then 125 μM H2O2)

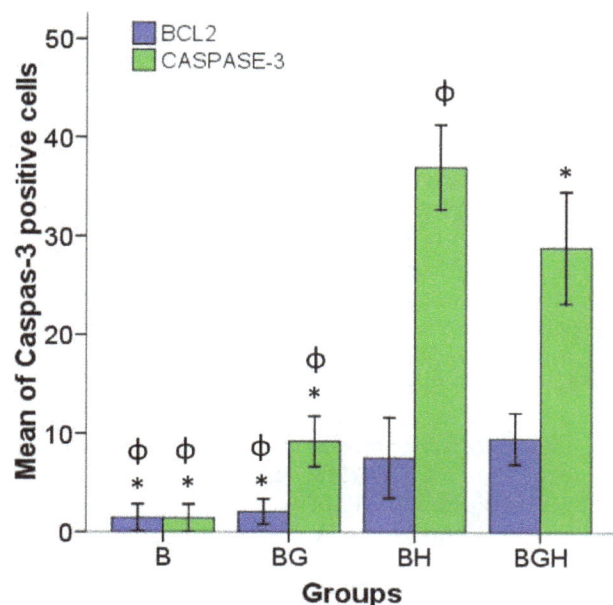

Figure 4. represents the histogram of the mean percentage of the Bcl-2 and Caspase-3 protein positive cells in the B, BG, BH and BGH experimental groups. The bars indicate the mean ± SEM; $P<0.05$,*(compared to BH group), Ω (compared to BGH group). B (untreated BMSCs), BH (BMSCs treated with 125 µM H2O2), BG (BMSCs treated with 100 µM ghrelin) and BGH (BMSCs treated with 100 µM ghrelin then 125 µM H2O2)

Discussion

According to the results of the current study, ghrelin (100µM) significantly decreased both gene expression and protein production of Caspase-3 in H2O2 suffered BMSCs. Ghrelin treatment also enhanced BCl2 production in these cells. As mentioned previously we have detected an antiapoptotic effect for ghrelin in BMSCs during similar condition.[18] Thus the presented results could justify our former finding. It has been proved that H2O2 induces apoptosis in BMSCs and this injury could be restored by melatonin via Bax/Bcl-2 ratio suppression and caspase-3 inactivation.[19] Our results are consistent with the following studies in the text however they have been performed in different cells and treatment situations.

It has been demonstrated by Baldanzi et al. that ghrelin inhibits cell death in cardiomyocytes and endothelial cells and they showed that this effect was through ERK1/2 and PI 3-kinase/AKT pathways.[20] As reported by Yang et al., ghrelin repressed apoptosis signal-regulating kinase 1 activity in PC12 cells and thus caspase 3 inhibitions through heat-shock protein 70 upregulation.[21] It has been shown that ghrelin inhibits apoptosis in pancreatic β cell line HIT-T15. This effect was achieved via activation of MAPK and Akt pathways. Ghrelin also increased Bcl-2, decreased Bax, and suppressed caspase-3 activation in this cell.[22] Moreover, it has been revealed that ghrelin (1000 ng/ml) in a dose-dependent manner inhibits TNF-alpha-induced apoptosis of vascular smooth muscle cells.[23] Previous studies have shown that ghrelin treatment diminishes diabetes-

induced cell death in lactotrophs through caspase-8 inhibition and increasing Bcl-2 levels.[24]

Bando and coworkers indicated that streptozotocin treated transgenic (RIP-GG Tg) mice, which have elevated pancreatic ghrelin levels, showed a significant elevation in pancreatic insulin mRNA expression. Furthermore, β-cell numbers increased in islets.[25] Han and colleagues have shown that ghrelin administration (10^{-8} M) combined with intramyocardial injection of adipose-derived mesenchymal stem cells (ADMSCs) inhibited cardiomyocyte apoptosis. Ghrelin increased ADMSCs survival under hypoxia/serum deprivation (H/SD) injury. It also decreased the proapoptotic protein Bax and increased the antiapoptotic protein Bcl-2 in vitro, and these effects were eliminated by PI3K inhibitor LY294002.[26] Furthermore, it has been reported that ghrelin could reverse rotenone-induced neurotoxicity in MES23.5 cells through improving the mitochondrial dysfunction and finally inhibition of caspase-3 activation and apoptosis.[27] In a study by Zhang and his group, ghrelin (0.1 µM) inhibited dexamethasone-induced apoptosis in INS-1 cells. It upregulated Bcl-2 and downregulated Bax expression, and decreased caspase-3 activity. Moreover, this protective effect of ghrelin was through GHS-R1a and the ERK and p38MAPKsignaling pathways.[28] HOXb4 is one of the factors that its upregulation, especially in hematopoietic cells, protects them against apoptosis.[29] Recently we have shown that ghrelin upregulates HOXB4 gene expression in the rat BMSCs.[30] These mentioned in vitro studies which imply the antiapoptotic effect of ghrelin are matching with some in vivo studies.[31-33] It has been identified that ghrelin causes an antiapoptotic effect in the renal tissue of chronic hypoxic rats by increasing the Bcl2/Bax ratio.[34]

A couple of studies have shown the therapeutic potential of BMSCs.[35] For example, BMSCs administration recovers neural tissue injury.[36,37] Their involvement in bone regeneration also has been identified.[38] Further investigations have shown the BMSCs beneficiary in renal injuries.[39,40] Ghrelin has been shown to be protective against multiple complications in various cells.[21-28] However, its effect on bone marrow stem cells has not been investigated prior to this study. We demonstrated that BMSCs treated with ghrelin are less vulnerable to oxidative stress.[18] The physiological function of endogenous ghrelin in BMSCs is not clear. In the present report, the authors suggest that ghrelin changes the expression of Bcl-2 and Caspase3 under H2O2-induced stress and this may regulate BMSCs survival. Since ghrelin is an endogenous peptide with the fewer side effects, its application as co-treatment in the medium could be valuable in developing the cell therapy strategies.

Conclusion

Ghrelin probably enhances BMSCs viability through regulation of pro- and antiapoptotic genes Caspase 3 and

Bcl2. However, the signaling pathway and in vivo application of this effect should be elucidated in future.

Acknowledgments

The results described in this paper were part of student thesis (Masoud Dadkhah) for MSc degree in physiology. The authors would like to thank the Vice-Chancellery for Research affairs of Zanjan University of Medical Sciences for financial support (grant no.A-10-141-7).

Ethical Issues

All the experiments were carried out under the ethical guidelines of Zanjan University of Medical Sciences (ZUMS.REC.1394.147).

Conflict of Interest

The authors report no conflicts of interest. The authors alone are responsible for the content and writing of the paper.

References

1. Kojima M, Hosoda H, Date Y, Nakazato M, Matsuo H, Kangawa K. Ghrelin is a growth-hormone-releasing acylated peptide from stomach. *Nature* 1999;402(6762):656-60. doi: 10.1038/45230

2. Albarran-Zeckler RG, Smith RG. The ghrelin receptors (GHS-R1a and GHS-R1b). *Endocr Dev* 2013;25:5-15. doi: 10.1159/000346042

3. Gnanapavan S, Kola B, Bustin SA, Morris DG, McGee P, Fairclough P, et al. The tissue distribution of the mRNA of ghrelin and subtypes of its receptor, GHS-R, in humans. *J Clin Endocrinol Metab* 2002;87(6):2988. doi: 10.1210/jcem.87.6.8739

4. Collden G, Tschop MH, Muller TD. Therapeutic potential of targeting the ghrelin pathway. *Int J Mol Sci* 2017;18(4). doi: 10.3390/ijms18040798

5. Omrani H, Alipour MR, Mohaddes G. Ghrelin improves antioxidant defense in blood and brain in normobaric hypoxia in adult male rats. *Adv Pharm Bull* 2015;5(2):283-8. doi: 10.15171/apb.2015.039

6. Frago LM, Baquedano E, Argente J, Chowen JA. Neuroprotective actions of ghrelin and growth hormone secretagogues. *Front Mol Neurosci* 2011;4:23. doi: 10.3389/fnmol.2011.00023

7. Krebsbach PH, Kuznetsov SA, Bianco P, Robey PG. Bone marrow stromal cells: Characterization and clinical application. *Crit Rev Oral Biol Med* 1999;10(2):165-81.

8. Bianco P, Riminucci M, Gronthos S, Robey PG. Bone marrow stromal stem cells: Nature, biology, and potential applications. *Stem Cells* 2001;19(3):180-92. doi: 10.1634/stemcells.19-3-180

9. Anthony BA, Link DC. Regulation of hematopoietic stem cells by bone marrow stromal cells. *Trends Immunol* 2014;35(1):32-7. doi: 10.1016/j.it.2013.10.002

10. Hu X, Yu SP, Fraser JL, Lu Z, Ogle ME, Wang JA, et al. Transplantation of hypoxia-preconditioned mesenchymal stem cells improves infarcted heart function via enhanced survival of implanted cells and angiogenesis. *J Thorac Cardiovasc Surg* 2008;135(4):799-808. doi: 10.1016/j.jtcvs.2007.07.071

11. Mahmood A, Lu D, Chopp M. Marrow stromal cell transplantation after traumatic brain injury promotes cellular proliferation within the brain. *Neurosurgery* 2004;55(5):1185-93.

12. Geng YJ. Molecular mechanisms for cardiovascular stem cell apoptosis and growth in the hearts with atherosclerotic coronary disease and ischemic heart failure. *Ann N Y Acad Sci* 2003;1010:687-97.

13. Zeng X, Yu SP, Taylor T, Ogle M, Wei L. Protective effect of apelin on cultured rat bone marrow mesenchymal stem cells against apoptosis. *Stem Cell Res* 2012;8(3):357-67. doi: 10.1016/j.scr.2011.12.004

14. Elmore S. Apoptosis: A review of programmed cell death. *Toxicol Pathol* 2007;35(4):495-516. doi: 10.1080/01926230701320337

15. Lee G, Kim J, Kim Y, Yoo S, Park JH. Identifying and monitoring neurons that undergo metamorphosis-regulated cell death (metamorphoptosis) by a neuron-specific caspase sensor (Casor) in drosophila melanogaster. *Apoptosis* 2018;23(1):41-53. doi: 10.1007/s10495-017-1435-6

16. Basu A, DuBois G, Haldar S. Posttranslational modifications of bcl2 family members--a potential therapeutic target for human malignancy. *Front Biosci* 2006;11:1508-21.

17. Abdanipour A, Tiraihi T, Noori-Zadeh A, Majdi A, Gosaili R. Evaluation of lovastatin effects on expression of anti-apoptotic Nrf2 and PGC-1α genes in neural stem cells treated with hydrogen peroxide. *Mol Neurobiol* 2014;49(3):1364-72. doi: 10.1007/s12035-013-8613-5

18. Abdanipour A, Shahsavandi B, Dadkhah M, Alipour M, Feizi H. The antiapoptotic effect of ghrelin in the H2O2 treated Bone Marrow-derived Mesenchymal Stem cells of rat. *J Zanjan Univ Med Sci Health Serv* 2017;25(113): 58-68.

19. Wang FW, Wang Z, Zhang YM, Du ZX, Zhang XL, Liu Q, et al. Protective effect of melatonin on bone marrow mesenchymal stem cells against hydrogen peroxide-induced apoptosis in vitro. *J Cell Biochem* 2013;114(10):2346-55. doi: 10.1002/jcb.24582

20. Baldanzi G, Filigheddu N, Cutrupi S, Catapano F, Bonissoni S, Fubini A, et al. Ghrelin and des-acyl ghrelin inhibit cell death in cardiomyocytes and endothelial cells through ERK1/2 and PI 3-kinase/AKT. *J Cell Biol* 2002;159(6):1029-37. doi: 10.1083/jcb.200207165

21. Yang M, Hu S, Wu B, Miao Y, Pan H, Zhu S. Ghrelin inhibits apoptosis signal-regulating kinase 1 activity via upregulating heat-shock protein 70. *Biochem Biophys Res Commun* 2007;359(2):373-8. doi: 10.1016/j.bbrc.2007.05.118

22. Zhang Y, Ying B, Shi L, Fan H, Yang D, Xu D, et al. Ghrelin inhibit cell apoptosis in pancreatic beta cell line hit-t15 via mitogen-activated protein kinase/phosphoinositide 3-kinase pathways. *Toxicology* 2007;237(1-3):194-202. doi: 10.1016/j.tox.2007.05.013

23. Zhan M, Yuan F, Liu H, Chen H, Qiu X, Fang W. Inhibition of proliferation and apoptosis of vascular smooth muscle cells by ghrelin. *Acta Biochim Biophys Sin (Shanghai)* 2008;40(9):769-76.

24. Granado M, Chowen JA, Garcia-Caceres C, Delgado-Rubin A, Barrios V, Castillero E, et al. Ghrelin treatment protects lactotrophs from apoptosis in the pituitary of diabetic rats. *Mol Cell Endocrinol* 2009;309(1-2):67-75. doi: 10.1016/j.mce.2009.06.006

25. Bando M, Iwakura H, Ariyasu H, Koyama H, Hosoda K, Adachi S, et al. Overexpression of intraislet ghrelin enhances β-cell proliferation after streptozotocin-induced β-cell injury in mice. *Am J Physiol Endocrinol Metab* 2013;305(1):E140-8. doi: 10.1152/ajpendo.00112.2013

26. Han D, Huang W, Ma S, Chen J, Gao L, Liu T, et al. Ghrelin improves functional survival of engrafted adipose-derived mesenchymal stem cells in ischemic heart through PI3K/Akt signaling pathway. *Biomed Res Int* 2015;2015:858349. doi: 10.1155/2015/858349

27. Yu J, Xu H, Shen X, Jiang H. Ghrelin protects mes23.5 cells against rotenone via inhibiting mitochondrial dysfunction and apoptosis. *Neuropeptides* 2016;56:69-74. doi: 10.1016/j.npep.2015.09.011

28. Zhang C, Li L, Zhao B, Jiao A, Li X, Sun N, et al. Ghrelin protects against dexamethasone-induced ins-1 cell apoptosis via erk and p38mapk signaling. *Int J Endocrinol* 2016;2016:4513051. doi: 10.1155/2016/4513051

29. Park SW, Won KJ, Lee YS, Kim HS, Kim YK, Lee HW, et al. Increased hoxb4 inhibits apoptotic cell death in pro-b cells. *Korean J Physiol Pharmacol* 2012;16(4):265-71. doi: 10.4196/kjpp.2012.16.4.265

30. Abdanipour A, Shahsavandi B, Alipour M, Feizi H. Ghrelin upregulates Hoxb4 gene expression in rat bone marrow stromal cells. *Cell J* 2018;20(2):183-7. doi: 10.22074/cellj.2018.5164

31. Rak A, Gregoraszczuk EL. Modulatory effect of ghrelin in prepubertal porcine ovarian follicles. *J Physiol Pharmacol* 2008;59(4):781-93.

32. Park JM, Kakimoto T, Kuroki T, Shiraishi R, Fujise T, Iwakiri R, et al. Suppression of intestinal mucosal apoptosis by ghrelin in fasting rats. *Exp Biol Med (Maywood)* 2008;233(1):48-56. doi: 10.3181/0706-rm-169

33. Koyuturk M, Sacan O, Karabulut S, Turk N, Bolkent S, Yanardag R, et al. The role of ghrelin on apoptosis, cell proliferation and oxidant-antioxidant system in the liver of neonatal diabetic rats. *Cell Biol Int* 2015;39(7):834-41. doi: 10.1002/cbin.10464

34. Almasi S, Shahsavandi B, Aliparasti MR, Alipour MR, Rahnama B, Feizi H. The antiapoptotic effect of ghrelin in the renal tissue of chronic hypoxic rats. *Physiol Pharmacol* 2015;19(2):114-20.

35. Brooke G, Cook M, Blair C, Han R, Heazlewood C, Jones B, et al. Therapeutic applications of mesenchymal stromal cells. *Semin Cell Dev Biol* 2007;18(6):846-58. doi: 10.1016/j.semcdb.2007.09.012

36. Bang OY, Lee JS, Lee PH, Lee G. Autologous mesenchymal stem cell transplantation in stroke patients. *Ann Neurol* 2005;57(6):874-82. doi: 10.1002/ana.20501

37. Wu J, Sun Z, Sun HS, Wu J, Weisel RD, Keating A, et al. Intravenously administered bone marrow cells migrate to damaged brain tissue and improve neural function in ischemic rats. *Cell Transplant* 2008;16(10):993-1005.

38. Zhang W, Zhu C, Wu Y, Ye D, Wang S, Zou D, et al. VEGF and BMP-2 promote bone regeneration by facilitating bone marrow stem cell homing and differentiation. *Eur Cell Mater* 2014;27:1-11; discussion -2.

39. Liu N, Patzak A, Zhang J. Cxcr4-overexpressing bone marrow-derived mesenchymal stem cells improve repair of acute kidney injury. *Am J Physiol Renal Physiol* 2013;305(7):F1064-73. doi: 10.1152/ajprenal.00178.2013

40. Bi L, Wang G, Yang D, Li S, Liang B, Han Z. Effects of autologous bone marrow-derived stem cell mobilization on acute tubular necrosis and cell apoptosis in rats. *Exp Ther Med* 2015;10(3):851-6. doi: 10.3892/etm.2015.2592

24

Application of Response Surface Method for Preparation, Optimization, and Characterization of Nicotinamide Loaded Solid Lipid Nanoparticles

Molood Alsadat Vakilinezhad[1], Shima Tanha[1], Hashem Montaseri[2], Rassoul Dinarvand[3], Amir Azadi[4], Hamid Akbari Javar[1]*

[1] *Department of Pharmaceutics, Faculty of Pharmacy, Tehran University of Medical Sciences, Tehran, Iran.*
[2] *Department of Quality Control, Faculty of Pharmacy, Shiraz University of Medical Sciences, Shiraz, Iran.*
[3] *Nanotechnology Research Centre, Faculty of Pharmacy, Tehran University of Medical Sciences, Tehran, Iran.*
[4] *Department of Pharmaceutics, School of Pharmacy, Shiraz University of Medical Sciences, Shiraz, Iran.*

Keywords:
· Nicotinamide
· Response surface method
· SLN
· Stearic acid

Abstract

Purpose: Solid lipid nanoparticles (SLNs) have been proven to possess pharmaceutical advantages. They have the ability to deliver hydrophilic drugs through lipid membranes of the body. However, the loading of such drugs into SLNs is challenging. Hydrophilic nicotinamide, a histone deacetylase inhibitor, is used to establish SLNs with enhanced encapsulation efficiency by using statistical design.

Methods: The possible effective parameters of these particles' characteristics were determined using pre-formulation studies and preliminary tests. Afterwards, the Response Surface Method (RSM) was utilized to optimize the preparation condition of SLNs. The effect of the amount of lipid, drug, surfactant, and the mixing apparatus were studied on particle size, zeta potential, and encapsulation efficiency of the obtained particles. The acquired particles were characterized in respect of their morphology, *in vitro* release profile, and cytotoxicity.

Results: According to this study, all the dependant variables could be fitted into quadratic models. Particles of 107 nm with zeta potential of about -40.9 and encapsulation efficiency of about 36% were obtained under optimized preparation conditions; i.e. with stearic acid to phospholipon® 90G ratio of 7.5 and nicotinamide to sodium taurocholate ratio of 14.74 using probe sonication. The validation test confirmed the model's suitability. The release profile demonstrated the controlled release profile following the initial burst release. Neither the nicotinamide nor the SLNs showed toxicity under the evaluated concentrations.

Conclusion: The acquired results suggested the suitability of the model for designing the delivery system with a highly encapsulated water soluble drug for controlling its delivery.

Introduction

Preparation of a controlled release drug delivery system for incorporation of hydrophilic drugs is a concern in the pharmaceutical field. Various investigations have been carried out for this purpose.[1,2] Solid lipid nanoparticles (SLNs) have attracted considerable attention in recent years due to their advantageous characteristics.[3-5] Their advantages include biocompatibility, safety, stability, ability to be control-released, and ease of large scale production.[6-8] SLNs have the ability of delivering hydrophilic drugs through lipid membranes of the body. However, the loading efficiency of hydrophilic drugs is negatively impacted due to their rapid dissolving within the aqueous phase.[9,10]

Nicotinamide (NA) has an aqueous solubility of 691-1000 mg/ml.[11] Considering its hydrophilic characteristics, it can benefit from the advantages of a controlled delivery system such as SLNs.

NA, the active form of niacin, is a histone deacetylase (HDAC) inhibitor. Histone acetylation plays an important role in chromatin condensation and gene expression. HDACs are among the key responsible enzymes characterizing cell fate. Some diseases such as cancer and neurodegenerative disorders are considered to be the consequence of deregulation in activity of HDACs.[12,13] In the field of neurophysiology, this deregulation leads to impaired learning and memory.[14,15] In recent years, NA has attracted scientists' attention for delaying the progression of Alzheimer's disease in preclinical studies.[16] Acquiring the high encapsulated system of this freely soluble compound not only benefits the controlled delivery of NA itself, but can also enunciate the possibility of delivering other hydrophilic drugs.

*Corresponding author: Hamid Akbari Javar, Email: akbarijo@tums.ac.ir

Numerous parameters affect the properties of a delivery system. The type of lipid used for preparation of SLNs can affect almost all characteristics of the particles, including the particle size and the drug encapsulation efficiency.[17,18] Various lipids had been evaluated for SLNs preparation. Of all the natural lipids that can be used, stearic acid (SA) and glyceryl monostearate (GMS) were among the most investigated ones. Given their chemical structures, it can be expected that the hydroxyl groups of GMS can undergo interaction with the amide group of NA. Furthermore, it can be expected that SLNs incorporating SA represent appropriate particle size and stability characteristics.[5,19]

Beside the lipid, there are various factors that affect the characteristics of SLNs. These include the concentrations and ratio of the polymer, drug, and surfactant, as well as the preparation situation, including the type of apparatus, mixing intensity, and mixing time.[20] In fact, providing an optimum preparation condition is a basic step in preparation of any particulate system.

In traditional methods for multi-factor optimization, the effect of one factor is studied at a time while the other factors remain constant. This requires numerous trials which cost a lot of time and expense. Moreover, since in this method the possible interactions between studied factors are not considered, several failures in prediction of the optimum situation can be observed. Mathematical modeling by providing rapid optimization of various influential variables could be considered as a useful replacement for this traditional method.[21-23]

The response surface method (RSM) was used commonly for optimizing the preparation condition, as well as predetermining the properties of the pharmaceutical preparation.[24,25] The purpose of this project is to design a SLN system with improved encapsulation efficiency of the hydrophilic drug using NA. The effect of different factors, including the type of lipid, the amount of drug and surfactants, and mixing situation were studied on particle size, size SPAN, zeta potential, and encapsulation efficiency of the obtained nanoparticles. Response surface test with D-optimal design was carried out to obtain nanoparticles with appropriate characteristics. The acquired SLNs were evaluated in respect of their morphology, drug release pattern, and cytotoxicity.

Materials and Methods

Stearic acid was provided from Merck, Germany. Phospholipon® 90G was purchased from Lipoid, Germany. The SH-SY5Y cell line was received from Pasteur institute, Iran; and essential cell culture media components were provided from Gibco, USA. The 3-(4,5-Dimethylthiazol-2-yl)-2,5-diphenyltetrazolium bromide, MTT, was purchased from Sigma-Aldrich, USA. All the others synthetic materials were provided in analytical grade from Sigma-Aldrich, Germany. Required solvents were procured from local suppliers.

Pre-formulation studies

Standard curves of NA were prepared in distilled water and n-octanol using UV spectrophotometric method in wavelength of 254 nm.

Solubility and partition coefficient of NA were determined using Organization for Economic Co-operation and Development Test Guideline 105 and 107 (OECD TG 105 and 107), respectively.[26,27]

Partitioning of NA in different lipids were determined (Table 1). Briefly, the stock solution of NA in distilled water was prepared. Tubes containing constant amount of melted lipid, i.e. SA or GMS, or their combinations in different ratio, were prepared separately. Known volume of stock was added to each tube. Tubes were shaken at almost 10 °C above the melting point of the containing lipid. Samples were then cooled and phases were separated by centrifuge. Both aqueous and lipid phases were analyzed for the NA amount contained therein. Lipid partition coefficient was determined using following equation:

$$Pc \left(\frac{SA \ and/or \ GMS}{water} \right) = \frac{Concentration \ of \ NA \ in \ SA \ and/or \ GMS}{Concentration \ of \ NA \ in \ water}$$

Possible interaction between NA and lipid(s) was determined by Fourier Transform Infra-Red Spectroscopy (FTIR) studies (VERTEX70 spectrophotometer, Bruker®, Germany). Samples were prepared as physical mixtures (NA mixed with lipid(s) at room temperature) and melted-cooled mixtures (NA mixed with melted lipid(s) and then cooled to room temperature). The spectrum of NA, lipids, their physical mixture (ratio of 1:1), and their melted-cooled mixture (ratio of 1:1) were obtained. All spectrums were conducted in range of 400-4000 cm⁻¹ and KBr was used for preparation of samples.

SLNs were prepared by microemulsification method using the top two lipid(s) mixtures with higher NA partitioning; i.e. SA, and mixture of SA and GMS with ratio of 2:1. The obtained particles were characterized in respect of their particle size, size SPAN and stability. The better lipid composition was chosen for the further evaluations.

Preparation of SLNs

SLNs were prepared using microemulsification method.[28] SA and phospholipon® 90G were used as the internal oil phase. The external water phase were composed of sodium taurocholate and ultrapure water. The oil phase was heated up to 70 ± 2 °C on a water bath with continues stirring. The water phase was also heated up to the same temperature separately. By adding the oil to the water phase under mixing situation, the primary oil-in-water microemulsion (O/W) was obtained. The microemulsion was dispersed in a cold ultrapure water and mixed for 5 minutes. The resulted aqueous dispersion of SLNs were filtered through Whatman® Puradisc Syringe Filter (0.2 μm), washed using cellulose dialysis bag (MWCO 12 KDa) and then lyophilized. To prepare

drug loaded SLNs, the aforementioned procedure was performed while NA was dispersed in the melted oil phase.

Table 1. Solubility, partition coefficient and lipid partitioning of nicotinamide.

Solubility				
		NA in water (mg/ml)	NA in n-octanol (mg/ml)	
Preliminary test		714.28	4.347	
Main test		735.10	4.61	
Partition Coefficient				
n-octanol:water		NA in water	NA in n-octanol	Partition coefficient
1:1	Test1	0.679	0.291	0.43
	Test2	0.692	0.277	0.40
1:2	Test1	0.787	0.370	0.47
	Test2	0.791	0.387	0.49
2:1	Test1	0.708	0.262	0.37
	Test2	0.717	0.258	0.36
Lipid Partitioning				
SA:GMS		PC lipid/water		
1:0		0.24		
0:1		0.14		
1:1		0.18		
2:1		0.26		
3:1		0.12		
1:2		0.16		
1:3		0.11		

*NA= Nicotinamide, SA=Stearic acid, GMS= Glyceryl monostearate, PC=Partition coefficient.

Preliminary tests

The first attempt for SLN preparation was based on the M. Gobbi et al. report; i.e. 0.35 mM SA, 0.07 mM phospholipon® 90G, and 0.037 mM sodium taurocholate using mechanical stirring (700-900 rpm).[28] Unfortunately, the reported particle size (45.7 ± 3 nm) could not be achieved.

To attain the proper particle size, different situations were explored. Differing values of SA, phospholipon® 90G, and sodium taurocholate, and also the rate of stirring, were evaluated. All experiments were carried out in triplicate. Table 2 shows the different conditions which were experimented. The suitable level of the corresponding factors were determined by these preliminary tryouts and used for designing the D-optimal test.

D-optimal design

Response surface D-optimal design was used to optimize the best experimental situation for SLN preparation. Stearic acid to Phospholipon® 90G ratio (SA/Phos), nicotinamide to sodium taurocholate ratio (NA/T), and mixing apparatus were considered as independent variables. The levels of these factors were determined through preliminary tests. SA/Phos ratio of 5 to 7.5, and NA/T ratio of 10 to 15 were evaluated. While oil phase was added slowly to water

phase, the effect of different mixing instruments - including stirrer (1200 rpm), bath sonication, and probe sonication- were studied on the characteristics of the prepared formulation. The optimum formulation was selected regarding the acquired particle size, size SPAN, zeta potential, and encapsulation efficiency.

The equations of the most accurate model were achieved and the best model that fitted the data was assessed. Design-Expert statistical software (version7, Stat-Ease Inc.) was used for this evaluation.

Outliers were determined using normal probability plot and Cook's distance. The suitability of the model was demonstrated using lack of fit and plot of the residuals versus predicted values. Response surfaces plots were studied to demonstrate the optimum condition of evaluated variables.

Characterization of SLNs

Size, size SPAN and zeta potential of SLNs

The obtained SLNs were well dispersed in deionized water and their particle size based on the number diameter was measured by laser diffraction technique using particle size analyzer (Shimadzu SALD-2101, Japan).

Table 2. The effect of different variables on particle size and size SPAN (preliminary tests)

Independent variables					Dependent variables	
Stearic acid (mM)	Phospholipon®90G (mM)	Sodium taurocholate (mM)	Mixing	Addition method	Particle size (μm)	Size SPAN
0.35	0.07	0.037	700rpm	Pour	7.1	4.62
0.35	0.07	0.037	900rpm	Pour	4.06	4.66
0.35	0.07	0.037	1200rpm	Pour	1.83	2.2
0.35	0.07	0.037	Bath sonic.*	Pour	1.88	3.87
0.35	0.07	0.037	Probe sonic.	Pour	0.705	1.95
0.5	0.07	0.037	1200rpm	Pour	0.806	3.01
0.5	0.07	0.037	Bath sonic.	Pour	0.91	2.48
0.5	0.07	0.037	Probe sonic.	Pour	0.64	0.89
0.75	0.07	0.037	Probe sonic.	Pour	12.83	6.37
1	0.07	0.037	Probe sonic.	Pour	Aggregation occurred	
0.5	0.07	0.025	Probe sonic.	Pour	9.53	3.19
0.5	0.07	0.03	Probe sonic.	Pour	0.38	0.77
0.5	0.07	0.045	Probe sonic.	Pour	1.96	2.05
0.5	0.07	0.037	1200rpm	Slowly added	0.52	0.375
0.5	0.07	0.037	Bath sonic.	Slowly added	0.59	0.59
0.5	0.07	0.037	Probe sonic.	Slowly added	0.23	0.41
0.5	0.07	0.037	1200rpm	injected	0.641	0.53
0.5	0.07	0.037	Bath sonic.	injected	1.47	0.717
0.5	0.07	0.037	Probe sonic.	injected	0.45	0.501

* Sonication

To evaluate the size dispersity of SLNs, SPAN value was measured using the diameters of 90%, 50% and 10% of SLNs, obtained by laser diffraction technique (Shimadzu SALD-2101, Japan), as indicated in the following formula:

$$SPAN = \frac{d(0.9) - d(0.1)}{d(0.5)}$$

The SLNs were dispersed in deionized water and their zeta potential were determined using NANO-flex® (Microtrac, USA) zeta potential analyzer.

Encapsulation Efficiency
Diethyl ether was added to the lyophilized SLNs and mixed for 10 minutes to dissolve SA. NA was dissolved by addition of deionized water. The mixture was aggressively vortexed and centrifuged. The NA amount was assayed from the supernatant sample. The encapsulation efficiency (EE) was calculated using the following equation:

$$\%EE = \frac{Amount\ of\ Loaded\ Drug}{Total\ amount\ of\ Drug} \times 100$$

NA assay was performed using high performance liquid chromatography (HPLC) method (A20 Shimadzu,

Japan). The system was consisted of analytical column of HRC-ODS (150×6.0mm), a pump-controller unit (A20 Shimadzu) and an injector that were equipped with 20μl loop. Mixture of phosphate buffer (pH=4.5), methanol and glacial acetic acid was used as the mobile phase with ratio of 63:32:5 v/v respectively. Flow rate was adjusted to 1.5 ml per minute. The UV detector's wavelength was set to 254 nm. Chromatograms was analyzed using Solution Software. NA standard solution was used for method development. Validation tests were performed completely on the developed method. All tests were done in triplicate.

Particle morphology
The morphology of the selected NA-loaded and blank formulations were characterized by scanning electron microscopy, SEM (Cambridge, S-360, U.K.). Samples were coated with gold using sputter coater (Fisons, model 7640, UK) and then captured.

In-vitro drug release
In vitro release of NA from SLNs were studied using dialysis bag diffusion technique. The selected formulation was placed in dialysis tube and suspended in continuously stirred medium of freshly prepared

phosphate buffer, PBS (pH 7.4) and incubated at 37 °C (JAL Tajhiz lab tech, JTSL 20, Iran). Samples (2 ml) were withdrawn at different time intervals (at the beginning of test, 5, 15 and 30 minutes and 1, 2, 4 and 6 hours) and replaced with the same volume of fresh PBS. The withdrawn samples were analyzed by HPLC and their NA amounts were calculated. All measurements were done in triplicates.

The NA release profile was plotted in zero-order, first-order and Higuchi models. The best fitted model was determined using the acquired linear regressions.[29]

In-vitro cytotoxicity study
Cytotoxicity assay was performed on SH-SY5Y human neuroblastoma cells using MTT cell viability test. Cells were cultivated in Dulbecco's modified Eagle's medium (DMEM) that were supplemented with 10% fetal bovine serum and 1% penicillin-streptomycin.

Cells were seeded in 96-well plates at concentration of 1×10^4 cells per well. The NA solution, and suspensions of the blank SLNs, and NA-loaded SLNs (150 µl) were incubated with cells. After 24 h incubation, the content of each well was replaced with the same volume of media containing MTT (5 mg/ml). Plates were incubated for another 4hours, then MTT was removed and replaced with 150 µl of DMSO. Using microplate reader (Anthos 2020, USA), cell viability was assessed at 570 nm. Control cells were assumed to have 100% viability.

Data analysis and statistics
The statistical model design was conducted using Design-Expert statistical software (version7, Stat-Ease Inc.). For other statistical analysis, ANOVA test were performed by SPSS® statistics 17.0 (windows based version). Statistical significant was considered to be *p* value <0.05.

Results
Pre-formulation studies
Linear correlation was found between UV absorption and NA concentration in water (1-100 mg/ml) and in n-octanol (0.1-5 mg/ml). NA solubility in water and n-octanol are reported in Table 1. Table 1 also demonstrates the calculated partition coefficient of duplicate runs of three different solvent ratios. The average partition coefficient was 0.42 ± 0.05. Negative LogP value of -0.37 confirms that NA is a naturally hydrophilic substance. The partitioning of NA in SA and GMS at different ratios is also reported in Table 1. Partitioning of NA in SA and also in the mixture of SA and GMS at the ratio of 2:1 was greater than at the other investigated ratios (Pc calculated to be 0.24 ± 0.17 and 0.26 ± 0.2, respectively).

The FTIR spectrum of NA and lipid(s) are shown in Figure 1. The -NH stretch peak of NA was shifted from 3259.1 cm⁻¹ to 3104.8 cm⁻¹ in NA-SA melted-cooled samples. No shift was observed for this bond at NA-SA physical mixture spectrum. The -C=O stretch peak was shifted from 1722.1 cm⁻¹ in NA to 1660.4 cm⁻¹ in NA-SA

physical mixture and to 1579.4 cm⁻¹ in NA-SA melted-cooled samples. No significant shifts were observed in either the NA-GMS physical mixture or their melted-cooled samples. The -C=O stretch peak was also shifted to 1635.5 cm⁻¹ in NA-SA-GMS physical mixture, and to 1579.4 cm⁻¹ in NA-SA-GMS in melted-cooled samples. Particle size, size SPAN and stability of the acquired particles with SA and also the mixture of SA and GMS (2:1), are reported in Figure 2. Using SA alone, stable nano-sized particles were achieved.

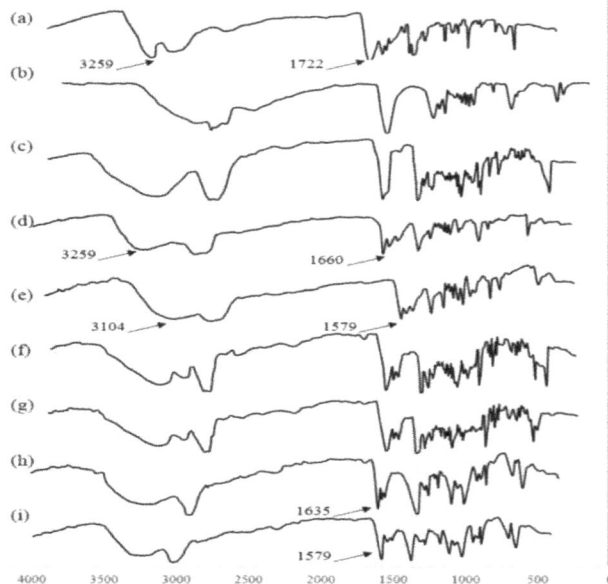

Figure 1. FTIR spectrums of (a) Nicotinamide, (b) Stearic acid, (c) Glyceryl monostearate, (d) physical mixture of Nicotinamide - Stearic acid, (e) melted-cooled sample of Nicotinamide - Stearic acid, (f) physical mixture of Nicotinamide - Glyceryl monostearate, (g) melted-cooled sample of Nicotinamide - Glyceryl monostearate, (h) physical mixture of Nicotinamide - Stearic acid - Glyceryl monostearate, and (i) melted-cooled sample of Nicotinamide - Stearic acid - Glyceryl monostearate.

Preparation of SLNs
Preliminary tests
As mentioned previously, SLNs were first prepared using 0.35 mM SA, 0.070 mM phospholipon® 90G, 0.037 mM sodium taurocholate and mechanical stirring of 700-900 rpm. Unlike the reported data (45.7 ± 3 nm),[28] the particle size in the micrometer range, i.e. 7.1 ± 4.62 µm and 4.06 ± 4.66 µm were obtained using the aforementioned stirring rates respectively (particle size was obtained before filtration).

To determine the most effective parameters affecting particle size, various factors such as mixing intensity, the amount of SA and sodium taurocholate, and the method of organic phase to the aqueous phase addition were investigated. Table 2 summarizes these results. The smallest particle size of 230 nm with SPAN value of 0.41 was acquired using the 0.5 mM SA, 0.07 mM phospholipon® 90G, and 0.037 mM sodium taurocholate while slowly adding the oil to water phase under probe sonication.

The appropriate range of SA, phospholipon® 90G, or sodium taurocholate concentrations was determined for further evaluation on the basis of these results.

D-optimal design

According to the preliminary tests, independent variables of SA/Phos ratio, NA/T ratio and mixing apparatus; and dependent responses of particle size, zeta potential and encapsulation efficiency were chosen for optimization

studies. Design and results of the D-optimal experiments are shown in Table 3. All the responses were polynomial and fitted to the quadratic model with no transformation except for the particle size, which transformed in base 10 log. Table 4 shows the analysis of variance for the models. These models were considered significant since their p-values are <0.05. The effect of these independent variables on corresponding responses is plotted in Figure 3.

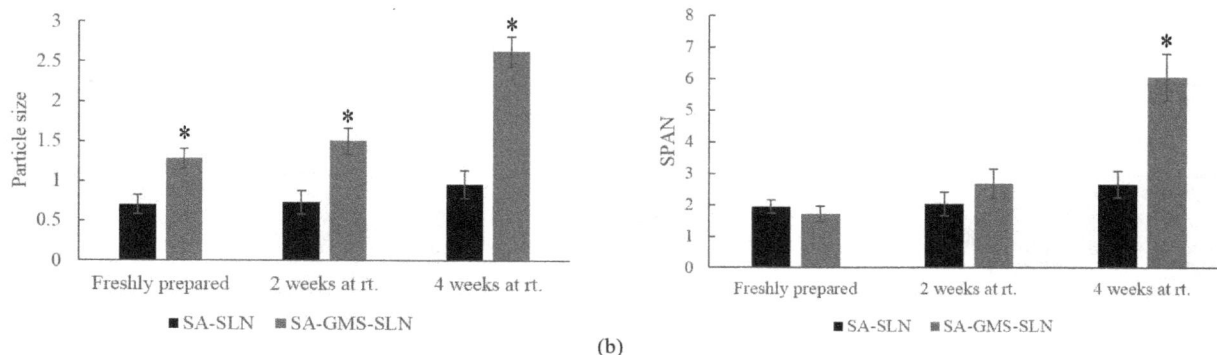

(a)   (b)

Figure 2. Characterization of SLNs prepared by stearic acid (SA-SLN) and mixture of stearic acid and Glyceryl monostearate with 2:1 ratio (SA-GMS-SLN). (a) Particle size and (b) size SPAN of freshly prepared particles and particles kept at room temperature for 2 and 4 weeks. (* p value <0.05).

Table 3. The dependent and Independent variables, experimental design matrix and results of D-optimal design.

Run	Independent variables			Dependent variables			
	A	B	C	Y1	Y2	Y3	Y4
	SA/Phos In range [a]	NA/T In range [a]	Mixing In range [a]	Particle size* Minimize [a]	Size SPAN	Zeta potential In range [a]	%EE Maximize [a]
1	6.80	12.50	bath	0.469	0.59	- 54.5	20.65
2	5.00	12.92	stirrer	0.63	3.61	- 71.2	19.54
3	5.00	12.92	stirrer	0.662	3.65	- 71.8	21.87
4	5.00	15.00	probe	0.389	1.59	- 51.5	26.43
5	6.45	15.00	stirrer	0.529	0.64	- 55.6	11.91
6	5.00	10.00	bath	0.07	0.73	- 49.1	21.59
7	7.19	10.00	stirrer	-	2.33	- 127.5	24.99
8	5.00	15.00	probe	0.435	0.55	- 51.1	28.66
9	6.03	10.00	stirrer	0.57	2.31	- 65.7	6.44
10	7.50	10.00	probe	1.976	3.76	- 83.6	22.68
11	6.25	10.00	bath	0.495	0.54	- 55.3	17.54
12	5.00	15.00	bath	0.577	1.35	- 65.5	16.29
13	6.25	12.50	probe	0.088	0.74	- 46.2	27.17
14	7.50	12.08	stirrer	0.608	4.19	- 68.1	17.05
15	5.31	10.63	probe	0.068	0.69	- 49.8	23.12
16	7.50	15.00	probe	0.112	0.69	- 41.5	37.24
17	6.25	12.39	stirrer	0.162	4.21	- 46.9	21.20
18	7.50	10.00	bath	6.701	0.64	- 91.4	21.22
19	6.45	15.00	stirrer	0.494	2.19	- 55.1	14.98
20	7.50	15.00	probe	0.095	0.75	- 40.3	33.41
21	7.50	15.00	bath	0.231	0.37	- 48.2	24.65
22	5.00	15.00	bath	0.547	0.83	- 62.4	13.40

SA/Phos (stearic acid to Phospholipon®90G ratio); NA/T (nicotinamide to sodium taurocholate ratio); %EE=%Encapsulation efficiency.
* reported in μm
[a] Constrains

Table 4. Analysis of variance for D-optimal refined models and the suggested independent variables for optimum preparation condition.

D-optimal design	Source of variation	Sum of Squares	Degree of freedom	Mean Square	F value	P>F	
Particle size	Model	4.55	9	0.41	32.14	<0.0001	Significant
	Residual	0.14	11	0.015			
	Pure Error	4.676E-003	5	9.352E-004			
Zeta potential	Model	6750.32	11	614.57	4.42	0.0132	Significant
	Residual	1391.86	10	139.19			
	Pure Error	5.91	5	1.18			
Entrapment efficiency	Model	806.01	11	73.27	3.46	0.0303	Significant
	Residual	212.00	10	21.20			
	Pure Error	21.47	5	4.29			

Suggested suituation							
				Observed	Predicted	% Observed to predicted ratio	
SA/Phos= 7.5			size	0.107	0.103	103.819	
NA/T= 14.74			Zeta Potential	-40.90	-40.30	101.489	
Mixing: Probe sonicaton			%EE	36.026	35.277	102.123	

SA/Phos (stearic acid to Phospholipon®90G ratio); NA/T (nicotinamide to sodium taurocholate ratio)

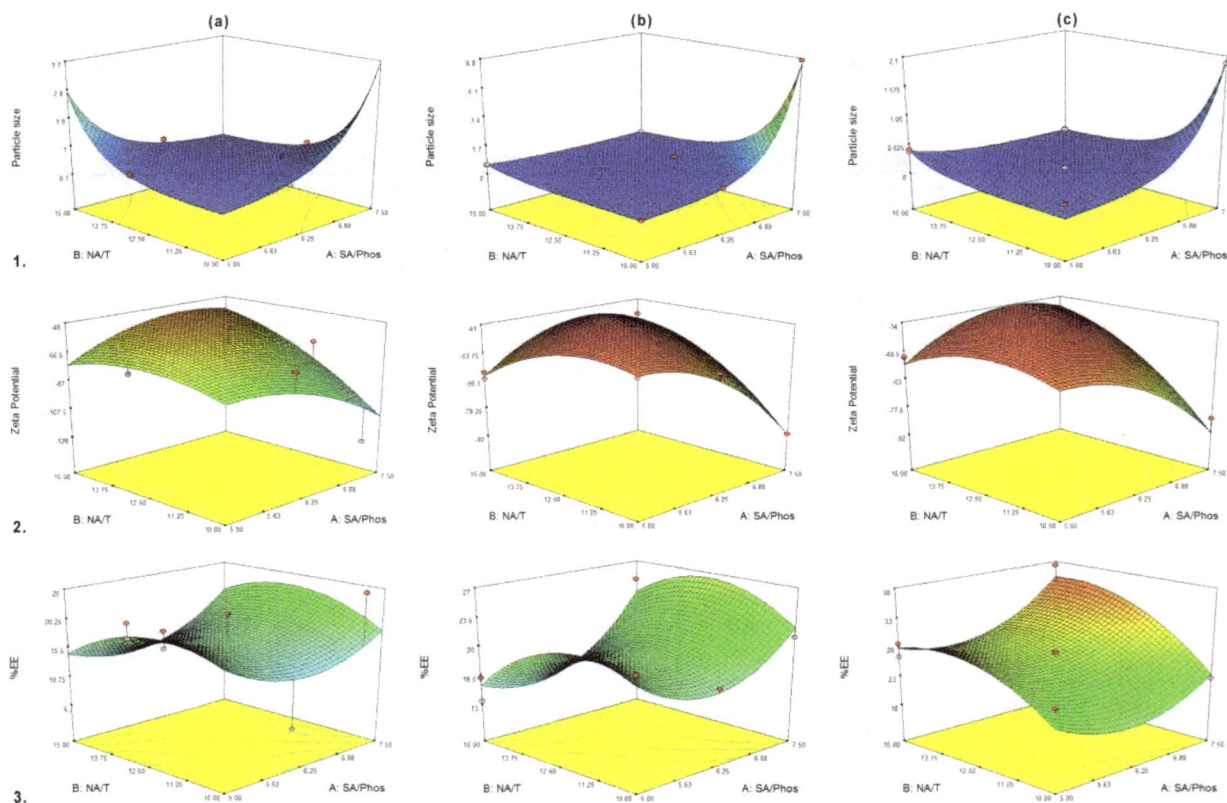

Figure 3. Response surface plots. Effect of Stearic acid to Phospholipon® 90G ratio (SA/Phos) and nicotinamide to sodium taurocholate ratio (NA/T) on (1) particle size, (2) zeta potential and (3) encapsulation efficiency (%EE) in different mixing situation of (a) stirrer, (b) bath sonication and (c) probe sonication.

Validation

The final equations in terms of coded factors were:

Log10(Particle size)= -0.75 +0.21× A -0.093× B +0.25× C[1] +0.039× C [2] -0.56× AB -0.24× AC[1] +0.21 ×AC [2] +0.15 ×A^2 +0.29 ×B^2

Zeta Potential= -46.98 -6.01 ×A +10.83 ×B -12.36 ×C[1] +3.74 ×C [2] +14.23 ×AB +1.74 ×AC[1] -1.35 ×AC [2] +3.72 ×BC[1] -4.50 ×BC [2] -11.42 ×A^2 -9.04 ×B^2

%EE= +21.17 +2.01 ×A +0.96 ×B -3.84 ×C[1] -1.47 ×C [2] +1.42 ×AB -0.58 ×AC[1] +0.39 ×AC [2] -1.45 ×BC[1] -2.04 ×BC [2] +4.31 ×A^2 -3.69 ×B^2

To be able to use the acquired equations confidently, validation tests were performed. It can be concluded from these results that the model can be fitted despite some contradictory data. The best situation according the

available data was achieved (Table 4). Plot of residuals versus predicted values demonstrates the suitability of the models (Figure 4).

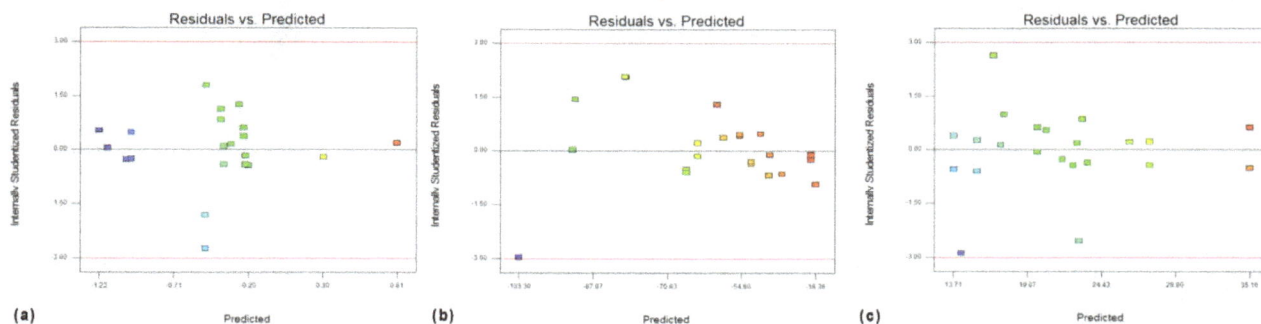

Figure 4. Residuals Vs. predicted graphs of (a) Particle size (b) zeta potential and (c) encapsulation efficiency.

Characterization of selected SLNs

Size, size SPAN and zeta potential of SLNs

The optimum preparation situation, i.e. SA/Phos ratio of 7.5 and NA/T ratio of 14.74 using probe sonication, was used to prepare blank SLNs and NA-loaded SLNs. Blank SLNs with size of 101 nm and zeta potential of -37.5 were acquired. NA-loaded SLNs of 107 nm with zeta potential of -40.9 were achieved.

Encapsulation Efficiency

NA assay was performed using the validated calibration curve (y=0.1385x + 0.0491 and r^2 0.9972) with acceptable precision and accuracy. In the optimum preparation condition, the encapsulation efficiency of 36% was achieved (Table 4).

Particle morphology

The final formulations were evaluated in respect of their morphologies (Figure 5). The SEM shows almost uni-

dispersed and spherical particles with agreeable sizes that were obtained by laser diffraction technique.

In-vitro drug release

The release profile of NA from the SLNs was studied (Figure 6). Approximately 50% of the drug was released in 4 h. It best fitted the Higuchi model, acquiring the highest r^2 value.

In-vitro cytotoxicity study

Figure 6 also demonstrates cytotoxicity of the acquired particles. According to the drug loading parameters, the amount of SLNs was calculated to represent NA concentrations of 120, 60, and 30 mg. The data shows that neither the NA nor the SLNs were toxic to the cells in the evaluated concentrations.

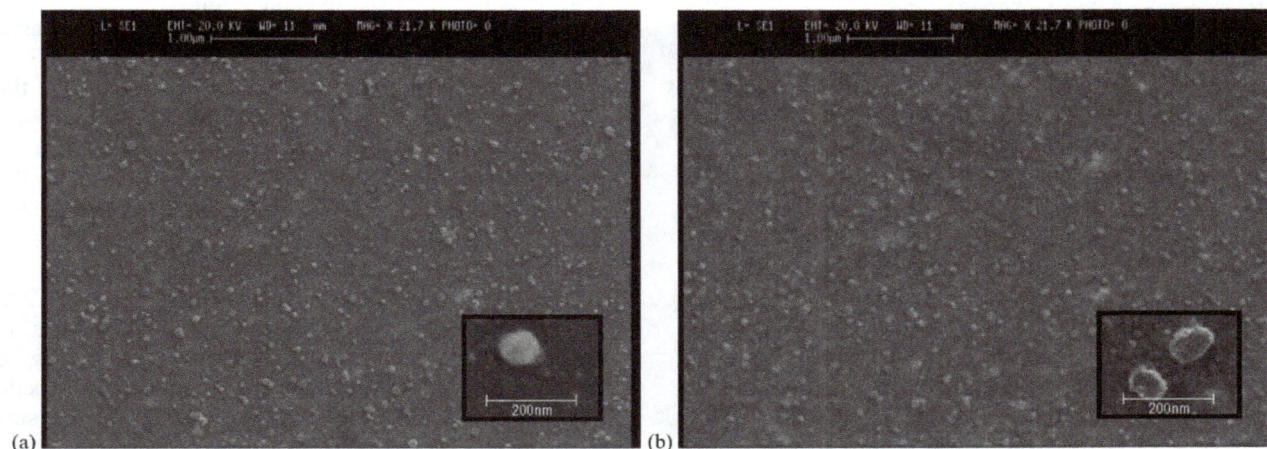

Figure 5. Scanning electron microscopy of the (a) Blank SLNs and (b) NA-loaded SLNs prepared in optimum condition; i.e. stearic acid to Phospholipon® 90G ratio (SA/Phos) of 7.5 and nicotinamide to sodium taurocholate ratio (NA/T) of 14.74 using probe sonication.

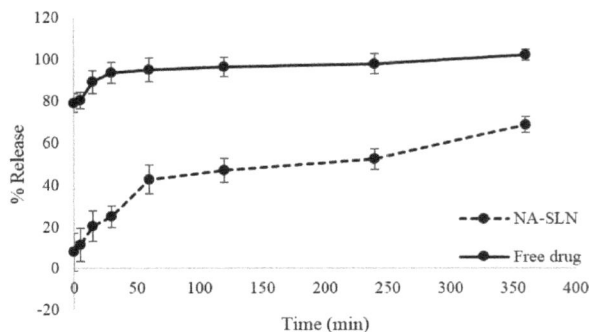
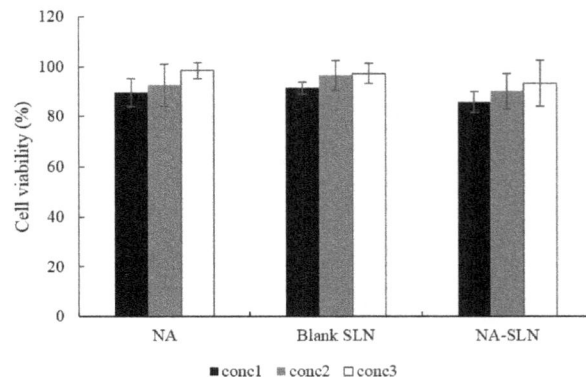

(a)   (b)

Figure 6. (a) The release profile of nicotinamide from SLNs (NA-SLN) and free drug; (b) Cytotoxicity evaluation of nicotinamide (NA), blank SLNs and NA-loaded SLNs (NA-SLN). Concentration 1, 2 and 3 represent the equivalent amounts of 120, 60 and 30mg NA (calculated based on the loading parameters).

Discussion

Biocompatible nano-particulate systems improve the controlled delivery of hydrophilic drugs to their sites of action, increase the therapeutic effect, and decrease the frequency of administration and thus the side effects of the drug. However, the low encapsulation efficiency of hydrophilic drugs in SLNs is a challenge in preparation of these pharmaceutical formulations. Through conducting proper pre-formulation studies and using statistical approaches such as D-optimal response surface tests, particulate systems with appropriate particle size, zeta potential, and encapsulation efficiency can be achieved. The present study aimed to achieve SLNs with efficient encapsulation of water soluble drugs possessing acceptable characteristics for sustained delivery.

NA is an HDAC inhibitor that could disrupt the progression of neurodegenerative disorders, like Alzheimer's disease. It could also play an important role in preserving the integrity of mitochondria by evolving in the electron transport chain. As a result, it could reduce the vulnerability of neurons to oxidative stresses.[30] Developing the high encapsulated system of such a freely soluble drug could benefit its delivery besides giving hope for the development of delivery systems for other soluble drugs.

The aqueous solubility of the drug directly affects its encapsulation efficiency into the SLNs. The solubility of NA in aqueous solvent ranges from 691 to 1000 mg/ml.[11] In the present investigation, NA had a solubility range of 735.1 mg/ml in water (Table 1). The acquired negative logP of -0.37 confirms that NA is a naturally hydrophilic substance. The variation of acquired logP at different ratios of water to n-octanol was within the reported acceptable limits of ± 0.3.[9]

The more the drug partitioned in the lipid(s), the higher was the encapsulation efficiency achieved. Therefore, the effects of partitioning of NA in SA, GMS, or their mixture at different ratios were investigated. Best partitioning was acquired in the mixture of SA to GMS with the ratio of 2:1. However, primary studies demonstrate that the particles obtained from this mixture are not stable in time (Figure 2). Hence, the second best lipid with high amount of NA partitioning, SA, was investigated instead. A stable particulate system with smaller particle size was achieved (0.7 μm in comparison to 1.3 μm in mixture of SA to GMS with ratio of 2:1).

Any interaction between the drug and the lipid lowers the affinity of the drug for leaving the primary microemulsion and, therefore, the SLNs. This improves the loading parameters.

The warmed primary microemulsion was poured into cold water to quench and solidify the particles during the preparation process. Considering this, the mixture of drug and lipid(s) was melted and then cooled to evaluate the solubility and possible interaction of the drug with lipids in the preparation process. The interaction was evaluated using FTIR studies.

The interactions between the functional groups were indicated through observation of shifting in the corresponding stretch bonds in the FTIR spectrum of the final compound. There was no significant shift in the presence of GMS; however the FTIR spectra showed obvious shifting for both -NH and -C=O peaks in NA-SA and NA-SA-GMS melted-cooled samples.

According to the results of these pre-formulation tests, SA was chosen for the further investigations.

The microemulsification method often results in the preparation of SLNs with reproducible sizes. However, there could be many parameters affecting the results. Various experiments were conducted to determine the most effective parameters regarding the size and also size SPAN as the size distribution indicator (Table 2).

Mixing intensity was among the studied parameters. In this matter, magnetic stirrer with a stirring rate of 1200 rpm was evaluated; bath sonication and probe sonication were also studied as mixing apparatuses. According to these results, nanoparticles prepared by using magnetic stirrer with a stirring rate of 1200 rpm had the same size as nanoparticles prepared by using bath sonication. However, size SPAN expanded in the bath sonication method. The data showed that mixing intensity is an important factor affecting both responses.

Different amounts of SA were also studied. Large particles formed or aggregation occurred at high amount (>0.75 mM).

Another factor affecting the characteristics of the final nanoparticles is the method of adding the organic phase to the aqueous phase. The organic phase can be added to the aqueous phase through pouring, injecting, or slow addition. Although the injection tip was warmed to inhibit the solidification of the lipid phase, narrow tips were not suitable due to the viscosity of the lipid. On the other hand, using the wider tips for injection resulted in larger particles. Slowly adding seems to be a more suitable method than the others since this results in smaller particle size and narrower particle size distribution.

The most assumingly effective independent variables for adjusting the preparation condition of SLNs were chosen considering these preliminary studies. Basically, by increasing the number of independent variables, the number of experiments needed to substantiate also increased exponentially. In this study the ratio of parameters, i.e. SA/Phos ratio and NA/T ratio, were considered to reduce the number of independent variables and subsequently the number of trials.

Response surface D-optimal design is a proven statistical method that can be used to optimize the best experimental situation for preparation of SLNs. It results in mathematical models for multifactor experiments. One could estimate the effect of the studied factors for a desired response.

The independent variables of SA/Phos ratio, NA/T ratio, and mixing apparatus, and dependent responses of particle size, zeta potential, and encapsulation efficiency were chosen for the optimization studies.

The p-value was used to indicate the statistical significance of the models. The p-value lower than 0.05 indicated that the model is significant with 95% confidence. All responses were fitted into the quadratic model and all the quadratic models were significant according to ANOVA results (Table 4).

Particle sizes were transformed in base 10 log. The smallest particle size of 68 nm was achieved with SA/Phos ratio of 5.31 and NA/T ratio of 10.63 by using the probe sonication (Table 3). Quadratic model suggested. Table 4 shows the result of the ANOVA test for the measured particle size. The F value of the model implies that this quadratic model is significant. All the variable factors had a significant effect on particle size: however, mixing apparatus was found to be the most effective one. Normally closed amounts of Predicted R-Squared to Adjusted R-Squared were expected. The "Pred. R-Squared" of 0.8433 is in reasonable agreement with the "Adj. R-Squared" of 0.9334. Signal to noise ratio was indicated by Adequate Precision. The resultant ratio of 23.508 showed the adequate signal. The effects of the independent variables on particle size are plotted in Figure 3. It was concluded that whenever the stirrer was used, particle size would increase due to increase in the SA/Phos ratio or increase in the NA/T ratio.

However, in cases where bath or probe sonication was used, increase in the SA/Phos ratio increased the particle size, although increase in the NA/T ratio did not significantly affect the particle size. This shows that mixing apparatus is the most effective parameter in this matter.

Table 4 also shows the results of the zeta potential modeling tests. No transformation was performed on the data. The 2FI model was suggested. However, the result of the ANOVA test showed that the quadratic model was also significant: this was preferable since it could exhibited the correlation in surface, and hence show the possible interaction between parameters. Although the mixing apparatus was significant in this model, NA/T ratio has the greatest influence. Further research should be undertaken to ensure that the model is fit. The effects of the independent variables on zeta potential are demonstrated in Figure 3. It can be concluded that no matter which apparatus is used for mixing, zeta potential will decrease due to increase in SA/Phos ratio or increase in the NA/T ratio. The only difference is the decreasing pattern.

No transformation was performed on encapsulation efficiency data. Linear model was suggested. For evaluating possible interactions between the parameters, data was fitted in the quadratic model. This was significant considering the results of ANOVA test (Table 4). The only significant term of this model is the mixing apparatus. Figure 3 demonstrates the effects of variables on encapsulation efficiency.

The results of the analytical tests were summed up in the final equations for every response. Positive and negative values show the synergistic and antagonistic effect on responses respectively. Each coefficient also represents the degree of effectiveness of that factor. These equations could be used to predict responses in imaginary situations.

In order to check the validity of models, validation test was performed. It can be concluded from the results that the model could be fitted despite contradictory data. The best situation according the available data seems to be the stearic acid to phospholipon® ratio of 7.5 and the nicotinamide to sodium taurocholate ratio of 14.74, using probe sonication as the mixing apparatus. In this condition, particle size of about 107 nm, zeta potential of about -40.9, and encapsulation efficiency of 36.02% was achieved.

The acquired zeta potential is comparable to the previously prepared SLNs.[28] Considering the solubility of NA, the acquired encapsulation efficiency seems to be suitable in comparison to the previously reported loading parameters of water soluble drugs.[2,10]

Considering the optimum situation for SLN preparation, final SLNs prepared and their morphological characteristics demonstrate the agreeable size with the acquired size by laser diffraction method. The particles were almost uni-dispersed and spherical (Figure 5).

The release profile of NA from the particles was also investigated. Considering the hydrophilicity of the drug, there was a primary fast rate of drug release, which could be attributed to the NA incorporated in the superficial lipid layer. In the studied formulation, almost 50% of the drug was released within the 4 h (Figure 6). The release rate then slowly continued for more than 10 h (data did not show), releasing the NA incorporated in the inner layer of particles. The recovery study shows that there is no interaction or barrier in the procedure that interferes in the detection of NA concentration.

It is often preferable that the delivery systems do not present cytotoxic effects. The cytotoxicity profile of NA, blank SLNs, and NA-loaded SLNs were evaluated. The results indicated that toxicity of NA and SLNs are negligible at investigated concentrations.

Conclusion

The present investigation demonstrates the benefits of pre-formulation and statistical studies in optimization of SLNs preparation and in improving the loading parameters of hydrophilic drugs into such carriers. Using the D-optimal surface response test, the effect of various parameters on particle size, zeta potential, and %EE were evaluated. All the responses fitted to the quadratic model and all models were considered pharmaceutically suitable. Using the suggested optimum situation with stearic acid to phospholipon ratio of 7.5 and nicotinamide to sodium taurocholate ratio of 14.74, and probe sonication as the mixing apparatus, 107 nm particles with zeta potential of about -40.9 and encapsulation efficiency of about 36% were obtained. Although the obtained particles had initial burst release, they could control the drug release afterwards. Their toxicity was considered negligible on the evaluated cell line. Overall, the acquired SLN system could be beneficial for delivery of nicotinamide. Besides, the suggested optimum situation for SLN preparation could be useful for designing the delivery systems for other hydrophilic drugs which is an ongoing work in our laboratory.

Acknowledgments

This study is part of PhD thesis supported by Tehran University of Medical Sciences (TUMS); Grant no. 94-02-33-29374.

Authors would like to acknowledge Dr. Ali-Mohammad Tamaddon from School of Pharmacy and Research Center for Nanotechnology in Drug Delivery, Shiraz University of Medical Sciences for his consult and cooperation throughout the study.

Ethical Issues

Not applicable.

Conflict of Interest

The authors report no declarations of interest.

References

1. Liu D, Chen L, Jiang S, Zhu S, Qian Y, Wang F, et al. Formulation and characterization of hydrophilic drug diclofenac sodium-loaded solid lipid nanoparticles based on phospholipid complexes technology. *J Liposome Res* 2014;24(1):17-26. doi: 10.3109/08982104.2013.826241

2. Nair R, Vishnu Priya K, Arun Kumar KS, Badivaddin TM, Sevukarajan M. Formulation and Evaluation of Solid Lipid Nanoparticles of Water Soluble Drug: Isoniazid. *J Pharm Sci Res* 2011;3(5):1256-64.

3. Gandomi N, Varshochian R, Atyabi F, Ghahremani MH, Sharifzadeh M, Amini M, et al. Solid lipid nanoparticles surface modified with anti-Contactin-2 or anti-Neurofascin for brain-targeted delivery of medicines. *Pharm Dev Technol* 2017;22(3):426-35. doi: 10.1080/10837450.2016.1226901

4. Mosallaei N, Jaafari MR, Hanafi-Bojd MY, Golmohammadzadeh S, Malaekeh-Nikouei B. Docetaxel-Loaded Solid Lipid Nanoparticles: Preparation, Characterization, In Vitro, and In Vivo Evaluations. *J Pharm Sci* 2013;102(6):1994-2004. doi: 10.1002/jps.23522

5. Layegh P, Mosallaei N, Bagheri D, Jaafari MR, Golmohammadzadeh S. The efficacy of isotretinoin-loaded solid lipid nanoparticles in comparison to Isotrex® on acne treatment. *Nanomed J* 2013;1(1):38-47.

6. Müller RH, Mäder K, Gohla S. Solid lipid nanoparticles (SLN) for controlled drug delivery - a review of the state of the art. *Eur J Pharm Biopharm* 2000;50(1):161-77. doi: 10.1016/s0939-6411(00)00087-4

7. Sailaja AK, Amareshwar P, Chakravarty P. Formulation of solid lipid nanoparticles and their applications. *Curr Pharm Res* 2011;1(2):197-203.

8. Pizzol CD, Filippin-Monteiro FB, Restrepo JA, Pittella F, Silva AH, Alves de Souza P, et al. Influence of Surfactant and Lipid Type on the Physicochemical Properties and Biocompatibility of Solid Lipid Nanoparticles. *Int J Environ Res Public Health* 2014;11(8):8581-96. doi: 10.3390/ijerph110808581

9. Rohit B, Pal KI. A Method to Prepare Solid Lipid Nanoparticles with Improved Entrapment Efficiency of Hydrophilic Drugs. *Curr Nanosci* 2013;9(2):211-20. doi: 10.2174/1573413711309020008

10. Singh S, Dobhal AK, Jain A, Pandit JK, Chakraborty S. Formulation and Evaluation of Solid Lipid Nanoparticles of a Water Soluble Drug: Zidovudine. *Chem Pharm Bull (Tokyo)* 2010;58(5):650-5. doi: 10.1248/cpb.58.650

11. 3-Pyridinecarboxamide (Nicotinamide). In: SIDS Initial Assessment Report For SIAM 15, CAS No: 98-92-0. 2002.

12. Timmermann S, Lehrmann H, Polesskaya A, Harel-Bellan A. Histone acetylation and disease. *Cell Mol Life Sci* 2001;58(5-6):728-36. doi: 10.1007/pl00000896

13. Haberland M, Montgomery RL, Olson EN. The many roles of histone deacetylases in development and physiology: implications for disease and therapy.

Nat Rev Genet 2009;10(1):32-42. doi: 10.1038/nrg2485

14. Peixoto L, Abel T. The Role of Histone Acetylation in Memory Formation and Cognitive Impairments. *Neuropsychopharmacology* 2013;38(1):62-76. doi: 10.1038/npp.2012.86

15. Stilling RM, Fischer A. The role of histone acetylation in age-associated memory impairment and Alzheimer's disease. *Neurobiol Learn Mem* 2011;96(1):19-26. doi: 10.1016/j.nlm.2011.04.002

16. Green KN, Steffan JS, Martinez-Coria H, Sun X, Schreiber SS, Thompson LM, et al. Nicotinamide Restores Cognition in Alzheimer's Disease Transgenic Mice via a Mechanism Involving Sirtuin Inhibition and Selective Reduction of Thr231-Phosphotau. *J Neurosci* 2008;28(45):11500-10. doi: 10.1523/JNEUROSCI.3203-08.2008

17. Das S, Ng WK, Kanaujia P, Kim S, Tan RB. Formulation design, preparation and physicochemical characterizations of solid lipid nanoparticles containing a hydrophobic drug: effects of process variables. *Colloids Surf B Biointerfaces* 2011;88(1):483-9. doi: 10.1016/j.colsurfb.2011.07.036

18. Garud A, Singh D, Garud N. Solid Lipid Nanoparticles (SLN): Method, Characterization and Applications. *Int Curr Pharm J* 2012;1(11):384-93. doi: 10.3329/icpj.v1i11.12065

19. Li M, Zahi MR, Yuan Q, Tian F, Liang H. Preparation and stability of astaxanthin solid lipid nanoparticles based on stearic acid. *Eur J Lipid Sci Technol* 2016;118(4):592-602. doi: 10.1002/ejlt.201400650

20. U.S. Department of Health and Human Services. FDA guidance of industry, ICH Q8 pharmaceutical development. Available from: http://www.fda.gov/CbER/gdlns/ichq8pharm.pdf.

21. Aboutaleb E, Atyabi F, Khoshayand MR, Vatanara AR, Ostad SN, Kobarfard F, et al. Improved brain delivery of vincristine using dextran sulfate complex solid lipid nanoparticles: Optimization and in vivo evaluation. *J Biomed Mater Res A* 2014;102(7):2125-36. doi: 10.1002/jbm.a.34890

22. Gheshlaghi R, Scharer JM, Moo-Young M, Douglas PL. Medium Optimization for Hen Egg White Lysozyme Production by Recombinant Aspergillus niger Using Statistical Methods. *Biotechnol Bioeng* 2005;90(6):754-60. doi: 10.1002/bit.20474

23. Kalil SJ, Maugeri F, Rodrigues MI. Response surface analysis and simulation as a tool for bioprocess design and optimization. *Process Biochem* 2000;35(6):539-50. doi: 10.1016/S0032-9592(99)00101-6

24. Azadi A, Hamidi M, Khoshayand MR, Amini M, Rouini MR. Preparation and optimization of surface-treated methotrexate-loaded nanogels intended for brain delivery. *Carbohydr Polym* 2012;90(1):462-71. doi: 10.1016/j.carbpol.2012.05.066

25. Ko JA, Park HJ, Park YS, Hwang SJ, Park JB. Chitosan microparticle preparation for controlled drug release by response surface methodology. *J Microencapsul* 2003;20(6):791-7. doi: 10.1080/0265204031000160051 4

26. OECD GUIDELINE FOR THE TESTING OF CHEMICALS 105: Water Solubility. OECD; 1995.

27. OECD GUIDELINE FOR THE TESTING OF CHEMICALS 107: Partition Coefficient (n-octanol/water): Shake Flask Method. OECD; 1995.

28. Gobbi M, Re F, Canovi M, Beeg M, Gregori M, Sesana S, et al. Lipid-based nanoparticles with high binding affinity for amyloid-beta1-42 peptide. *Biomaterials* 2010;31(25):6519-29. doi: 10.1016/j.biomaterials.2010.04.044

29. Vakilinezhad MA, Alipour S, Montaseri H. Fabrication and in vitro evaluation of magnetic PLGA nanoparticles as a potential Methotrexate delivery system for breast cancer. *J Drug Deliv Sci Technol* 2018;44:467-74. doi: 10.1016/j.jddst.2018.01.002

30. Liu D, Pitta M, Jiang H, Lee JH, Zhang G, Chen X, et al. Nicotinamide forestalls pathology and cognitive decline in Alzheimer mice: evidence for improved neuronal bioenergetics and autophagy procession. *Neurobiol Aging* 2013;34(6):1564-80. doi: 10.1016/j.neurobiolaging.2012.11.020

25

The Cytotoxic and Antimigratory Activity of Brazilin-Doxorubicin on MCF-7/HER2 Cells

Riris Istighfari Jenie[1,2] iD, Sri Handayani[2,3] iD, Ratna Asmah Susidarti[1,2], Linar Zalinar Udin[3], Edy Meiyanto[1,2]* iD

[1] Departement of Pharmaceutical Chemistry, Faculty of Pharmacy, Universitas Gadjah Mada, Indonesia.
[2] Cancer Chemoprevention Research Center, Faculty of Pharmacy, Universitas Gadjah Mada, Indonesia.
[3] Research Center for Chemistry, Indonesian Institute of Sciences (LIPI), Indonesia.

Keywords:
· Brazilin
· Doxorubicin
· Cytotoxic effect
· Migration
· MCF-7/HER2 cells

Abstract

Purpose: Breast cancer cells with overexpression of HER2 are known to be more aggressive, invasive, and resistant to chemotherapeutic agent. Brazilin, the major compound in the *Caesalpinia sappan* L. (CS) heartwood, has been studied for it's anticancer activity. The purpose of this study was to investigate the cytotoxic and antimigratory activity of brazilin (Bi) in combination with doxorubicin (Dox) on MCF-7/HER2 cells.

Methods: Cytotoxic activities of Bi individually and in combination with Dox were examined by MTT assay. Synergistic effects were analyzed by combination index (CI). Apoptosis and cell cycle profiles were observed by using flow cytometry. Migrating and invading cells were observed by using a Boyden chamber assay. Levels of MMP2 and MMP9 activity were observed by using a gelatin zymography assay. Levels of HER2, Bcl-2, Rac1, and p120 protein expression were observed by using an immunoblotting assay.

Results: The results of the MTT assay showed that Bi inhibited MCF-7/HER2 cell growth in a dose-dependent manner with an IC_{50} of 54 ± 3.7 µM. Furthermore, the combination of Bi and Dox showed a synergistic effect (CI <1). Flow cytometric analysis of Bi and its combination with Dox showed cellular accumulation in the G_2/M phase and induction of apoptosis through suppression of Bcl-2 protein expression. In the Boyden chamber assay, gelatin zymography, and subsequent immunoblotting assay, the combination Bi and Dox inhibited migration, possibly through downregulation of MMP9, MMP2, HER2, Rac1, and p120 protein expression.

Conclusion: We conclude that Bi enhanced cytotoxic activity of Dox and inhibited migration of MCF-7/HER2 cells. Therefore, we believe that it has strong potential to be developed for the treatment of metastatic breast cancer with HER2 overexpression.

Introduction

Metastasis is the latest stage of cancer progression and is difficult to overcome.[1] Metastasis is the process by which cancer cells leave the primary tumor and form secondary tumors at new sites. Several steps are involved in the metastasis process, including angiogenesis, loss of cell–cell adhesion, migration, invasion, and growth at the target organ site.[2] Although much research has been focused on the discovery of agents that have a role in metastasis, the effectiveness of the agents remains limited[3] and needs to be further explored.

Targeting drug discovery on the basis of molecular markers at every step of the metastatic cascade escalates the effectiveness of cancer treatment. ErbB2/HER2 (human epidermal growth factor receptor 2) is one of the important protein targets for cancer treatment. HER2 is a member of the epidermal growth factor receptor family that is overexpressed in many human cancers, especially breast cancer, and is related to invasiveness, drug resistance, and poor prognosis.[4] Overexpression of HER2 induces proliferation, migration, and invasion of cancer cells through its downstream signaling pathway. Overexpression of this protein increases Src synthesis and activates Vav2, followed by activation of Ras homolog-Guanosine Triphosphate-ases (Rho-GTPases) such as Rac1, cell division cycle 42 (Cdc42), and Ras homolog A (RhoA) and modulation of cell migration.[5] However, to activate HER2 signaling-induced migration, p120 catenin (p120) is needed as a Vav2 substrate.

Overexpression HER2 also has a role in increasing of the activation of matrix metalloproteases (MMPs), including MMP9 and MMP2.[5] Invasive cancer cells secrete MMPs, which have the ability to degrade components of the basal matrix and the extracellular matrix (ECM), followed by invasion of cells to other sites. The expression and activation of MMPs have an important role in tumor growth and invasion.[2] Many agents are studied for HER2-targeted therapy. Trastuzumab (Herceptin; Genentech, South San Francisco, CA) is an agent that competitively binds to the extracellular domain of HER2 and inhibits the HER2 signaling

*Corresponding author: Edy Meiyanto, Email: edy_meiyanto@ugm.ac.id

pathway.[6] Flavonoids hesperetin and naringenin inhibit the HER2 activation pathway through the same action as lapatinib as a tyrosine kinase inhibitor.[7] However, resistance of cancer cells to HER2-targeted agent was reported.[6,8] It is important to investigate alternative agents that have a role in the HER2 pathway.

Caesalpinia sappan L. is a promising medicinal plant that is targeted at the metastasis stage. Several studies revealed the potential of this plant and its compounds, such as brazilin and brazilein, for use in cancer treatment.[9–11] Brazilin (Figure 1) induces cell cycle arrest and inhibits MMP9 on cancer cells by suppressing nuclear factor (NF)-κB activation.[12] Brazilein inhibits migration and invasion through suppression of Rac1 protein expression, as well as MMP2 and MMP9 activation and expression, on metastatic cancer cells.[13,14] Because HER2 involves NF-κB, Rac1, and MMP protein upregulation, the potential cytotoxic and antimetastatic effect of brazilin on HER2 pathway and brazilin's potency as a co-chemotherapeutic agent need to be explored.

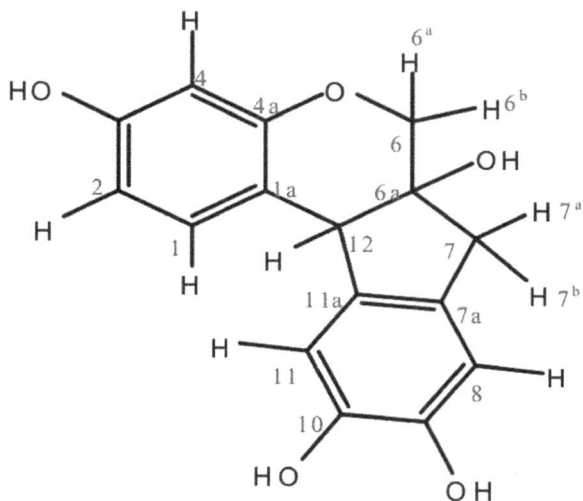

Figure 1. Chemical structure of brazilin

Doxorubicin is a well-known chemotherapeutic agent for treatment of metastatic cancer. Unfortunately, on one hand, this agent causes many side effects, such as resistance of tumor cells and toxicity in normal cells. On the other hand, HER2-positive breast cancer cells cause a phosphoinositide 3-kinase (PI3K)-dependent activation of Akt and NF-κB. This mechanism is associated with increased resistance of the cells to multiple chemotherapeutic agents, including doxorubicin.[15,16] To resolve these side effects, combination regimens have been developed to improve the effectiveness of cancer treatment.[17] One of the benefits of combination therapy is reduction of the concentration of the chemotherapeutic agent, which may reduce its toxicity. Surprisingly, a low concentration of doxorubicin induces epithelial-to-mesenchymal transition (EMT) followed by an increase instead of inhibition of cancer metastasis.[18,19] Therefore, brazilin has potential to be developed as a co-chemotherapeutic agent to counter doxorubicin-induced migration and invasion on HER2-overexpressing cancer

cells. The goal of this study was to understand the role of the HER2 pathway as a mechanism of the cytotoxic and migration-inhibitory effect of brazilin and the combination of brazilin with doxorubicin on HER2 breast cancer cells (MCF-7/HER2).

Materials and Methods
Preparation of Samples
Doxorubicin was purchased from Sigma-Aldrich (St. Louis, MO). Dried heartwood powder of *Caesalpinia sappan* L. was obtained from B2P2TOOT (Tawangmangu, Indonesia). Dried powder was extracted in methanol by maceration to get the methanol extract. The methanol extract was diluted as 4:1 methanol/water and then partitioned with hexane. The aqueous layer was fractioned with ethyl acetate and concentrated with a vacuum rotary evaporator to get the ethyl acetate fraction. Brazilin (0.245 g) (Figure 1) was obtained by separation of ethyl acetate fractions using Sephadex G-15 column (Sigma-Aldrich) chromatography (15 × 7 cm) with gradient polarity of the mobile phase (CHCl₃:MeOH) and was collected using thin-layer chromatography.

Identification of Brazilin
High-Performance Liquid Chromatography
The profile of brazilin was obtained using a high-performance liquid chromatography (HPLC) instrument (Shimadzu LC-10; Shimadzu, Kyoto, Japan) under the following conditions: reversed-phase C-18 column (RP-18 LiChroCART 125-4; Millipore Sigma, Burlington, MA) with methanol/water (30:70 vol/vol) as a mobile phase with a flow rate of 1 ml/min.

Fourier Transform Infrared
Infrared spectra were obtained using the KBr pellet method with a Fourier transform infrared (FTIR) instrument (Spectrum 100; PerkinElmer, Waltham, MA). Infrared spectra of our brazilin showed a band of –OH bond at 3371 cm⁻¹, a band of aliphatic C=C bond at 2928 cm⁻¹, and a band of aromatic C=C bond at 1610 cm⁻¹. The absence of carbonyl group (C=O) spectra at 1700 cm⁻¹ on brazilin is the main difference between brazilin and brazilein.

Liquid Chromatography-Mass Spectrometry
Liquid chromatography-mass spectrometry (LC-MS) (Mariner Biospectrometry workstation [McKinley Scientific, Sparta, NJ], Hitachi L-6200 [Hitachi, Tokyo, Japan]) was performed using a Supelco reversed-phase C-18 column (250 mm × 2 mm, 5 µm; Sigma-Aldrich) with an electrospray ionization (ESI) system (positive ion mode). The ESI mass spectrum was presented at 287 mass-to-charge ratio, corresponding to the [M+H]⁺ of brazilin (molecular weight, 286 g/mol).

H-NMR and C-NMR
Analysis was also carried out using nuclear magnetic resonance (NMR) spectrometry (JNM-ECA 500

spectrometer; JEOL, Tokyo, Japan) with proton nuclear magnetic resonance (^{1}H-NMR) and carbon nuclear magnetic resonance (C-NMR). The NMR data of the C-isolate showed ^{1}H-NMR (500 MHz, in acetone-d$_6$) 7.19 (^{1}H, d, J = 8.43 Hz, H-1), 6.49 (^{1}H, dd, J = 2.6 and 8.43 Hz, H-2), 6.31 (^{1}H, d, J = 2.6 Hz, H-4), 3.94 (^{1}H, d, J = 11.03 Hz, H-6^a), 3.71 (^{1}H, d, J = 11.03 Hz, H-6^b), 3.01 (^{1}H, d, J = 15.6 Hz, H-7^a), 2.81 (^{1}H, d, J = 15.6 Hz, H-7^b), 6.76 (^{1}H, s, H-8), 6.65 (^{1}H, s, H-11), and 3.97 (^{1}H, s, H-12); and ^{13}C-NMR (125 MHz, in acetone-d$_6$) 132.0 (C-1), 109.6 (C-2), 155.5 (C-3), 104,0 (C-4), 157.6 (C-4a), 70.8 (C-6), 77.8 (C-6a), 42.9 (C-7), 131.5 (C-7a), 112.7 (C-8), 144.8 (C-9), 144.6 (C-10), 112.4 (C-11), 137.4 (C-11a), and 51.1 (C-12). Based on comparison of the HPLC, FTIR, LC-MS, and NMR data, our findings for brazilin were similar to previously reported data.[20]

Cell Culture

The MCF-7/HER2 and MCF-7/empty vector (MCF-7/Mock) cell lines were kindly provided by Prof. Yoshio Inouye, mediated by Prof. Dr. Masashi Kawaichi (Nara Institute of Science and Technology). These cells were cultured in Dulbecco's modified Eagle's medium (Thermo Fisher Scientific, Waltham, MA) with 10% fetal bovine serum (FBS) (Thermo Fisher Scientific), 1.5% penicillin-streptomycin (Thermo Fisher Scientific), and 0.5% amphotericin B (Thermo Fisher Scientific).

Cytotoxic Assay with Individual Samples and Combination Samples

The cells (1 × 10^4/well) in 96-well plates were treated with various concentrations of the different treatment groups. After 24-h incubation, culture medium was removed and cells were washed in phosphate-buffered saline (PBS) (Sigma-Aldrich). Then, cells were incubated for 4 h with 100 μL of culture medium and 10 μL of 3-(4,5-dimethylthiazol-2-yl)-2,5-diphenyltetrazolium bromide (MTT) (Sigma-Aldrich) with 5 mg/mL in every well. The MTT reaction was stopped using sodium dodecyl sulfate (SDS) reagent (10% SDS in 0.01 M HCl; Millipore Sigma) and incubated overnight. The absorbance was measured with a microplate reader (Bio-Rad Laboratories, Hercules, CA) at 595 nm. The combination index (CI) was calculated using CompuSyn software (version 1.0; ComboSyn, Paramus, NJ).

Cell Cycle Distribution

A propidium iodide (PI) staining kit (BD Biosciences, San Jose, CA) was used to analyze DNA content. Cells were seeded into 24-well plates with 5 × 10^4 cells/well and treated with various concentrations of samples alone and in combination. After a 24-h treatment, cells were harvested, fixed with 70% ethanol, labeled with PI/RNase stain (2 μg/mL), and incubated at room temperature (RT) in the dark for 10 minutes. The DNA content was analyzed using flow cytometry (BD Biosciences) and Flowing software (version 2.5.1; Cell Imaging Core, Turku Centre for Biotechnology, Turku, Finland).

Apoptosis Detection

Populations of apoptotic cells were determined by PI-annexin V assay (Annexin V-FITC Apoptosis Detection Kit; Roche Mannheim, Germany). Cells (5 × 10^4/well) were seeded into a 24-well plate and treated with various concentrations of samples, alone and in combination. After a 24-h treatment, cells were harvested, added to 1× binding buffer, labeled with PI-annexin V, and incubated at RT in the dark for 5 minutes. Then, the cell suspension was analyzed using flow cytometry (BD Biosciences).

Migration and Invasion Assay

Cell migration and invasion were assayed in accordance with CytoSelect™ cell migration and invasion assay protocol (Cell Biolabs, San Diego, CA). Cells were serum-starved for 24 h, harvested, and suspended in 0.5% FBS/DMEM. Cells (3 × 10^5 cells/well) were seeded into the upper compartment of an insert chamber with or without samples on both migration and invasion compartments. The 10% FBS/DMEM medium was placed in the lower chamber. After a 24-h incubation at 37°C, nonmigrating cells on the upper side of the membrane were wiped off the upper compartment, and migrating cells on the lower side of the membrane were stained using the CytoSelect™ staining kit for 10 min at RT. After being gently washed and dried, cells were dissolved with extraction solution. The absorbance was measured using a microplate reader (SH-1000; Corona Electric Co., Hitachinaka, Japan) at 560 nm.

Gelatin Zymography

Secretion of MMP9 and MMP2 in the medium was assayed by gelatin zymography. Cells (1 × 10^6) were seeded into each well of a 6-well plate and incubated at 37°C in a CO$_2$ incubator for 24 h. Cells were incubated with a quarter of the half maximal inhibitory concentration (¼ IC$_{50}$) of samples, alone and in combination, in serum-free medium for 24 h. The medium was collected and subjected to polyacrylamide gel electrophoresis (PAGE) on 10% SDS-PAGE gel containing 0.1% gelatin and run in the SDS running buffer. The gels were washed in renaturing solution containing 2.5% Triton X-100 for 30 minutes, then incubated with incubation buffer (50 mM Tris-HCl, 150 mM NaCl, 10 mM CaCl$_2$) for 20 h at 37°C. The gels were stained using 0.5% Coomassie Brilliant Blue and incubated for 30 min at RT and destained with destaining solution (10% v/v methanol and 5% v/v acetic acid). Gels were then scanned and documented.

Immunoblotting Assay

Cells (1 × 10^6) were seeded into a 10-cm culture dish and incubated at 37°C in a CO$_2$ incubator for 24 h. Cells were incubated with ¼ IC$_{50}$ of samples, alone and in combination, for 24 h. Cells were collected with radioimmunoprecipitation assay (RIPA) buffer (25 mM Tris-HCl, pH 7.6, 150 mM NaCl, 1% Nonidet P-40, 1% deoxycholic acid-Na, 0.1% SDS, protease and phosphatase inhibitor cocktail). Protein concentrations were determined using the Bradford assay method, measured using a microplate reader (SH-1000; Corona Electric Co.). Then, samples were separated by electrophoresis on 7–15% SDS-PAGE gels and electrotransferred onto PVDF transfer membranes (Immobilon; Millipore Sigma). After being blocked with 1× NET gelatin buffer, the membranes were probed with antibodies for Rac1 (ab33186; Abcam, Cambridge, UK), HER2 (sc-52439), p120 (sc-13957), Bcl-2 (sc-7382), and β-actin (sc-47778; Santa Cruz Biotechnology, Dallas, TX) and then exposed to horseradish peroxidase-conjugated secondary antimouse (sc-2031; Santa Cruz Biotechnology) or antirabbit (7074P2, Cell Signaling Technology, Danvers, MA) antibodies. Protein expression was detected using an Amersham enhanced chemiluminescence system (GE Healthcare Life Sciences, Marlborough, MA).

Immunofluorescence Microscopy

Cells (5×10^4) were seeded onto coverslips in 24-well plates and incubated at 37°C in a CO_2 incubator for 24 h. Cells were incubated with a half of IC_{50} (½ IC_{50}) of samples, alone and in combination, for 24 h. Cells were washed with PBS, and after fixation with 70% cold ethanol and blocking with 1% bovine serum albumin (BSA), they were incubated with primary antibody for HER2 (sc-52439) followed by Alexa Fluor 488 secondary antibody. Then, cells were washed and incubated with 4′,6-diamidino-2-phenylindole (DAPI). Coverslips were moved into object glass and analyzed using a fluorescence microscope (Zeiss MC 80; Carl Zeiss Microscopy, Jena, Germany) equipped with blue argon (for DAPI) and green argon (for Alexa Fluor 488) lasers.

Statistical Analysis

Statistical analysis was performed using Student's t test (Excel 2013 software; Microsoft, Redmond, WA). P values less than 0.05 were considered significant. Effects of combinations on growth inhibition were analyzed using the CI equation developed by Reynolds and Maurer.[21] Gelatin zymography results were calculated by using ImageJ software (National Institutes of Health, Bethesda, MD).

Results and Discussion

Cytotoxic Assay of Samples Alone and in Combination

Brazilin was reported to have anticancer activity by inducing cell cycle arrest.[12] Therefore, we performed cytotoxic assays to confirm the potency of brazilin as an anticancer agent. The cytotoxic effect of brazilin and doxorubicin was measured by MTT assay. After 24-hour incubation, doxorubicin inhibited MCF-7/Mock and MCF-7/HER2 cell growth with similar IC_{50} values (3 µM) (Figures 2A and 2B), whereas brazilin inhibited MCF-7/Mock and MCF-7/HER2 cell growth in a dose-dependent manner with IC_{50} values of 44 ± 2.4 µM and 54 ± 3.7 µM, respectively (Figures 2C and 2D). These results show that brazilin possessed moderate cytotoxic

activity but that it has potential to be developed as a co-chemotherapeutic agent.

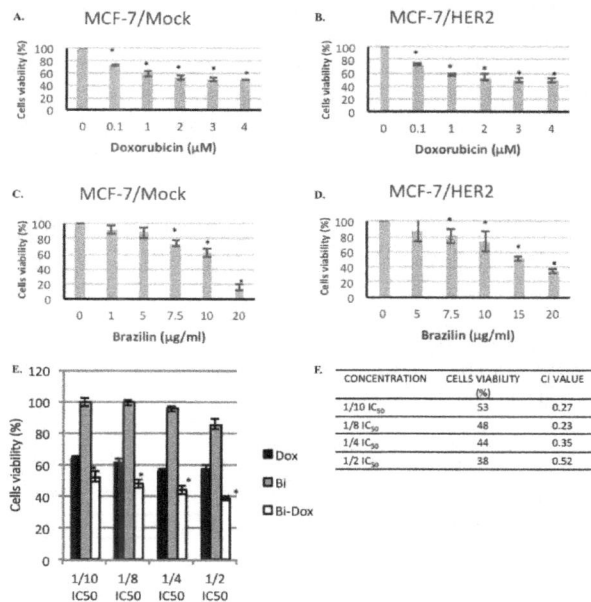

Figure 2. Cytotoxic activity of treatment with brazilin alone and its combination with doxorubicin on MCF-7/HER2 cells. Effects of treatment of MCF-7/Mock (A) and MCF-7/HER2 (B) with doxorubicin alone and treatment of MCF-7/Mock (C) and MCF-7/HER2 (D) with brazilin alone are shown. The combination of brazilin and doxorubicin (1/10-1/2 IC_{50}) (E) and the combination index value of the combination of brazilin and doxorubicin (F) effects on MCF-7/HER2 cells are also depicted. Cells were treated with various concentrations of samples for 24 h before assessment by MTT assay. Error bar represents standard deviation (n = 3, *$P < 0.05$ by Student's t test)

Next, to confirm whether brazilin enhanced the cytotoxic activity of doxorubicin, we analyzed the synergistic combination by using the CI. Combinations of 1/10, ⅛, ¼, and ½ IC_{50} of brazilin/doxorubicin showed a synergistic effect on inhibition of MCF-7/HER2 cell growth (CI <1) (Figures 2E and 2F). The combination of ½ IC_{50} brazilin/doxorubicin inhibited cell viability up to 62% compared with untreated cells. The findings regarding the combination of brazilin and doxorubicin indicated promise as a compound for HER2-positive breast cancer treatment. The synergistic cytotoxic activity may occur as a result of inhibition of cell cycle modulation or apoptosis induction. Accordingly, we observed the effect of brazilin and its combination with doxorubicin on cell cycle modulation and apoptosis in further experiments.

Cell Cycle and Apoptosis Modulation

Flow cytometric analysis for cell cycle showed that a single treatment of ½ IC_{50} brazilin or ½ IC_{50} doxorubicin caused a G_2/M phase accumulation compared with untreated cells (Figures 3A and 3B). Combination treatment with ½ IC_{50} brazilin and ½ IC_{50} doxorubicin induced G_2/M phase accumulation compared with either treatment alone (Figures 3A and 3B). Moreover, flow cytometric analysis for apoptosis showed that after 24-h incubation, treatment with either ½ IC$_{50}$ doxorubicin or ½ IC$_{50}$ brazilin alone induced apoptosis up to 9% and 12%, respectively, compared with untreated cells (Figures 3C and 3D). Combination of ½ IC$_{50}$ brazilin and ½ IC$_{50}$ doxorubicin increased necrosis rather than apoptosis (Figures 3C and 3D). We hypothesized that the necrosis event occurred after apoptosis induction. In *in vitro* studies, apoptosis leading to necrosis is the normal phenomenon of cell death owing to the absence of

phagocytic cells.[22] Next, to confirm our hypothesis, we observed the level of Bcl-2 protein expression. The result showed that brazilin alone and in combination with doxorubicin decreased the level of Bcl-2 protein expression (Figure 3E). Therefore, combination of brazilin and doxorubicin inhibited proliferation possibly by inducing apoptosis and cellular accumulation in G$_2$/M phase.

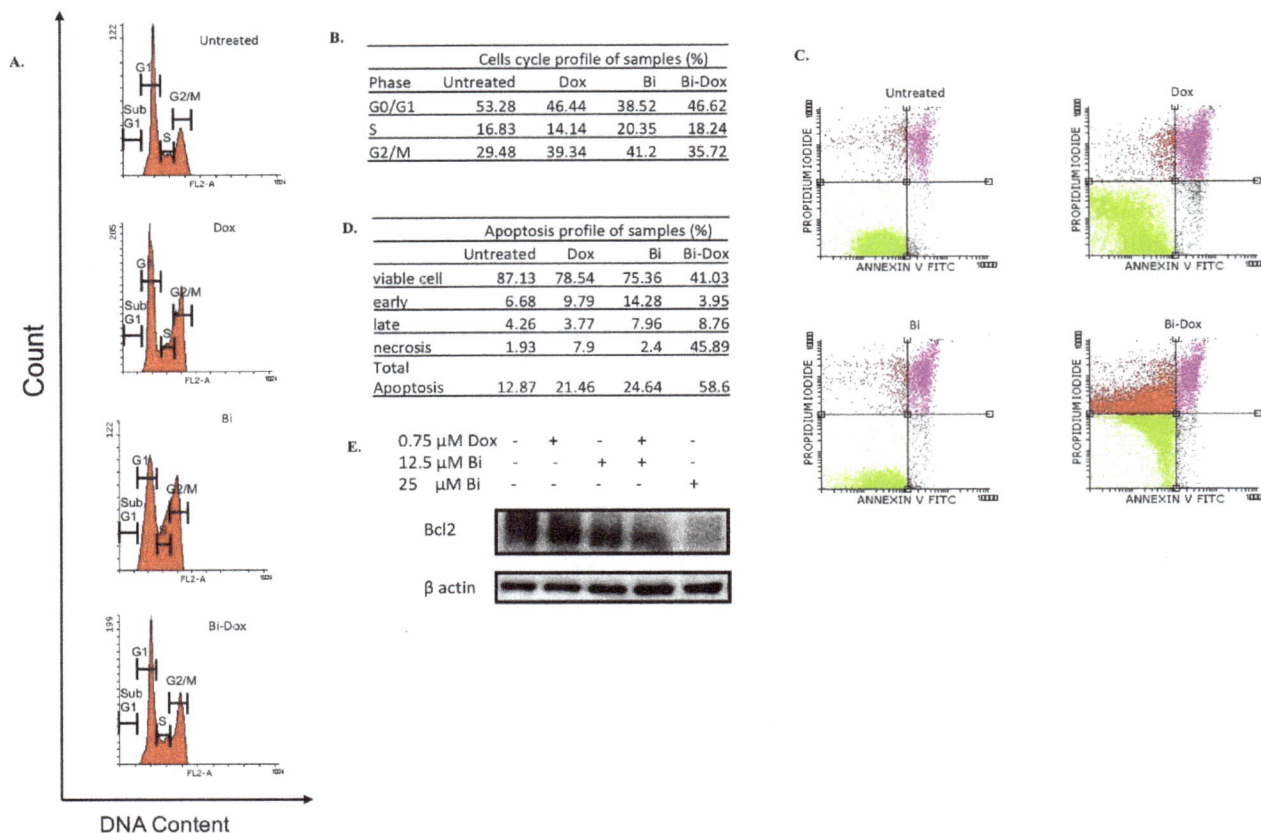

Figure 3. The effect of treatment with brazilin alone and its combination with doxorubicin on MCF-7/HER2 cell cycle profiles and apoptosis. Cells were treated with vehicle (untreated), 1.5 µM (½ IC$_{50}$) doxorubicin, 25 µM (½ IC$_{50}$) brazilin, and the combination of ½ IC$_{50}$ brazilin and ½ IC$_{50}$ doxorubicin for 24 h, then stained with PI/RNase for cell cycle analysis (A) or with PI-annexin V for apoptosis analysis (C). The analysis of cell cycle and apoptosis were conducted by using flow cytometry as described in the Materials and Methods; and quantified by using Flowing software (B and D). Cells were treated with brazilin alone and in combination with doxorubicin for 24 h, and the Bcl-2 protein levels (E) were observed by immunoblotting assay

Inhibition of Migration and Invasion

To study whether the combination of brazilin and doxorubicin had an antimetastatic effect on MCF-7/HER2 cells, we first tested the effect of each agent alone and in combination as ¼ IC$_{50}$ of brazilin/doxorubicin by migration and invasion assay. On one hand, the result showed that treatment with 0.75 µM doxorubicin alone increased migration and invasion of MCF-7/HER2 cells up to 11% and 16%, respectively. On the other hand, treatment with 12.5 µM brazilin alone, inhibited migration (up to 16%) but not invasion compared with untreated cells. Interestingly, the addition of brazilin to doxorubicin treatment inhibited migration and invasion up to 44% and 18%, respectively, compared with doxorubicin alone (Figures 4A and 4B).

Inhibition of MMP2, MMP9, HER2, p120, and Rac1 Protein Expression

Metastasis is a set of complex processes comprising internal and external molecular events. The high expression of proteinases such as MMP9 and MMP2 in the microenvironment of cancer cells is an example of external molecular events known to be involved in the degradation of the ECM and to play a critical role in tumor invasion and metastasis.[23] To understand the molecular mechanism that plays a role in inhibition of MCF-7/HER2 cell migration and invasion as a result of the treatments, we thus tested the effect of brazilin and its combination with doxorubicin on alteration of MMP2 and MMP9 protein expression according to gelatinolytic activity by using gelatin zymography. The results indicated that ¼ IC$_{50}$ brazilin alone and in combination with doxorubicin decreased MMP2 and MMP9 protein levels on MCF-7/HER2 cells (Figures 4C and 4D).

The HER2 pathway has an important role in the migration and invasion of cancer cells. In the present study, we observed the effect of brazilin and its combination with doxorubicin on modulation of HER2 protein expression on MCF-7/HER2 and MCF-7/Mock cells. The results showed that treatment with brazilin alone decreased HER2 protein levels (Figure 4E). This result was confirmed with immunofluorescence data that showed a downtrend of protein expression by the combination of brazilin and doxorubicin (Figure 4F). We also observed the effect of the combination of brazilin and doxorubicin on modulation of p120 and Rac1

proteins that have a role in HER2 overexpression and cell migration. The combination of brazilin and doxorubicin indicated a downtrend of p120 and Rac1 protein levels compared with untreated cells (Figure 4E). Estrogen receptor-α (ERα) is upregulated during HER2 therapy.[24] Then, we also checked the effect of brazilin treatment on ERα protein levels. The results showed that treatment of brazilin and its combination with doxorubicin did not affect ERα protein expression (Figure 4E). The combination of brazilin and doxorubicin showed a downtrend of HER2, p120, and Rac1 protein levels compared with untreated cells (Figures 4E and 4F).

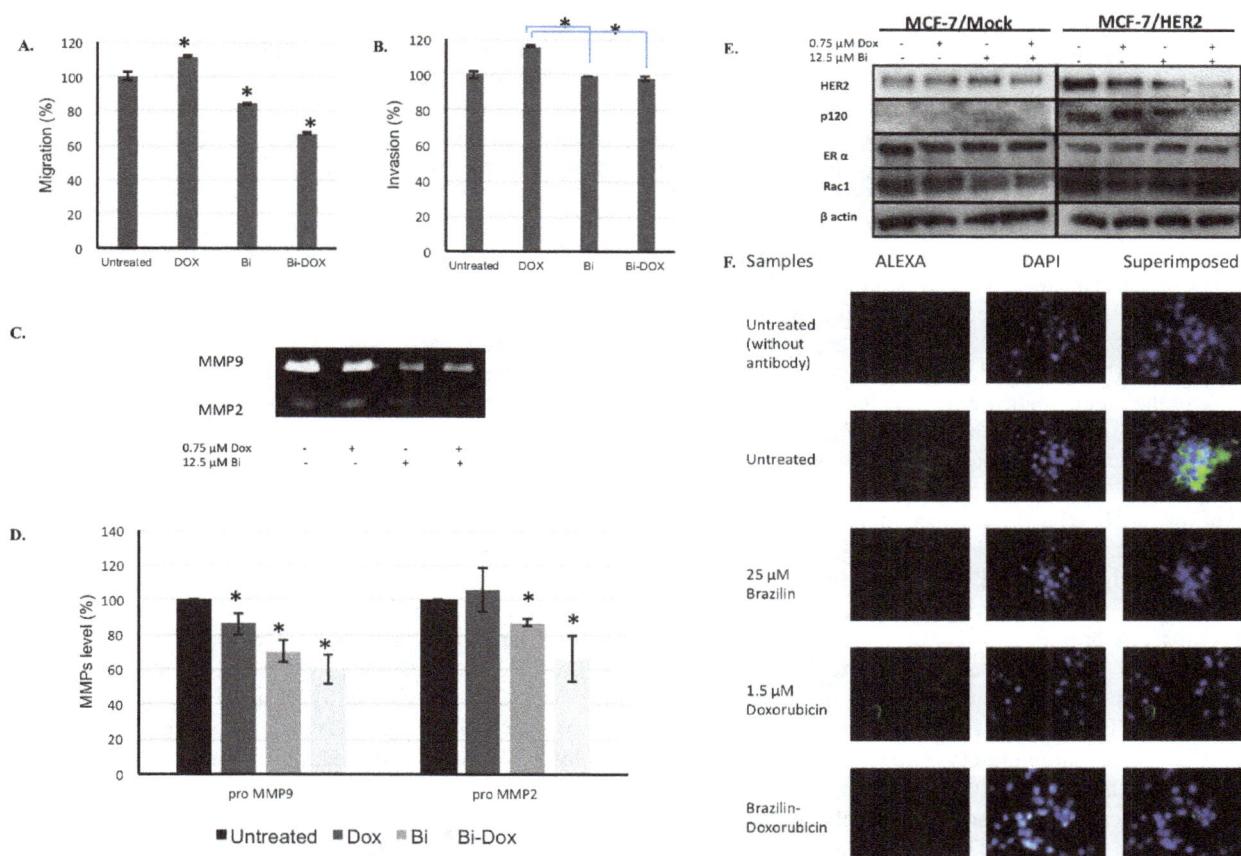

Figure 4. The effect of treatment with brazilin alone and its combination with doxorubicin on MCF-7/HER2 cell migration and invasion. Cells were incubated with ¼ IC$_{50}$ of brazilin or doxorubicin, alone and in combination, for 24 h in low serum concentration. Then, migration (A) and invasion (B) of cells under the chamber were measured using the migration and invasion assay. Cells were treated with ¼ IC$_{50}$ of brazilin or doxorubicin, alone and in combination, for 24 h. Then, the levels of the MMP protein bands were observed by gelatin zymography (C) and calculated by using ImageJ software (D). The levels of the HER2, p120, ERα, and Rac1 protein bands were observed by immunoblotting assay (E). Cells were treated with ½ IC$_{50}$ of brazilin or doxorubicin, alone and in combination, for 24 h and were observed according to the immunofluorescence method to visualize the alteration of HER2 expression resulting from treatment (F). Error bar represents standard deviation (n = 3, *$P < 0.05$ by Student's t test)

Migration and invasion are the basic metastatic stages of breast cancer. Importantly, overexpression of HER2 protein worsens the prognosis of metastatic cancer.[25] This study shows that the isoflavone brazilin has synergistic cytotoxic effects when combined with doxorubicin against MCF-7/Mock as well as MCF-7/HER2 cells. The flavonoids apigenin, hesperetin, and naringenin sensitize HER2-positive breast cancer cells,

leading to cell death.[7,26] Wighteone, an isoflavone derived from *Erythrina suberosa*, inhibits the proliferation of MCF-7 HER2-positive breast cancer cells.[27] Combination of polyphenols, including flavonoids, with other anticancer drugs increases the antitumor effects more than treatment using only one of the compounds.[17] The present study reveals the potency of brazilin as a co-chemotherapeutic agent for treatment of HER2-overexpressing breast cancer.

In order to confirm the mechanism that has a role in the synergistic cytotoxic effect of brazilin and doxorubicin on MCF-7/HER2 cells, studies of cell cycle modulation and apoptosis need to be done. We found that brazilin, doxorubicin, and their combination induce G_2/M accumulation (Figures 3A and 3B). On one hand, doxorubicin induces G_2/M arrest through its action as a type II topoisomerase inhibitor.[28] On the other hand, this study also confirms the finding of Kim et al.[12] that brazilin causes G_2/M arrest on U266 myeloma cells. Several isoflavones, such as genistein and DW532, induce G_2/M accumulation through binding on tubulin and leading to depolymerization of microtubules.[29,30] Because brazilin has an isoflavone structure, the effect of G_2/M accumulation by brazilin may travel the same pathway. Thus, brazilin and doxorubicin synergistically induce G_2/M arrest through different pathways.

This study also reveals that brazilin and its combination with doxorubicin induces apoptosis on MCF-7/HER2 cells by decreasing of Bcl-2 protein expression (Fig. 3E). Because the apoptotic mechanism of doxorubicin induces apoptosis through the FAS/FAS ligand,[31] the decrease in Bcl-2 seen in this study may be mainly attributable to brazilin. Decreasing Bcl-2 expression is followed by activation of caspases, leading to apoptosis.[32] Brazilin induces apoptosis through a caspase-dependent pathway.[33] HER2 overexpression activates the NF-κB transcription factor, which is involved with transcription of many genes, including *Bcl2*.[34] Jeon et al. reported that brazilin inhibits activation of NF-κB.[35] The flavonoid curcumin and its analog sensitized doxorubicin through inhibition of HER2 and activation of NF-κB.[36] Inactivation of NF-κB via the HER2 pathway may have a role in the induction of apoptosis by brazilin.

Migration and invasion are the important parts of the metastatic process.[2] This study reveals the inhibition of cell migration by brazilin (Figures 4A and 4B). Previous studies revealed antimigratory effects of the flavonoids brazilein and baicalein.[13,14,37] Secretion of MMP protein in the tumor microenvironment has a role in supporting migration and invasion of cancer cells through ECM degradation.[23] Our study shows the downregulation of MMP2 and MMP9 protein levels by treatment with brazilin alone and its combination with doxorubicin on HER2-overexpressing cells (Figures 4C and 4D). These data are in line with previous studies which showed that brazilein inhibits MMP2 on MDA-MB-231 cells and that its combination with cisplatin showed downregulation of MMP9 on 4T1 cells.[13,14] Other flavonoids, such as 7,7″-dimethoxyagastisflavone, luteolin, quercetin, and a curcumin analog (potassium pentagamavunon-0, K PGV-0), inhibit metastasis through suppression of MMP secretion.[38-40] Because NF-κB transcripts MMP protein[41] and HER2 protein has a role on NF-κB protein activation,[42] we drew an inference about the effect of inhibitory effects on migration and invasion by brazilin

and its combination with doxorubicin on MCF-7/HER2 cells probably being related to the HER2/NF-κB pathway. Furthermore, we confirmed our hypothesis that brazilin and its combination with doxorubicin would suppress HER2 protein expression (Figures 4E and 4F). Many studies found the HER2-inhibitory effect of flavonoids on cancer cells. Berberine, apigenin, and amentoflavone inhibit cell growth by downregulating HER2 protein expression.[43-45] Other proteins that are well known as key regulators of cell migration through the HER2 pathway are Rac1 and p120 catenin protein.[5] Rac1 expression induces migration and increases the resistance mechanism of anti-HER2 therapies.[46] This study shows downregulation of Rac1 protein expression by brazilin. Curcumin and wogonin inhibit cell migration by suppressing Rac1 protein expression.[47,48] Brazilein and its combination with cisplatin were revealed to downregulate Rac1 but not p120 protein expression on 4T1, a triple-negative breast cancer cell.[14] Interestingly, this study proves that the combination of brazilin with doxorubicin downregulates HER2, Rac1, and p120 protein expression on HER2-overexpressing cancer cells (Figure 4E). The expression of p120 is needed for migration and invasion of HER2-positive breast cancer cells.[5] However, the mechanism that has a role in inhibition of p120 expression by brazilin was not previously clearly understood. It probably is associated with its action on inactivation of NF-κB/Snail. Researchers in a previous study reported that apigenin inhibits EMT via inhibiting the NF-κB/Snail pathway.[49] Expression of Snail mediated by NF-κB activation increases splicing of the 120 kD isoform of p120 catenin.[50] Snail is known to have an important role on EMT induced by doxorubicin. On one hand, we hypothesized that brazilin-sensitized migration cells may increase via doxorubicin through this mechanism. On the other hand, Johnson et al.[5] reported that activation of Rho-GTPases, including Rac1, correlate with p120 levels in HER2-expressing cells. Thus, brazilin may suppress not only Rac1 expression but also its activation. However, further investigation is needed.

Cross-talk between ERα and HER2 induced HER2-resistant cancer cells.[51] The presence of ERα may interfere with agents that target the HER2 receptor.[24] To obtain additional data, we confirmed that brazilin and its combination with doxorubicin did not affect ERα expression. This means that suppression of HER2 expression by brazilin may not interfere with expression of ERα. Nevertheless, further studies are needed to confirm the mechanism that has a role in cytotoxic and migration-inhibitory effects of brazilin in combination with doxorubicin on HER2-overexpressing breast cancer cells. Brazilin has potential to be developed as a co-chemotherapeutic agent for metastatic cancer with HER2 overexpression.

Conclusion

This study shows that brazilin and doxorubicin work synergistically in inducing cytotoxicity in MCF-7/HER-2 cells, as shown by the CI value less than 1. The mechanisms involved were cell cycle arrest at the G_2/M phase and apoptosis induction by suppressing Bcl-2 expression. Moreover, we found that brazilin inhibited migration and invasion of MCF-7/HER-2 cells, whereas doxorubicin increased it. The mechanism involved was downregulation of the expression of HER2, p120, MMP2, and MMP9. Thus, brazilin has potential to be developed in combination with chemotherapeutic agents to increase cytotoxicity and to inhibit migration and invasion toward HER2-overexpressing breast cancer cells.

Acknowledgments
We thank to PUPT 2015-2016 from Indonesian Ministry of Research and Technology and High Education for the project grant. We also thank to Dr. Ahmad Darmawan for the NMR identification and Dra. Puspa Dewi Narrij Lotulung, M. Eng from Indonesian Institute of Sciences (LIPI) for LC/MS identification and thank Prof. Masashi Kawaichi, MD, Ph.D. from Nara Institute of Science and Technology, Japan, for providing the cell lines and for the technical assistance in this project.
Some parts of the data in this publication were used in the thesis dissertation of Dr. Sri Handayani

Ethical Issues
Not applicable.

Conflict of Interest
We declare that we have no conflict of interest.

References
1. Chakraborty S, Rahman T. The difficulties in cancer treatment. *Ecancermedicalscience* 2012;6. doi: 10.3332/ecancer.2012.ed16
2. Brooks SA, Lomax-Browne HJ, Carter TM, Kinch CE, Hall DM. Molecular interactions in cancer cell metastasis. *Acta Histochem* 2010;112(1):3-25. doi: 10.1016/j.acthis.2008.11.022
3. Weber GF. Why does cancer therapy lack effective anti-metastasis drugs? *Cancer Lett* 2013;328(2):207-11. doi: 10.1016/j.canlet.2012.09.025
4. Brix DM, Bundgaard Clemmensen KK, Kallunki T. When good turns bad: Regulation of invasion and metastasis by ErbB2 receptor tyrosine kinase. *Cells* 2014;3(1):53-78. doi: 10.3390/cells3010053
5. Johnson E, Seachrist DD, DeLeon-Rodriguez CM, Lozada KL, Miedler J, Abdul-Karim FW, et al. HER2/ErbB2-induced breast cancer cell migration and invasion require p120 catenin activation of Rac1 and Cdc42. *J Biol Chem* 2010;285(38):29491-501. doi: 10.1074/jbc.M110.136770
6. Ahmad S, Gupta S, Kumar R, Varshney GC, Raghava GPS. Herceptin resistance database for understanding mechanism of resistance in breast cancer patients. *Sci Rep* 2014;4. doi: 10.1038/srep04483
7. Chandrika BB, Steephan M, Kumar TRS, Sabu A, Haridas M. Hesperetin and naringenin sensitize HER2 positive cancer cells to death by serving as HER2

tyrosine kinase inhibitors. *Life Sci* 2016;160:47-56. doi: 10.1016/j.lfs.2016.07.007
8. Liu L, Greger J, Shi H, Liu Y, Greshock J, Annan R, et al. Novel mechanism of lapatinib resistance in HER2-positive breast tumor cells: Activation of Axl. *Cancer Res* 2009;69(17):6871-8. doi: 10.1158/0008-5472.can-08-4490
9. Kim EC, Hwang YS, Lee HJ, Lee SK, Park MH, Jeon BH, et al. Caesalpinia sappan induces cell death by increasing the expression of p53 and p21WAF1/CIP1 in head and neck cancer cells. *Am J Chin Med* 2005;33(3):405-14. doi: 10.1142/s0192415x05003016
10. Tao LY, Li JY, Zhang JY. Brazilein, a compound isolated from caesalpinia sappan linn., induced growth inhibition in breast cancer cells via involvement of GSK-3beta/beta-catenin/cyclin D1 pathway. *Chem Biol Interact* 2013;206(1):1-5. doi: 10.1016/j.cbi.2013.07.015
11. Handayani S, Susidarti RA, Jenie RI, Meiyanto E. Two active compounds from caesalpinia sappan L. in combination with cisplatin synergistically induce apoptosis and cell cycle arrest on WiDr cells. *Adv Pharm Bull* 2017;7(3):375-80. doi: 10.15171/apb.2017.045
12. Kim B, Kim SH, Jeong SJ, Sohn EJ, Jung JH, Lee MH, et al. Brazilin induces apoptosis and G2/M arrest via inactivation of histone deacetylase in multiple myeloma U266 cells. *J Agric Food Chem* 2012;60(39):9882-9. doi: 10.1021/jf302527p
13. Hsieh CY, Tsai PC, Chu CL, Chang FR, Chang LS, Wu YC, et al. Brazilein suppresses migration and invasion of MDA-MB-231 breast cancer cells. *Chem Biol Interact* 2013;204(2):105-15. doi: 10.1016/j.cbi.2013.05.005
14. Handayani S, Susidarti RA, Udin Z, Meiyanto E, Jenie RI. Brazilein in Combination with Cisplatin Inhibit Proliferation and Migration on Highly Metastatic Cancer Cells, 4T1. *Indones J Biotechnol* 2016;21(1):38-47. doi:10.22146/ijbiotech.26106
15. Kang HJ, Yi YW, Hong YB, Kim HJ, Jang YJ, Seong YS, et al. Her2 confers drug resistance of human breast cancer cells through activation of NRF2 by direct interaction. *Sci Rep* 2014;4:7201. doi: 10.1038/srep07201
16. Knuefermann C, Lu Y, Liu B, Jin W, Liang K, Wu L, et al. HER2/PI-3k/Akt activation leads to a multidrug resistance in human breast adenocarcinoma cells. *Oncogene* 2003;22(21):3205-12. doi: 10.1038/sj.onc.1206394
17. Fantini M, Benvenuto M, Masuelli L, Frajese GV, Tresoldi I, Modesti A, et al. In vitro and in vivo antitumoral effects of combinations of polyphenols, or polyphenols and anticancer drugs: Perspectives on cancer treatment. *Int J Mol Sci* 2015;16(5):9236-82. doi: 10.3390/ijms16059236
18. Chen WC, Lai YA, Lin YC, Ma JW, Huang LF, Yang NS, et al. Curcumin suppresses doxorubicin-induced epithelial-mesenchymal transition via the inhibition of

TGF-β and PI3k/AKT signaling pathways in triple-negative breast cancer cells. *J Agric Food Chem* 2013;61(48):11817-24. doi: 10.1021/jf404092f

19. Yang J, Guo W, Wang L, Yu L, Mei H, Fang S, et al. Notch signaling is important for epithelial-mesenchymal transition induced by low concentrations of doxorubicin in osteosarcoma cell lines. *Oncol Lett* 2017;13(4):2260-8. doi: 10.3892/ol.2017.5708

20. Nirmal NP, Rajput MS, Prasad RG, Ahmad M. Brazilin from caesalpinia sappan heartwood and its pharmacological activities: A review. *Asian Pac J Trop Med* 2015;8(6):421-30. doi: 10.1016/j.apjtm.2015.05.014

21. Reynolds CP, Maurer BJ. Evaluating response to antineoplastic drug combinations in tissue culture models. *Methods Mol Med* 2005;110:173-83. doi: 10.1385/1-59259-869-2:173

22. Ouyang L, Shi Z, Zhao S, Wang FT, Zhou TT, Liu B, et al. Programmed cell death pathways in cancer: A review of apoptosis, autophagy and programmed necrosis. *Cell Prolif* 2012;45(6):487-98. doi: 10.1111/j.1365-2184.2012.00845.x

23. Hua H, Li M, Luo T, Yin Y, Jiang Y. Matrix metalloproteinases in tumorigenesis: An evolving paradigm. *Cell Mol Life Sci* 2011;68(23):3853-68. doi: 10.1007/s00018-011-0763-x

24. Giuliano M, Hu H, Wang YC, Fu X, Nardone A, Herrera S, et al. Upregulation of ER signaling as an adaptive mechanism of cell survival in HER2-positive breast tumors treated with anti-HER2 therapy. *Clin Cancer Res* 2015;21(17):3995-4003. doi: 10.1158/1078-0432.ccr-14-2728

25. Nahta R. Molecular mechanisms of trastuzumab-based treatment in HER2-overexpressing breast cancer. *ISRN Oncol* 2012;2012:428062. doi: 10.5402/2012/428062

26. Seo HS, Jo JK, Ku JM, Choi HS, Choi YK, Woo JK, et al. Induction of caspase-dependent extrinsic apoptosis by apigenin through inhibition of signal transducer and activator of transcription 3 (STAT3) signalling in HER2-overexpressing BT-474 breast cancer cells. *Biosci Rep* 2015;35(6). doi: 10.1042/bsr20150165

27. Cao ZW, Zeng Q, Pei HJ, Ren LD, Bai HZ, Na RN. HSP90 expression and its association with wighteone metabolite response in HER2-positive breast cancer cells. *Oncol Lett* 2016;11(6):3719-22. doi: 10.3892/ol.2016.4488

28. Minotti G, Menna P, Salvatorelli E, Cairo G, Gianni L. Anthracyclines: Molecular advances and pharmacologic developments in antitumor activity and cardiotoxicity. *Pharmacol Rev* 2004;56(2):185-229. doi: 10.1124/pr.56.2.6

29. Mukherjee S, Acharya BR, Bhattacharyya B, Chakrabarti G. Genistein arrests cell cycle progression of A549 cells at the G(2)/M phase and depolymerizes interphase microtubules through

binding to a unique site of tubulin. *Biochemistry* 2010;49(8):1702-12. doi: 10.1021/bi901760d

30. Peng T, Wu JR, Tong LJ, Li MY, Chen F, Leng YX, et al. Identification of Dw532 as a novel anti-tumor agent targeting both kinases and tubulin. *Acta Pharmacol Sin* 2014;35(7):916-28. doi: 10.1038/aps.2014.33

31. Zhao L, Zhang B. Doxorubicin induces cardiotoxicity through upregulation of death receptors mediated apoptosis in cardiomyocytes. *Sci Rep* 2017;7:44735. doi: 10.1038/srep44735

32. Czabotar PE, Lessene G, Strasser A, Adams JM. Control of apoptosis by the BCL-2 protein family: Implications for physiology and therapy. *Nat Rev Mol Cell Biol* 2014;15(1):49-63. doi: 10.1038/nrm3722

33. Lee DY, Lee MK, Kim GS, Noh HJ, Lee MH. Brazilin inhibits growth and induces apoptosis in human glioblastoma cells. *Molecules* 2013;18(2):2449-57. doi: 10.3390/molecules18022449

34. Merkhofer EC, Cogswell P, Baldwin AS. Her2 activates NF-kappaB and induces invasion through the canonical pathway involving ikkalpha. *Oncogene* 2010;29(8):1238-48. doi: 10.1038/onc.2009.410

35. Jeon J, Lee JH, Park KA, Byun HS, Lee H, Lee Y, et al. Brazilin selectively disrupts proximal Il-1 receptor signaling complex formation by targeting an IKK-upstream signaling components. *Biochem Pharmacol* 2014;89(4):515-25. doi: 10.1016/j.bcp.2014.04.004

36. Meiyanto E, Putri DD, Susidarti RA, Murwanti R, Sardjiman, Fitriasari A, et al. Curcumin and its analogues (PGV-0 and PGV-1) enhance sensitivity of resistant MCF-7 cells to doxorubicin through inhibition of HER2 and NF-kB activation. *Asian Pac J Cancer Prev* 2014;15(1):179-84.

37. Shang D, Li Z, Zhu Z, Chen H, Zhao L, Wang X, et al. Baicalein suppresses 17- β-estradiol-induced migration, adhesion and invasion of breast cancer cells via the G protein-coupled receptor 30 signaling pathway. *Oncol Rep* 2015;33(4):2077-85. doi: 10.3892/or.2015.3786

38. Lin YC, Tsai PH, Lin CY, Cheng CH, Lin TH, Lee KP, et al. Impact of flavonoids on matrix metalloproteinase secretion and invadopodia formation in highly invasive A431-III cancer cells. *PLoS One* 2013;8(8):e71903. doi: 10.1371/journal.pone.0071903

39. Lin CM, Lin YL, Ho SY, Chen PR, Tsai YH, Chung CH, et al. The inhibitory effect of 7,7"-dimethoxyagastisflavone on the metastasis of melanoma cells via the suppression of F-actin polymerization. *Oncotarget* 2016;8(36):60046-59. doi: 10.18632/oncotarget.10960

40. Putri H, Jenie RI, Handayani S, Kastian RF, Meiyanto E. Combination of potassium pentagamavunon-0 and doxorubicin induces apoptosis and cell cycle arrest and inhibits metastasis in breast cancer cells. *Asian Pac J Cancer Prev* 2016;17(5):2683-8.

41. Yeh CB, Hsieh MJ, Hsieh YH, Chien MH, Chiou HL, Yang SF. Antimetastatic effects of norcantharidin on

hepatocellular carcinoma by transcriptional inhibition of MMP-9 through modulation of NF-kB activity. *PLoS One* 2012;7(2):e31055. doi: 10.1371/journal.pone.0031055

42. Siddiqa A, Long LM, Li L, Marciniak RA, Kazhdan I. Expression of HER-2 in MCF-7 breast cancer cells modulates anti-apoptotic proteins survivin and Bcl-2 via the extracellular signal-related kinase (ERK) and phosphoinositide-3 kinase (PI3K) signalling pathways. *BMC Cancer* 2008;8:129. doi: 10.1186/1471-2407-8-129

43. Lee JS, Sul JY, Park JB, Lee MS, Cha EY, Song IS, et al. Fatty acid synthase inhibition by amentoflavone suppresses HER2/neu (erbB2) oncogene in SKBR3 human breast cancer cells. *Phytother Res* 2013;27(5):713-20. doi: 10.1002/ptr.4778

44. Way TD, Kao MC, Lin JK. Degradation of HER2/neu by apigenin induces apoptosis through cytochrome c release and caspase-3 activation in HER2/neu-overexpressing breast cancer cells. *FEBS Lett* 2005;579(1):145-52. doi: 10.1016/j.febslet.2004.11.061

45. Kuo HP, Chuang TC, Yeh MH, Hsu SC, Way TD, Chen PY, et al. Growth suppression of HER2-overexpressing breast cancer cells by berberine via modulation of the HER2/PI3K/AKT signaling pathway. *J Agric Food Chem* 2011;59(15):8216-24. doi: 10.1021/jf2012584

46. Bid HK, Roberts RD, Manchanda PK, Houghton PJ. RAC1: An emerging therapeutic option for targeting cancer angiogenesis and metastasis. *Mol Cancer Ther* 2013;12(10):1925-34. doi: 10.1158/1535-7163.mct-13-0164

47. Zhao K, Wei L, Hui H, Dai Q, You QD, Guo QL, et al. Wogonin suppresses melanoma cell B16-F10 invasion and migration by inhibiting ras-medicated pathways. *PLoS One* 2014;9(9):e106458. doi: 10.1371/journal.pone.0106458

48. Chen QY, Zheng Y, Jiao DM, Chen FY, Hu HZ, Wu YQ, et al. Curcumin inhibits lung cancer cell migration and invasion through Rac1-dependent signaling pathway. *J Nutr Biochem* 2014;25(2):177-85. doi: 10.1016/j.jnutbio.2013.10.004

49. Qin Y, Zhao D, Zhou HG, Wang XH, Zhong WL, Chen S, et al. Apigenin inhibits NF-kappab and snail signaling, EMT and metastasis in human hepatocellular carcinoma. *Oncotarget* 2016;7(27):41421-31. doi: 10.18632/oncotarget.9404

50. Ohkubo T, Ozawa M. The transcription factor snail downregulates the tight junction components independently of E-cadherin downregulation. *J Cell Sci* 2004;117(Pt 9):1675-85. doi: 10.1242/jcs.01004

51. Chen Z, Wang Y, Warden C, Chen S. Cross-talk between ER and HER2 regulates c-MYC-mediated glutamine metabolism in aromatase inhibitor resistant breast cancer cells. *J Steroid Biochem Mol Biol* 2015;149:118-27. doi: 10.1016/j.jsbmb.2015.02.004

26

A Molecular Study on Drug Delivery System Based on Carbon Nanotube Compared to Silicon Carbide Nanotube for Encapsulation of Platinum-Based Anticancer Drug

Zahra Khatti[1], Seyed Majid Hashemianzadeh[2], Seyed Ali Shafiei[3]*

[1] *Department of Chemistry, Iran University of Science and Technology, Tehran, Iran.*
[2] *Molecular Simulation Research Laboratory, Department of Chemistry, Iran University of Science and Technology, Tehran, Iran.*
[3] *Neurology and Neuroscience Research Center, Qom University of Medical Sciences, Qom, Iran.*

Keywords:
· Molecular Dynamic Simulation
· Carbon nanotube
· Silicon Carbide nanotube
· Platinum-based anticancer drug

Abstract

Purpose: Drug delivery has a critical role in the treatment of cancer, in particular, carbon nanotubes for their potential use in various biomedical devices and therapies. From many other materials which could be more biocompatible and biodegradable and which could form single-walled nanotubes, silicon carbide was selected.

Methods: To compare two drug delivery systems based on single-walled nanotubes, molecular dynamic simulations were applied and encapsulation behavior of the drug carboplatin was investigated inside the silicon carbide nanotube and the carbon nanotube.

Results: Localization of the carboplatin inside the nanotubes indicated that the carboplatin moves throughout the tubes and possesses a greater probability of finding the drug molecule along the nanotubes in the first quarter of the tubes. The energy analysis exhibited the lowest free energy of binding belongs to the encapsulation of the drug carboplatin in the silicon carbide nanotube, about -145 Kcal/mol.

Conclusion: The results confirmed that the silicon carbide nanotube is a more suitable model than the carbon nanotube for drug delivery system based on nanotubes as a carrier of platinum-based anticancer drugs.

Introduction

Carbon nanotubes (CNTs), due to their unique atomic configuration, mechanical, optical and electronic properties, have been envisioned in designing biomedical devices and therapies on novel delivery platforms.[1-5] The physicochemical versatility of carbon nanotubes is related to their high surface-area-to-volume ratios and facile functionalization along the nanotube axis and a great inner content that can be filled with the desired drug molecules.[6-8] Additionally, the ability of single-walled carbon nanotubes (SWCNT) to incorporate inside cells has been proven, independent of cell type and functional groups linked to the nanotubes.[9,10] In vivo assays have demonstrated that SWCNTs as carriers have no obvious toxicity,[11] and in animal models have demonstrated the efficacy of drug-loaded CNTs through targeting tumors.[6,12] Whereas water is the main component in biological systems and CNTs are hydrophobic, heterogeneous CNTs could be considered including silicon carbide nanotube (SiCNT) in aqueous media.[13] In previous studies, several advantages have been shown for SiCNTs compared to CNTs. First, there is the relative stability increase from the CNTs to SiCNTs when the ratio of Si over C is 50:50, due to alternative sp2 and sp3 hybridization bond structures that

are more stable than a smooth-walled tube.[14] Additionally, the external surface of SiCNTs has higher reactivity than that of CNTs to facilitate aimed side wall functionalization.[15,16] Furthermore, the experimental results prove the biocompatibility of silicon nanotubes and hence an alternative option for applications in nanomedicine.[17,18] Platinum-based anticancer drugs are used to treat many types of solid tumors via binding to DNA and inducing cellular apoptosis, despite their adverse side effects,[19,20] so that many of these side effects for healthy cells can be greatly reduced by nanoscale drug delivery. A fast and reliable tool to evaluate theoretically such systems is molecular modeling, which could interpret the details of the interaction between the drug and both the DNA and the nanostructures.[21] On the other hand, our previous study allowed the assessment of a drug delivery system caused by another nanotube apart from CNTs, as carrier on theoretical level for the first time.[22] Therefore, in the present study, molecular dynamics (MD) simulation was employed to investigate another so-named nanotube SiCNT as delivery system compared to CNT. Carboplatin (diammineplatinum(II) cyclobutane-1,1-dicarboxylate) was selected as a drug model because it

*Corresponding author: Seyed Ali Shafiei, Email sashafiei@muq.ac.ir

encompasses fewer adverse effects and has greater water solubility than other platinum agents.[23-25] Our simulations have been performed to assess the encapsulation behavior and localization of the anticancer drug carboplatin inside pristine CNT and SiCNT. For this purpose, the placement of the drug inside nanotubes and the free energy calculations were implemented to determine the preference between the two predicted drug delivery systems.

Materials and Methods
Systems preparation
In the present work, the zigzag open-ended single-walled nanotubes with 14 Å diameter and 40 Å length were considered, so (18, 0) carbon nanotube and (14, 0) silicon carbide nanotube were applied. Molecular dynamic simulations were applied for two systems; both of them containing a carboplatin molecule at a position along the CNT and SiCNT z-axis, i.e., drug_CNT and drug_SiCNT. Two systems were solvated in an aqueous solution. The parameters of CNT were modeled using the AMBER99SB force field.[26,27] All the Lennard-Jones parameters and partial charge values for the carbon and silicon atoms for SiCNT were obtained from density functional theory calculations, summarized in Table 1.[14,28] Other parameters were taken from the DREIDING force field and used in MD simulations. The structure of carboplatin was obtained from our previous works,[22,29] and the parameters were identified from the literature and the GAFF;[30,31] additionally, the carboplatins' partial charges using the RESP module of AMBER 12 were calculated. The desired structures were immersed in a periodic water box of octagonal shape with a minimal distance of 12 Å from the system surface. Two systems were solvated with a TIP3P solvation model.[32]

Table 1. Lennard-Jones parameters and partial charges for SiCNT atoms

Atom	ε (kcal/mol)	σ (Å)	Atomic Charge (e)
C	0.086	3.4	0.45
Si	0.469	3.7364	-0.45

Molecular dynamics simulations
Molecular dynamics simulations were performed by employing the AMBER 12 simulation package.[33] All simulations were conducted under the isothermal-isobaric ensemble at 1 atm and 300 K using the SANDER module in the AMBER 12 program. Constant temperature and pressure were maintained using Langevin dynamics.[34] Bond lengths containing hydrogen atoms were constrained using the SHAKE algorithm.[35] Periodic boundary conditions were applied and the long-range electrostatic interactions were handled with the particle mesh Ewald method; the nonbonded interactions were treated with cutoff at 12Å.[36] Each simulation in energy minimization stage included 5000 steps for solvent and 5000 steps for solute relaxation. All systems

were then heated from 0K to 300K for 120 ps and equilibrated at 300K for 200 ps. The production stages were run for 10 ns with a time step of 2 fs, and the trajectories for structural coordinates were saved every 1 ps for data analysis. Configuration analysis of the trajectories was performed with the ptraj module included in AmberTools14. Additionally, binding free energies were evaluated using the MM/PBSA (molecular mechanics/Poisson-Boltzmann surface area) method by previous experiment.[29,37] The analysis of the interaction energies between the nanotubes and the drug was accomplished with AmberTools14 and implementation of MMPBSA.py script.

Results
The results from MD simulations of the two systems revealed that throughout the simulation time, both encapsulated carboplatin molecules resided inside the CNT and SiCNT cavity. Time-averaged radial distribution functions (RDF) were calculated to assess the localization of carboplatin inside the nanotubes (Figure 1), also RMSD plots were illustrated the drug movement inside the carbon and silicon carbide nanotubes (Figure 2). Moreover, MM/PBSA analysis of the trajectories was performed to estimate the binding free energy of the drug_CNT and the drug_SiCNT. Binding and absolute free energies of molecules are evaluated using this attractive method:

$$\Delta G_{binding} = [G_{complex}] - [G_{drug}] - [G_{CNT}]$$

Additionally, separation of the total free energy of binding into the van der Waals, electrostatic, and solute-solvent interactions, and discussion of each of the terms can be allowed and is calculated from:

$$\Delta G_{tot} = \Delta E_{MM} + \Delta G_{solv} - T\Delta S$$

$$\Delta E_{MM} = E_{int} + E_{vdW} + E_{ele}$$

$$\Delta G_{solv}^{PBSA} = \Delta G_{solv}^{nonpolar} + \Delta G_{solv}^{electrostatic}$$

where the molecular mechanics energy of the molecule (ΔE_{MM}) includes the van der Waals (E_{vdW}), internal energy (bonds, angles and dihedrals) (E_{int}) and the electrostatic energy (E_{ele}) terms. The solvation energy (G_{solv}) containing the polar and nonpolar parts is obtained from an implicit solvent description. Table 2 summarizes all energy terms for the two simulated systems in order to evaluate binding free energy using the MM/PBSA method.

Discussion
Localization of carboplatin inside the CNT and SiCNT
To assess the localization of carboplatin inside the nanotubes, time-averaged radial distribution functions (RDF) were calculated. Figure 1a illustrates the RDF plot between the carboplatin center of mass and the carbon atoms of the CNT. In addition, Figure 1b illustrates the RDF plot between the carboplatin center of mass and the

carbon and silicon atoms of the SiCNT. Both plots indicate that the drug moves throughout the tubes and there is a greater probability of finding the drug along the CNT and SiCNT in the first quarter of the tubes. Since drug exposure at the end of the nanotube is an important

option for the drug molecules to release,[38] the encapsulation and the preferential position of the carboplatin inside the tubes have a significant contribution in drug delivery.

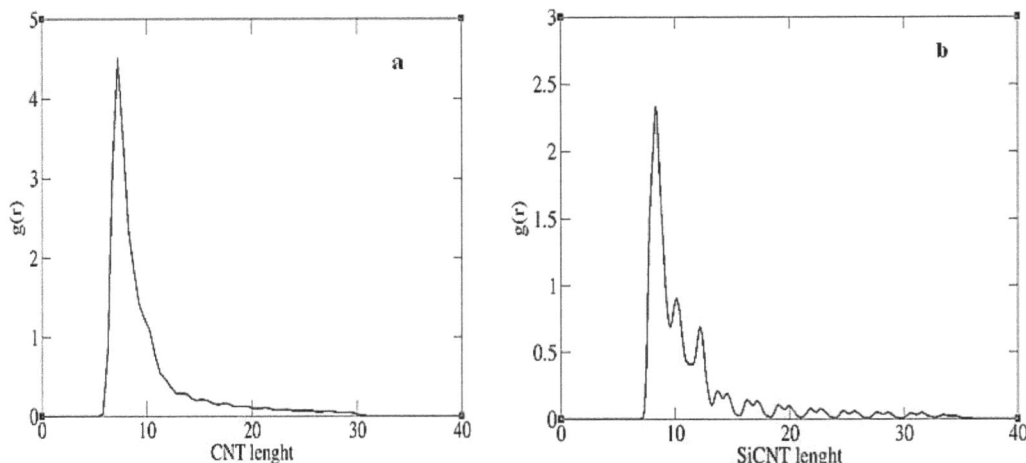

Figure 1. The RDF plot between the carboplatin center of mass and (a) the carbon atoms of the CNT, (b) the carbon and silicon atoms of the SiCNT

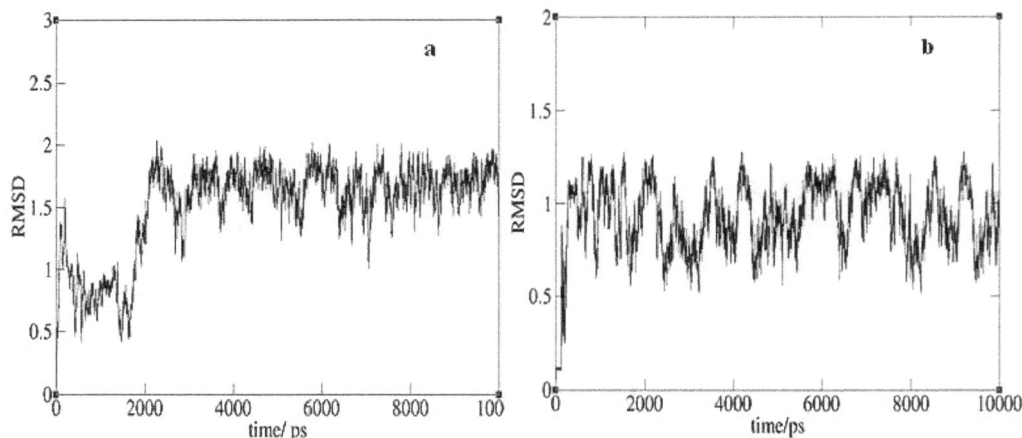

Figure 2. RMSD plots of encapsulation of the carboplatin inside the (a) CNT, (b) SiCNT.

Energy analysis
With regard to RMSD plots of drug movement inside the carbon and silicon carbide nanotubes (Figure 2), it is obvious that the two systems have stable equilibration, so it is possible to assess the thermodynamic properties of systems by sampling in simulation time and achieving the localization and the encapsulation behavior of the carboplatin inside the CNT and SiCNT. From the results of energy terms in Table 2, the total binding free energy in the drug_CNT system with an average of about −46 kcal mol^{-1} and the drug_SiCNT with −145 kcal mol^{-1} remains constant. It is derived that the dominant contribution of interactions is related to nonbonded van der Waals energy; evidently indicating that encapsulation of carboplatin inside the silicon carbide nanotube has stronger vdW interactions. The solvation free energies (G_{solv}^{PBSA}) have a positive and small contribution of the

binding free energy for both systems (Table 2), due to the hydrophobic structures of nanotubes; however, this is slightly reduced in the drug_SiCNT system. Whereas the partial charge on carbon atoms of CNT is zero, this reduction of solvation free energies can be related to partial charges on carbon and silicon atoms of the silicon carbide nanotube's structure. Regard these results, the larger van der Waals value belongs to the drug_SiCNT, so the carboplatin drug has stronger interaction inside the SiCNT than it does inside the carbon nanotube. Comparison of these energy profiles reveals that the carboplatin molecule prefers to spend more time inside the SiCNT until it reaches the target cell. Consequently, using SiCNT nanotube as a platinum drug carrier can be the more suitable option for drug delivery with this type of nanostructure.

Table 2. Energy values for encapsulation of drug inside the nanotubes

Complex	drug_CNT	drug_SiCNT
E_{vdW}	-50.7566	-147.1443
E_{ele}	-0.9297	-2.9051
G_{solv}^{ele}	7.0830	6.0232
$G_{solv}^{nonpolar}$	-1.7366	-1.0369
E_{MM}	-51.6863	-150.0495
G_{solv}^{PBSA}	5.3464	4.9863
$\Delta G_{binding}$	**-46.3399**	**-145.0631**

All values in this table are in kcal/mol.

Conclusion

Molecular dynamic simulations to investigate the encapsulation behavior of the drug carboplatin inside the silicon carbide nanotube were applied as a comparison with the carbon nanotube as an anticancer drug delivery system based on single-walled nanotubes. The RDF plots show the localization of carboplatin inside the nanotubes, indicating that the drug moves throughout the tubes and has a greater probability of finding the carboplatin along the CNT and SiCNT in the first quarter of the tubes. Additionally, the binding free energy profiles in the encapsulation of drug inside both systems were investigated. The results confirmed that the appropriate drug delivery system for platinum drug is the use of SiCNTs to CNTs. Since the free energy of binding in the silicon carbide nanotube is about three times that of the carbon nanotube, the length of time remaining for the drug in this system will be greater, and the probability of releasing the drug will be less than with carbon nanotube, before reaching the target cells.

Acknowledgments

The authors give special thanks to S. Skies for editing this manuscript.

Ethical Issues

Not applicable.

Conflict of Interest

The authors declare no conflict of interests.

References

1. Baughman RH, Zakhidov AA, de Heer WA. Carbon nanotubes--the route toward applications. *Science* 2002;297(5582):787-92. doi: 10.1126/science.1060928

2. Sharma A, Jain N, Sareen R. Nanocarriers for diagnosis and targeting of breast cancer. *BioMed Res Int* 2013;2013:960821. doi: 10.1155/2013/960821

3. Wong CH, Vijayaraghavan V. Compressive characteristics of single walled carbon nanotube with water interactions investigated by using molecular dynamics simulation. *Phys Lett A* 2014;378(5-6):570-6. doi: 10.1016/j.physleta.2013.12.026

4. Adeli M, Hakimpoor F, Ashiri M, Kabiri R, Bavadi M. Anticancer drug delivery systems based on noncovalent interactions between carbon nanotubes and linear-dendritic copolymers. *Soft Matter* 2011;7(8):4062-70. doi: 10.1039/c0sm01550d

5. Madani SY, Mandel A, Seifalian AM. A concise review of carbon nanotube's toxicology. *Nano Reviews* 2013;4. doi: 10.3402/nano.v4i0.21521

6. McDevitt MR, Chattopadhyay D, Kappel BJ, Jaggi JS, Schiffman SR, Antczak C, et al. Tumor targeting with antibody-functionalized, radiolabeled carbon nanotubes. *J Nucl Med* 2007;48(7):1180-9. doi: 10.2967/jnumed.106.039131

7. Liu Z, Chen K, Davis C, Sherlock S, Cao Q, Chen X, et al. Drug delivery with carbon nanotubes for in vivo cancer treatment. *Cancer Res* 2008;68(16):6652-60. doi: 10.1158/0008-5472.CAN-08-1468

8. Castle AB, Gracia-Espino E, Nieto-Delgado C, Terrones H, Terrones M, Hussain S. Hydroxyl-functionalized and N-doped multiwalled carbon nanotubes decorated with silver nanoparticles preserve cellular function. *ACS Nano* 2011;5(4):2458-66. doi: 10.1021/nn200178c

9. Kang B, Chang S, Dai Y, Yu D, Chen D. Cell response to carbon nanotubes: Size-dependent intracellular uptake mechanism and subcellular fate. *Small* 2010;6(21):2362-6. doi: 10.1002/smll.201001260

10. Kostarelos K, Lacerda L, Pastorin G, Wu W, Wieckowski S, Luangsivilay J, et al. Cellular uptake of functionalized carbon nanotubes is independent of functional group and cell type. *Nat Nanotechnol* 2007;2(2):108-13. doi: 10.1038/nnano.2006.209

11. Schipper ML, Nakayama-Ratchford N, Davis CR, Kam NW, Chu P, Liu Z, et al. A pilot toxicology study of single-walled carbon nanotubes in a small sample of mice. *Nat Nanotechnol* 2008;3(4):216-21. doi: 10.1038/nnano.2008.68

12. Liu Z, Cai W, He L, Nakayama N, Chen K, Sun X, et al. In vivo biodistribution and highly efficient tumour targeting of carbon nanotubes in mice. *Nat Nanotechnol* 2007;2(1):47-52. doi: 10.1038/nnano.2006.170

13. Lee C, Drelich J, Yap Y. Superhydrophobicity of boron nitride nanotubes grown on silicon substrates. *Langmuir* 2009;25(9):4853-60. doi: 10.1021/la900511z

14. Mavrandonakis A, Froudakis GE, Schnell M, Mühlhäuser M. From pure carbon to silicon–carbon nanotubes: An Ab-initio study. *Nano Lett* 2003;3(11):1481-4. doi: 10.1021/nl0343250

15. Wu IJ, Guo GY. Optical properties of SiC nanotubes: An ab initio study. *Phys Rev B* 2007;76(3):035343.

16. Miyamoto Y, Yu BD. Computational designing of graphitic silicon carbide and its tubular forms. *Appl Phys Lett* 2002;80(4):586-8. doi: 10.1063/1.1445474

17. Mu C, Zhao Q, Xu D, Zhuang Q, Shao Y. Silicon nanotube array/gold electrode for direct electrochemistry of cytochrome c. *J Phys Chem B* 2007;111(6):1491-5. doi: 10.1021/jp0657944

18. Sahu T, Ghosh B, Pradhan SK, Ganguly T. Diverse role of silicon carbide in the domain of nanomaterials. *Int J Electrochem* 2012;2012:271285. doi: 10.1155/2012/271285

19. Wang D, Lippard SJ. Cellular processing of platinum anticancer drugs. *Nat Rev Drug Discov* 2005;4(4):307-20. doi: 10.1038/nrd1691

20. McWhinney SR, Goldberg RM, McLeod HL. Platinum neurotoxicity pharmacogenetics. *Mol Cancer Ther* 2009;8(1):10-6. doi: 10.1158/1535-7163.MCT-08-0840

21. Sargolzaei M, Nikoofard H, Afshar M. DNA binding mode and affinity of antitumor drugs of 2-aroylbenzofuran-3-ols: Molecular dynamics simulation study. *Pharm Chem J* 2016;50(3):137-42. doi: 10.1007/s11094-016-1411-4

22. Khatti Z, Hashemianzadeh SM. Boron nitride nanotube as a delivery system for platinum drugs: Drug encapsulation and diffusion coefficient prediction. *Eur J Pharm Sci* 2016;88:291-7. doi: 10.1016/j.ejps.2016.04.011

23. Kelland L. The resurgence of platinum-based cancer chemotherapy. *Nat Rev Cancer* 2007;7(8):573-84. doi: 10.1038/nrc2167

24. Arlt M, Haase D, Hampel S, Oswald S, Bachmatiuk A, Klingeler R, et al. Delivery of carboplatin by carbon-based nanocontainers mediates increased cancer cell death. *Nanotechnology* 2010;21(33):335101. doi: 10.1088/0957-4484/21/33/335101

25. Negureanu L, Salsbury FR Jr. Non-specificity and synergy at the binding site of the carboplatin-induced DNA adduct via molecular dynamics simulations of the mutsα-DNA recognition complex. *J Biomol Struct Dyn* 2014;32(6):969-92. doi: 10.1080/07391102.2013.799437

26. Cornell WD, Cieplak P, Bayly CI, Gould IR, Merz KM, Ferguson DM, et al. A second generation force field for the simulation of proteins, nucleic acids, and organic molecules. *J Am Chem Soc* 1995;117(19):5179-97. doi: 10.1021/ja00124a002

27. Hummer G, Rasaiah JC, Noworyta JP. Water conduction through the hydrophobic channel of a carbon nanotube. *Nature* 2001;414(6860):188-90. doi: 10.1038/35102535

28. Taghavi F, Javadian S, Hashemianzadeh SM. Molecular dynamics simulation of single-walled silicon carbide nanotubes immersed in water. *J Mol Graph Model* 2013;44:33-43. doi: 10.1016/j.jmgm.2013.04.012

29. Khatti Z, Hashemianzadeh SM. Investigation of thermodynamic and structural properties of drug delivery system based on carbon nanotubes as a carboplatin drug carrier by molecular dynamics simulations. *J Incl Phenom Macrocycl Chem* 2015;83(1-2):131-40. doi: 10.1007/s10847-015-0549-0

30. Yao S, Plastaras JP, Marzilli LG. A molecular mechanics amber-type force field for modeling platinum complexes of guanine derivatives. *Inorg Chem* 1994;33(26):6061-77. doi: 10.1021/ic00104a015

31. Cundari TR, Fu W, Moody EW, Slavin LL, Snyder LA, Sommerer SO, et al. Molecular mechanics force field for platinum coordination complexes. *J Phys Chem* 1996;100(46):18057-64. doi: 10.1021/jp961240x

32. Jorgensen WL, Chandrasekhar J, Madura JD, Impey RW, Klein ML. Comparison of simple potential functions for simulating liquid water. *J Chem Phys* 1983;79(2):926-35. doi: 10.1063/1.445869

33. Case D, Darden T, Cheatham III T, Simmerling C, Wang J, Duke R, et al. Amber 12. San Francisco: University of California; 2012.

34. Cerutti DS, Duke R, Freddolino PL, Fan H, Lybrand TP. Vulnerability in popular molecular dynamics packages concerning langevin and andersen dynamics. *J Chem Theory Comput* 2008;4(10):1669-80. doi: 10.1021/ct8002173

35. Miyamoto S, Kollman PA. Settle: An analytical version of the SHAKE and RATTLE algorithm for rigid water models. *J Comput Chem* 1992;13(8):952-62. doi: 10.1002/jcc.540130805

36. Essmann U, Perera L, Berkowitz ML, Darden T, Lee H, Pedersen LG. A smooth particle mesh ewald method. *J Chem Phys* 1995;103(19):8577-93. doi: 10.1063/1.470117

37. Kollman PA, Massova I, Reyes C, Kuhn B, Huo S, Chong L, et al. Calculating structures and free energies of complex molecules: Combining molecular mechanics and continuum models. *Acc Chem Res* 2000;33(12):889-97.

38. Hampel S, Kunze D, Haase D, Kramer K, Rauschenbach M, Ritschel M, et al. Carbon nanotubes filled with a chemotherapeutic agent: A nanocarrier mediates inhibition of tumor cell growth. *Nanomedicine (Lond)* 2008;3(2):175-82. doi: 10.2217/17435889.3.2.175

Permissions

All chapters in this book were first published in APB, by Tabriz University of Medical Sciences; hereby published with permission under the Creative Commons Attribution License or equivalent. Every chapter published in this book has been scrutinized by our experts. Their significance has been extensively debated. The topics covered herein carry significant findings which will fuel the growth of the discipline. They may even be implemented as practical applications or may be referred to as a beginning point for another development.

The contributors of this book come from diverse backgrounds, making this book a truly international effort. This book will bring forth new frontiers with its revolutionizing research information and detailed analysis of the nascent developments around the world.

We would like to thank all the contributing authors for lending their expertise to make the book truly unique. They have played a crucial role in the development of this book. Without their invaluable contributions this book wouldn't have been possible. They have made vital efforts to compile up to date information on the varied aspects of this subject to make this book a valuable addition to the collection of many professionals and students.

This book was conceptualized with the vision of imparting up-to-date information and advanced data in this field. To ensure the same, a matchless editorial board was set up. Every individual on the board went through rigorous rounds of assessment to prove their worth. After which they invested a large part of their time researching and compiling the most relevant data for our readers.

The editorial board has been involved in producing this book since its inception. They have spent rigorous hours researching and exploring the diverse topics which have resulted in the successful publishing of this book. They have passed on their knowledge of decades through this book. To expedite this challenging task, the publisher supported the team at every step. A small team of assistant editors was also appointed to further simplify the editing procedure and attain best results for the readers.

Apart from the editorial board, the designing team has also invested a significant amount of their time in understanding the subject and creating the most relevant covers. They scrutinized every image to scout for the most suitable representation of the subject and create an appropriate cover for the book.

The publishing team has been an ardent support to the editorial, designing and production team. Their endless efforts to recruit the best for this project, has resulted in the accomplishment of this book. They are a veteran in the field of academics and their pool of knowledge is as vast as their experience in printing. Their expertise and guidance has proved useful at every step. Their uncompromising quality standards have made this book an exceptional effort. Their encouragement from time to time has been an inspiration for everyone.

The publisher and the editorial board hope that this book will prove to be a valuable piece of knowledge for researchers, students, practitioners and scholars across the globe.

List of Contributors

Ali Mohammadi, Samira Goldar, Dariush Shanehbandi, Leila Mohammadnejad, Elham Baghbani, Tohid Kazemi, Saeed Kachalaki and Behzad Baradaran
Immunology Research Center, Tabriz University of Medical Sciences, Tabriz, Iran

Behzad Mansoori
Immunology Research Center, Tabriz University of Medical Sciences, Tabriz, Iran
Student Research Committee, Tabriz University of Medical Sciences, Tabriz, Iran

Mayank Chaturvedi
Department of Pharmaceutics, Rajiv Academy for Pharmacy, Chattikkara, Mathura, India

Manish Kumar Shailendra Bhatt and Vipin Saini
Department of Pharmaceutics, M M College of Pharmacy, Maharishi Markandeshwar University, Mullana, Ambala-133207, Haryana, India

Kamla Pathak
Department of Pharmaceutics, Pharmacy College Saifai, Uttar Pradesh University of Medical sciences, Saifai, Etawah, 206130, Uttar Pradesh, India

Roghiyeh Pashaei-Asl
Department of Anatomy, Medical School, Iran University of Medical Science, Tehran, Iran
Cellular and Molecular Research Center, Iran University of Medical Sciences, Tehran, Iran

Fatima Pashaei-Asl
Molecular Biology Laboratory, Biotechnology Research Center, Tabriz University of Medical Sciences, Tabriz, Iran

Parvin Mostafa Gharabaghi
Women's Reproductive Health Research Center, Tabriz University of Medical Sciences Tabriz, Iran

Maryam Pashaiasl
Women's Reproductive Health Research Center, Tabriz University of Medical Sciences Tabriz, Iran
Drug Applied Research Center, Tabriz University of Medical Sciences, Tabriz, Iran
Department of Anatomical Sciences, Faculty of Medicine, Tabriz University of Medical Sciences, Iran

Khodadad Khodadadi
Genetic Research Theme, Murdoch Children's Research Institute, Royal Children's Hospital, The University of Melbourne, Melbourne, Australia

Mansour Ebrahimi
Department of Biology, University of Qom, Qom, Iran

Esmaeil Ebrahimie
Institute of Biotechnology, Shiraz University, Shiraz, Iran
School of Biological Sciences, Faculty of Science and Engineering, Flinders University, Adelaide, Australia
School of Information Technology and Mathematical Sciences, Division of Information Technology, Engineering and the Environment, The University of South Australia, Adelaide, Australia
School of Animal and Veterinary Science, The University of Adelaide, Australia

Elias Adikwu
Department of Pharmacology, Faculty of Basic Medical Sciences, University of Port Harcourt, Choba, Rivers State, Nigeria

Bonsome Bokolo
Department of Pharmacology, Faculty of Basic Medical Sciences, Niger Delta University Wilberforce Island, Bayelsa State, Nigeria

Hashem Montaseri and Elham Khezri
Department of quality control, Faculty of pharmacy, Shiraz University of Medical Science, Shiraz, Iran

Zahra Sobhani
Department of quality control, Faculty of pharmacy, Shiraz University of Medical Science, Shiraz, Iran
Center for nanotechnology in drug delivery, Faculty of pharmacy, Shiraz University of Medical Science, Shiraz, Iran

Soliman Mohammadi Samani
Department of pharmaceutics, Faculty of pharmacy, Shiraz University of Medical Science, Shiraz, Iran

Maryam Hassan Famian
Department of molecular biology, Ahar Branch, Islamic Azad University, Ahar, Iran.

Soheila Montazer Saheb and Azadeh Montaseri
Stem Cell Research Center, Tabriz University of Medical Sciences, Tabriz, Iran

Atinderpal Kaur, Sonal Gupta, Reema Gabrani and Shweta Dang
1Department of Biotechnology, Jaypee Institute of Information Tehnology, A-10, Sector 62, Noida, UP 201307, India

Amit Tyagi
Department of Nuclear Medicine, Institute of Nuclear Medicine and Allied Sciences, Brig SK Mazumdar Marg, Delhi, 110054, India

Rakesh Kumar Sharma
Division of CBRN Defence, Institute of Nuclear Medicine and Allied Sciences, Brig SK Mazumdar Marg, Delhi, 110054, India

Javed Ali
Faculty of Pharmacy, Jamia Hamdard, Hamdard Nagar, New Delhi, 110062, India

Ali Akbar Alizadeh
Biotechnology Research Center, Tabriz University of Medical Sciences, Tabriz, Iran

Maryam Hamzeh-Mivehroud, Mehdi Sharifi and Siavoush Dastmalchi
Biotechnology Research Center, Tabriz University of Medical Sciences, Tabriz, Iran
School of Pharmacy, Tabriz University of Medical Sciences, Tabriz, Iran

Behzad Jafari
Biotechnology Research Center, Tabriz University of Medical Sciences, Tabriz, Iran
School of Pharmacy, Tabriz University of Medical Sciences, Tabriz, Iran
Students Research Committee, Tabriz University of Medical Sciences, Tabriz, Iran

Niloofar Bazazzadegan, Mehdi Banan and Hamid Reza Khorram Khorshid
Genetics Research Center, University of Social Welfare and Rehabilitation Sciences, Tehran, Iran

Marzieh Dehghan Shasaltaneh, Reza Nazari and Gholam Hossein Riazi
Laboratory of Neuro-organic Chemistry, Institute of Biochemistry and Biophysics (IBB), University of Tehran, Tehran, Iran

Kioomars Saliminejad and Koorosh Kamali
Reproductive Biotechnology Research Center, Avicenna Research Institute, ACECR, Tehran, Iran

Zead Helmi Abudayeh and Loay Khaled Hassouneh
Faculty of Pharmacy, Isra University, Amman, Jordan

Qais Ibrahim Abualassal
Faculty of Pharmacy, Isra University, Amman, Jordan
Department of Drug Sciences, University of Pavia, Italy

Khaldun Mohammad Al Azzam
Preparatory Year Department, Al-Ghad International Colleges for Applied Medical Sciences, 11451 Riyadh, Kingdom of Saudi Arabia

Anahita Mohammadian§, Elahe Naderali§, Seyedeh Momeneh Mohammadi, Aliakbar Movasaghpour, Behnaz Valipour, Mohammad Nouri and Hojjatollah Nozad Charoudeh
Stem Cell Research Center, Tabriz university of Medical Sciences, Tabriz, Iran

Akbar Mohammad Hoseini, Ali Mohammadi, Vahid Khaze Shahgoli and Behzad Baradaran
Immunology Research Center, Tabriz University of Medical Sciences, Tabriz, Iran

Saiedeh Razi Soofiyani
Immunology Research Center, Tabriz University of Medical Sciences, Tabriz, Iran
Department of Molecular Medicine, Faculty of Advanced Biomedical Sciences, Tabriz University of Medical Sciences, Tabriz, Iran

Mohammad Saeid Hejazi
Molecular Medicine Research Center, Tabriz University of Medical Sciences, Tabriz, Iran
Department of Molecular Medicine, Faculty of Advanced Biomedical Sciences, Tabriz University of Medical Sciences, Tabriz, Iran

Reza Vajdi-Hokmabad
Department of veterinary, Miyaneh branch, Islamic Azad University, Miyaneh, Iran

Mojtaba Ziaee
Medicinal Plant Research Center, Institute of Medicinal Plants, ACECR, Karaj, Iran

Saeed Sadigh-Eteghad and Javad Mahmoudi
Neurosciences Research Center (NSRC), Tabriz University of Medical Sciences, Tabriz, Iran

Siamak Sandoghchian Shotorbani
Department of Immunology, Tabriz Branch, Islamic Azad University, Tabriz, Iran

Ali Kamal Attia, Nisreen Farouk Abo-Talib and Marwa Hosny Tammam
National Organization for Drug Control and Research, Cairo, Egypt

Rana Refaat Makar
Faculty of Pharmacy, Ahram Canadian University, Egypt

Randa Latif and Omaima Naim El Gazayerly
Faculty of Pharmacy, Department of Pharmaceutics, Cairo University, Cairo, Egypt

Ehab Ahmed Hosni
Faculty of Pharmacy, Russian University, Egypt

Jafar Majidi and Behzad Baradaran
Immunology Research Center, Tabriz University of Medical Sciences, Tabriz, Iran

Dariush Shanehbandi, Tohid Kazemi and Leili Aghebati-Maleki
Immunology Research Center, Tabriz University of Medical Sciences, Tabriz, Iran
Student Research Committee, Tabriz University of Medical Sciences, Tabriz, Iran

Farzaneh Fathi
Student Research Committee, Tabriz University of Medical Sciences, Tabriz, Iran
Research Center for Pharmaceutical Nanotechnology, Tabriz University of Medical Sciences, Tabriz, Iran

Jafar Ezzati Nazhad Dolatabadi
Research Center for Pharmaceutical Nanotechnology, Tabriz University of Medical Sciences, Tabriz, Iran

Narjes Khavasi and Seyyed Muhammad Bagher Fazljou
Department of Traditional Medicine, Faculty of Traditional Medicine, Tabriz University of Medical Sciences, Tabriz, Iran

Mohammad Hosein Somi and Elnaz Faramarzi
Department of liver and Gastrointestinal Diseases Research Center, Tabriz University of Medical sciences, Tabriz, Iran

Ebrahim Khadem and Mohammad Hossein Ayati
Department of Traditional Medicine, School of Traditional Medicine, Tehran University of Medical Sciences, Tehran, Iran

Mohammadali Torbati
Department of Food Science and Technology, Faculty of nutrition, Tabriz University of Medical Sciences, Tabriz, Iran

Naime Majidi Zolbanin and Alireza Mohajjel Nayebi
Drug Applied Research Center, Tabriz University of Medical Sciences, Tabriz, Iran
Pharmacology and Toxicology Department, School of Pharmacy, Tabriz University of Medical Sciences, Tabriz, Iran

Reza Jafari
Department of Immunology, Faculty of Medicine, Mashhad University of Medical Sciences, Mashhad, Iran
Immunology Research Center, Inflammation and Inflammatory Diseases Division, School of Medicine, Mashhad University of Medical Sciences, Mashhad, Iran

Leili Aghebati-Maleki and Dariush Shanehbandi
Immunology Research Center, Tabriz University of Medical Sciences, Tabriz, Iran

Jafar Majidi, Mehdi Yousefi and Farhad Jadidi-Niaragh
Immunology Research Center, Tabriz University of Medical Sciences, Tabriz, Iran
Department of Immunology, School of Medicine, Tabriz University of Medical Sciences, Tabriz, Iran

Mohammad-Sadegh Soltani Zangbar
Department of Immunology, School of Medicine, Tabriz University of Medical Sciences, Tabriz, Iran

Fatemeh Atyabi
Department of Pharmaceutics, Faculty of Pharmacy, Tehran University of Medical Sciences, Tehran, Iran
Nanotechnology Research Centre, Faculty of Pharmacy, Tehran University of Medical Sciences, Tehran, Iran

Mohammad Alizadeh and Elham Mirtaheri
Nutrition Research Center, Faculty of Nutrition, Tabriz University of Medical Sciences, Tabriz, Iran.

Nazli Namazi
Nutrition Research Center, Faculty of Nutrition, Tabriz University of Medical Sciences, Tabriz, Iran
Diabetes Research Center, Endocrinology and Metabolism Clinical Sciences Institute, Tehran University of Medical Sciences, Tehran, Iran

Nafiseh Sargheini
Molecular Biomedicine, University of Bonn, Bonn, Germany

Sorayya Kheirouri
Department of Nutrition, Tabriz University of Medical Sciences, Tabriz, Iran

Arezou Khezerlou and Maryam Azizi-Lalabadi
Student Research Committee, Department of Food Sciences and Technology, Faculty of Nutrition and Food Sciences, Tabriz University of Medical Sciences, Tabriz, Iran

Mahmood Alizadeh-Sani
Student Research Committee, Department of Food Sciences and Technology, Faculty of Nutrition and Food Sciences, Tabriz University of Medical Sciences, Tabriz, Iran
Drug Applied Research Center, Tabriz University of Medical Sciences, Tabriz, Iran

Hamed Hamishehkar
Drug Applied Research Center, Tabriz University of Medical Sciences, Tabriz, Iran

Yaghob Azadi
Drug Applied Research Center, Tabriz University of Medical Sciences, Tabriz, Iran
Student Research Committee, Tabriz University of Medical Sciences, Tabriz, Iran

Elyas Nattagh-Eshtivani, Mehdi Fasihi, Abed Ghavami and Aydin Aynehchi
Student Research Committee, Faculty of Nutrition and Food Sciences, Tabriz University of Medical Sciences, Tabriz, Iran

Ali Ehsani
Department of Food Sciences and Technology, Faculty of Nutrition and Food Sciences, Tabriz University of Medical Sciences, Tabriz, Iran

Arun Kumar, Sandeep Kumar and Arun Nanda
Department of Pharmaceutical Sciences, Maharshi Dayanand University, Rohtak-124001, India

Roshanak Ghods and Ali Ghobadi
Research Institute for Islamic and Complementary Medicine, Iran University of Medical Sciences, Tehran, Iran
School of Persian Medicine, Iran University of Medical Sciences, Tehran, Iran

Manouchehr Gharouni
Faculty of Medicine, Tehran University of Medical Sciences, Tehran, Iran.

Massoud Amanlou and Niusha Sharifi
Department of Medicinal Chemistry, Faculty of Pharmacy, Tehran University of Medical Sciences, Tehran, Iran

Gholamreza Amin
Department of Pharmacognosy, Faculty of Pharmacy, Tehran University of Medical Sciences, Tehran, Iran

Alireza Abdanipour
Department of Anatomical Sciences, Faculty of Medicine, Zanjan University of Medical Sciences, Zanjan, Iran

Masoud Dadkhah, Mohsen Alipour and Hadi Feizi
Department of Physiology and Pharmacology, Faculty of Medicine, Zanjan University of Medical Sciences, Zanjan, Iran

Molood Alsadat Vakilinezhad, Shima Tanha and Hamid Akbari Javar
Department of Pharmaceutics, Faculty of Pharmacy, Tehran University of Medical Sciences, Tehran, Iran

Hashem Montaseri
Department of Quality Control, Faculty of Pharmacy, Shiraz University of Medical Sciences, Shiraz, Iran

Rassoul Dinarvand
Nanotechnology Research Centre, Faculty of Pharmacy, Tehran University of Medical Sciences, Tehran, Iran

Amir Azadi
Department of Pharmaceutics, School of Pharmacy, Shiraz University of Medical Sciences, Shiraz, Iran

Riris Istighfari Jenie, Ratna Asmah Susidarti and Edy Meiyanto
Departement of Pharmaceutical Chemistry, Faculty of Pharmacy, Universitas Gadjah Mada, Indonesia

Sri Handayani
Cancer Chemoprevention Research Center, Faculty of Pharmacy, Universitas Gadjah Mada, Indonesia
Research Center for Chemistry, Indonesian Institute of Sciences (LIPI), Indonesia

Linar Zalinar Udin
Research Center for Chemistry, Indonesian Institute of Sciences (LIPI), Indonesia

Zahra Khatti
Department of Chemistry, Iran University of Science and Technology, Tehran, Iran

Seyed Majid Hashemianzadeh
Molecular Simulation Research Laboratory, Department of Chemistry, Iran University of Science and Technology, Tehran, Iran

Seyed Ali Shafiei
Neurology and Neuroscience Research Center, Qom University of Medical Sciences, Qom, Iran

Index